Techniques in Musculoskeletal Rehabilitation:

Companion Handbook

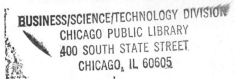

Paul Goodyer
Brockville Physiotherapy
and Sports Injuries Clinic
Brockville, Ontario
Canada

McGRAW-HILL
Medical Publishing Division
New York   Chicago   San Francisco   Lisbon   London   Madrid
Mexico City   Milan   New Delhi   San Juan   Seoul   Singapore
Sydney   Toronto

McGraw-Hill

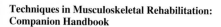

*A Division of The **McGraw·Hill** Companies*

**Techniques in Musculoskeletal Rehabilitation:
Companion Handbook**

Copyright © 2001 by The **McGraw-Hill Companies,** Inc. All rights reserved. Printed in the United States of America. Except as permitted under the United States Copyright Act of 1976, no part of this publication may be reproduced or distributed in any form or by any means, or stored in a data base or retrieval system, without the prior written permission of the publisher.

1234567890DOC/DOC0987654321

ISBN 0-07-135497-2

This book was set in Times by Circle Graphics, Inc.
The editors were Stephen Zollo and Barbara Holton.
The production manager was Clare Stanley.
The index was prepared by Jerry Ralya.

R. R. Donnelley & Sons, Inc. was printer and binder.

This book is printed on acid-free paper.

Library of Congress Cataloging-in–Publication-Data

Goodyer, Paul.
    Techniques in musculoskeletal rehabilitation : companion handbook/ author, Paul Goodyer.
        p. ; cm.
    Companion v. to: Techniques in musculoskeletal rehabilitation / William E. Prentice, Michael L. Voight. c2001.
    ISBN 0-07-135497-2
    1. Physical therapy—Handbooks, manuals, etc. 2. Orthopedics—Handbooks, manuals, etc. 3. Musculoskeletal system—Diseases—Patients—Rehabilitation—Handbooks, manuals, etc. I. Prentice, William E. Techniques in musculoskeletal rehabilitation. II. Title.
    [DNLM: 1. Musculoskeletal Diseases—diagnosis—Handbooks. 2. Musculoskeletal Diseases—therapy—Handbooks. 3. Physical Examination—methods—Handbooks. WE 39 G658t 2001]
RM701 .G665 2001
616.7′062—dc21

                                 00-053282

Techniques in Musculoskeletal Rehabilitation:

Companion Handbook

Notice

Medicine is an ever-changing science. As new research and clinical experience broaden our knowledge, changes in treatment and drug therapy are required. The authors and the publisher of this work have checked with sources believed to be reliable in their efforts to provide information that is complete and generally in accord with the standards accepted at the time of publication. However, in view of the possibility of human error or changes in medical sciences, neither the authors nor the publisher nor any other party who has been involved in the preparation or publication of this work warrants that the information contained herein is in every respect accurate or complete, and they disclaim all responsibility for any errors or omissions or for the results obtained from use of the information contained in this work. Readers are encouraged to confirm the information contained herein with other sources. For example and in particular, readers are advised to check the product information sheet included in the package of each drug they plan to administer to be certain that the information contained in this work is accurate and that changes have not been made in the recommended dose or in the contraindications for administration. This recommendation is of particular importance in connection with new or infrequently used drugs.

Dedication

To My Wife Alison
The Wind Beneath My Wings

Table of Contents

Preface xiii

CHAPTER 1   **ORTHOPAEDIC PHYSICAL THERAPY ASSESSMENT**... 1

Subjective Examination... 2
    Question 1: Onset 2
    Question 2: Duration 3
    Question 3: Frequency..................................... 3
    Question 4: Area of Symptoms 4
    Question 5: Type of Symptoms 4
    Question 6: Miscellaneous 5
Objective Examination.. 5
    Observation... 6
    Active Movements... 7
    Passive Movements 8
    Resisted Movements.. 9
    Palpation.. 10
    Specific Tests... 10
    Posture 10
    Gait 13
Possible Causes of Concern................................... 14

CHAPTER 2   **SHOULDER AND UPPER ARM ASSESSMENT**.. 21

Tables of Test Movements 21
    Active Movements of the Shoulder 21
    Passive Movements of the Shoulder................. 23
    Resisted Movements of the Shoulder 25
    Resisted Movements of the Shoulder Girdle 27
Table of Examination Findings Related to
    Specific Conditions... 28
    Onset.. 28
    Typical Age Ranges 28
    Duration... 29
    Frequency 29
    Area of Symptoms 30
    Type of Symptoms 30
    Observations... 31
    Active Movements... 31
    Passive Movements 32
    Resisted Movements....................................... 33
    Palpation.. 33
Palpation of the Shoulder and Upper Arm 34
Specific Tests for the Shoulder and Arm 37

Shoulder and Upper Arm Conditions 40
    Acute Rotator Cuff Tendonitis 40
    Chronic Rotator Cuff Tendonitis 44
    Rotator Cuff Tear 48
    Adhesive Capsulitis.. 52
    Bicipital Tendonitis 55
    Chronic Instability of Shoulder Joint.............. 58
    Acromioclavicular Joint Injury........................ 62
    Acromioclavicular Joint Irritation 65
    Pectoral Muscle Tear.. 67
    Subacromial Bursitis 70

CHAPTER 3   **ELBOW, WRIST, AND**
                 HAND ASSESSMENT...................................... **76**
    Table of Test Movements 76
    Active Movements of the
        Elbow and Forearm 76
    Active Movements of the Wrist....................... 77
    Active Movements of the Hand........................ 78
    Passive Movements of the
        Elbow and Forearm 80
    Passive Movements of the Wrist and Hand...... 82
    Resisted Movements of the
        Elbow and Forearm 84
    Resisted Movements of the Wrist and Hand 84
    Table of Examination Findings Related to
        Specific Conditions 86
        Onset.. 86
        Typical Age Ranges 86
        Duration... 87
        Frequency 87
        Area of Symptoms.. 88
        Type of Symptoms 88
        Observations.. 89
        Active Movements.. 90
        Passive Movements 91
        Resisted Movements..................................... 91
        Palpation.. 92
    Palpation of the Elbow, Wrist and Hand 93
    Specific Tests for Elbow, Wrist and Hand.......... 100
    Elbow, Wrist, and Hand Conditions 102
    Lateral Epicondylitis 102
    Medial Epicondylitis 107
    Olecranon Bursitis 111
    Ulnar Nerve Entrapment (Cubital Tunnel
        Syndrome) 114

Median Nerve Entrapment.............................. 117
Carpal Tunnel Syndrome................................ 119
Wrist Extensor Tendonitis............................. 122
de Quervains Tenosynovitis 126
Metacarpophalangeal Joint Injury
    of the Thumb 130
Osteoarthritis of the Carpometacarpal
    Joint of the Thumb................................. 133
Trigger Finger.. 136
Wrist Flexor Tendonitis................................. 139
Dupytren's Contracture 142
Wrist Sprain.. 145

**CHAPTER 4   CERVICAL AND THORACIC SPINE
    ASSESSMENT.. 151**
Tables of Test Movements 151
    Active Movements of the Cervical Spine....... 151
    Passive Movements of the Cervical Spine..... 153
    Resisted Movements of the Cervical Spine.... 154
    Active Movements of the Shoulder Girdle..... 155
    Active Movements of the Thoracic Spine 156
Table of Examination Findings Related to
    Specific Conditions... 157
    Onset.. 157
    Typical Age Range 157
    Duration... 158
    Frequency 158
    Area of Symptoms 159
    Type of Symptoms 160
    Observation... 161
    Active Movements... 162
    Passive Movements 164
    Resisted Movements..................................... 165
    Palpation.. 166
Palpation of the Thoracic and Cervical Spine 167
Specific Tests of the Cervical
    and Thoracic Region....................................... 173
Cervical and Thoracic Conditions 178
    Cervical Disc (no Radiculopathy) 178
    Cervical Disc (with Radiculopathy) 183
    Cervical Facet Joint Irritation
        (no Radiculopathy) 188
    Cervical Facet Joint Irritation
        (with Radiculopathy)..................................... 191
    Cervical Postural Strain................................. 195
    Upper Trapezius Muscle Strain 199

Latisimus Dorsi Muscle Strain 203
Cervical Facet Joint Locking 206
Thoracic Facet Joint Locking 209
Thoracic Outlet Syndrome 212
Whiplash... 215
Cervical Spondylosis 220

CHAPTER 5   **LOW BACK AND PELVIS**
ASSESSMENT.. 227
Tables of Test Movements 227
   Active Movements of the Low Back 227
   Resisted Movements of the Low Back 228
Table of Examination Findings Related to
   Specific Conditions... 230
   Onset... 230
   Typical Age Ranges 230
   Duration.. 231
   Frequency 231
   Area of Symptoms 232
   Type of Symptoms 233
   Observation.. 234
   Active Movements... 235
   Passive Movements 236
   Resisted Movements.. 237
   Palpation.. 238
Palpation of the Low Back and Pelvis.............. 239
Specific Tests for the Low Back and Pelvis 245
Back and Pelvis Conditions............................. 247
   Lumbar Disc (no Radiculopathy) 247
   Lumbar Disc (with Radiculopathy) 251
   Lumbar Facet Joint Irritation
     (no Radiculopathy) 257
   Sacroiliac Joint Strain.................................... 261
   Lumbar Muscle Strain 266
   Low Back Postural Strain 270
   Lumbar Facet Joint Irritation
     (with Radiculopathy)..................................... 274
   Lumbar Facet Joint Strain.............................. 278
   Combined Disc/Facet Joint Problem 282
   Spinal Stenosis.. 286
   Chronic Spinal Instability.............................. 290

CHAPTER 6   **HIP AND KNEE ASSESSMENT** 296
Tables of Test Movements 296
   Active Movements of the Hip 296
   Passive Movements of the Hip 298

Resisted Movements of the Hip...................... 300
Active Movements of the Knee 302
Passive Movements of the Knee..................... 303
Passive Movements of the Patella 304
Resisted Movements of the Knee 305
Table of Examination Findings Related to
  Specific Conditions.. 306
  Onset.. 306
  Typical Age Ranges 306
  Duration... 307
  Frequency 307
  Area of Symptoms... 308
  Type of Symptoms 309
  Observation... 310
  Active Movements.. 311
  Passive Movements 312
  Resisted Movements.. 313
  Palpation... 314
Palpation of the Hip and Knee........................... 315
Specific Tests of the Hip and Knee.................... 323
Hip and Knee Conditions 329
  Trochanteric Bursitis 329
  Osteoarthritis of the Hip 333
  Adductor Tendonitis of the Hip...................... 338
  Psoas Bursitis... 341
  Groin Strain 344
  Piriformis Syndrome 347
  Iliotibial Band Friction Syndrome 351
  Hamstring Muscle Tear 354
  Hamstring Tendonitis 358
  Quadriceps Muscle Tear.................................. 361
  Quadriceps Tendon Tear 365
  Collateral Ligament Strain of Knee................ 368
  Patella Femoral Syndrome 373
  Osteoarthritis of the Knee.............................. 377

CHAPTER 7   **LOWER LEG AND FOOT ASSESSMENT.. 384**
Tables of Test Movements 384
  Active Movements of the Foot and Ankle...... 384
  Passive Movements of the Foot and Ankle 385
  Resisted Movements of the Foot and Ankle... 387
Table of Examination Findings Related to
  Specific Conditions.. 389
  Onset.. 389
  Typical Age Ranges 389
  Duration... 390

Frequency 390
Area of Symptoms... 391
Type of Symptoms 392
Observation.. 393
Active Movements... 394
Passive Movements 395
Resisted Movements.. 396
Palpation 397
Palpation of the Lower Leg and Foot 398
Specific Tests for the Lower Leg and Foot......... 408
Lower Leg and Foot Conditions 410
Ankle Ligament Strain/Tear 410
Recurrent Ankle Instability 416
Gastrocnemius Muscle/Tendon Tear............. 420
Achilles Tendonitis... 424
Plantar Fasciitis 428
Peroneal Tenosynovitis 432
Posterior Tibial Tenosynovitis 436
Anterior Tibial Tendonitis............................... 440
Shin Splints... 444
Morton's Neuroma 447
Tarsal Tunnel Syndrome 450

Index 457

Preface

To a great extent this book came about through feedback from students on clinical placement. They wanted something simple and easy to read that covered both assessment and treatment for orthopaedic outpatients. The concept of the book was therefore a handy pocketbook, the sort of thing that can be easily read on a bus or in the corridor before an exam. This necessitates the book being small, so detail has been sacrificed in order to maintain brevity.

With the students in mind the first section of this book covers general aspects of orthopaedic assessment and some specific detail on gait and posture. There is also a separate section dealing with "red-flag" warning signs, which may require the patient to be referred to the doctor or for more caution to be exercised during treatment of the patient.

Subsequent chapters deal with each body area in turn, and each one of these chapters starts with a selection of tables. The first group of tables cover the active, passive, and resisted movements for the specific body area discussed within that chapter. These tables are followed by a description of palpation techniques accompanied by photographs, which enable the reader to identify anatomical structures related to the conditions covered in the chapter. This is followed by a description of special tests that are of diagnostic significance in the assessment of that body area. Here again brevity has been a watchword, as there are countless tests that can be used. I have made a selection of the ones that I use most often, and which in some cases may be of singular importance in arriving at a diagnosis.

The second set of tables in each chapter are, I believe, unique to this book, because the "traditional" way of looking at an orthopaedic condition is to name the condition and then follow this with a description of the signs and symptoms. I feel that in assessment of patients this situation is reversed. As we examine the patient we gradually build up a picture of the underlying problem. In this way each sign or symptom, or each group of signs and symptoms, leads us along a given path. Therefore the tables list commonly found signs and symptoms, and the related conditions that may possibly produce them. There is, of course, overlap between conditions; however, the tables are a useful and effective means of stimulating the form of deductive reasoning that applies to analysis of findings during the assessment procedure. The use of these tables is discussed in greater detail at the end of the first chapter.

The greater proportion of each chapter still deals with conditions in the "traditional" manner, with the signs and symptoms for each condition presented in a sequence that should closely approximate the order in which the information is received during the assessment process. I would like to think that the reader will be able to move back and forth between the tables and the text, just as in the assessment we repeatedly review, analyze, and re-review the information we receive before coming to a final conclusion. The assessment findings are, in general, related to current standard texts; however, there is always some healthy disagreement between authors as to the relevance of particular findings and their diagnostic significance. So, when in doubt I have used my own clinical experience as my main guide, and in a few of the conditions as my only guide when review of the literature revealed an overall lack of consensuses of opinion.

After the assessment of each condition I have included a section that I have called Treatment Ideas. Treatment of patients with any specific condition or impairment is certainly more controversial than the analysis of assessment findings. Here again I have used a selection of standard texts as the main referencing, but I must admit to a major bias towards my own clinical practice, which I feel is natural and normal. We are each a product of our education, environment, and experience, and I believe that in treating patients we have to trust our own knowledge and instincts. I have used the heading Treatment *Ideas* because it is impossible to give hard and fast rules on treatment of any one patient for any given condition, as treatment varies from patient to patient. What I hope to do is provide a framework for ideas. In the clinic we always encourage students to be imaginative in their treatment planning. This enables us to learn from them—many of my most successful treatment ideas have been born in this way.

The treatment ideas also give an overview of progression of treatment for each condition. It has been my experience that students have their greatest difficulty with initiation and progression of treatment. When this occurs we try to give the student ideas, rather than just telling them what to do, and I have approached treatment for each condition in this same manner. I have also tried to include some of the "hints and wrinkles" that I have learned over the years, which have helped me to treat some recalcitrant problems with reasonable success. In this way, if when treating a patient the reader comes up against what seems to be a brick wall, then one or two of the ideas may help them circumvent the problem. I have tried to keep the description of assessment as brief as possible, while still having enough detail to be useful. On the other hand I have deliberately kept the treatment ideas more discursive in nature, as I hope to recreate the conversational approach of discussion of treatment, which I have personally found to be very helpful when supervising students on clinical placement, or in consultation with fellow clinicians during daily practice.

Choice of conditions to be covered in this book was also dictated by my own clinical experience, in that I have stayed with those conditions that form the bulk of my caseload, as well as those of the physical therapists with whom I work. In some cases the conditions are quite "rare"; however, I seem to see a few of them every year. One the other hand I have not included some conditions that other people may think common, simply because I have not seen them on a regular basis. This somewhat arbitrary selection of conditions was necessary in order to keep the book small in size. One particular area that I have left out altogether is fractures, as I feel coverage of this area would require delving into complete and separate pathophysiology, and a more detailed coverage of treatment options. This I believe to be beyond the scope of this book, and may well warrant a book of its own.

I hope the book will fit the epithet: small but useful, and prove to be an effective aide-memoire for both students and clinicians. As it is a first attempt, any and all feedback would be more than welcome. I am always particularly interested in the personal experiences of other clinicians in assessing and treating orthopaedic conditions.

Acknowledgements

I feel that I have been tremendously lucky having McGraw-Hill as my publisher. In particular I would like to thank Stephen Zollo my editor, without whose advice and encouragement I am sure the book would never have been completed. Barbara Holton, the editing supervisor has also been wonderful providing expert technical advice and moral support. The book could also not have been completed if it were not for the help of all the staff in the Brockville Clinic, in particular Dawn-Marie Chevrier who did all the hard work typing, retyping, correcting and typing some more. Last, but certainly not least I have to thank my wife Alison for putting up with me during the trials and tribulations of writing the book and also for providing the majority of the artwork.

The aims of an assessment are to establish a diagnosis, formulate a prognosis, and determine a plan of care. The diagnosis is simply nomenclature describing the collection of signs and symptoms that the patient presents to you the therapist. The prognosis is your best guess as to how much better your patient will be, and in what time period. Your plan of care is the series of steps you and the patient will have to take to reach your goal. This may seem to be a somewhat simplistic way of looking at the process but it is not meant to be. Patients are human beings and as such they come in a wonderful variety of shapes, sizes, and personalities. In real life this means that although any two patients may have the same diagnosis, the treatments you use and the outcomes of those treatments can vary quite dramatically. Some therapists find the prospect of this variation in outcomes daunting; I think that it is one of the most rewarding aspects of our profession. If we could give the same treatment to all patients with the same diagnosis and get the same result each time, then our job would be simple and, I believe, boring.

The assessment should produce a diagnosis. Patients virtually demand that we put a name to their problem, but the naming of the problem should not be your prime concern. Identification of the anatomical structure or structures at fault should be the fundamental goal of the assessment process. When you have identified the source of the problem you have to assess the extent of the damage to estimate how long it will take you and the patient to overcome it. The type and degree of damage that a body structure has sustained will also determine the degree of recovery that can be achieved. The patients' personality, mental state, home environment, occupational status, and a host of other factors will also influence your treatment outcome.

In this book the process of assessing a patient is not covered at great depth. Instead, the fundamentals of assessment as they relate to the commonest problems that are encountered in outpatient clinical practice are discussed. In general, you will find that the conditions presented in this book will account for the signs and symptoms of over 80% of your orthopaedic outpatients.

A full assessment of any patient can include any or all of the following components:

The history: This can cover history of the present condition, family history, past medical history, demographics, occupation and occupational status, medications, results of tests, social habits/living environment, health status, and growth and development.

Review of systems: This can include determining the physiological and anatomical status of the musculoskeletal, cardiopulmonary, neuromuscular, and integumentary systems.

Tests and measures: This can include assessment and analysis of pain, joint integrity and mobility, muscle performance, range of motion, posture, assistive devices, orthotics, splints, gait, locomotion, balance, ergonomics, and body mechanics.

You will not carry out all the elements of an assessment for every patient you see. Which areas you choose to assess and to what depth will depend on the patient's problem, their age, stage of recovery, point that they are at in the rehabilitation process, and any other relevant factors. In this book I have tried to cut away to the bare bones of the examination (no pun intended). In order to simplify the assessment process I want you to consider those areas of assessment that are generic to the most common orthopaedic conditions, those being the conditions that I tend to see most frequently in clinical practice. The first division that can be made in the assessment process is between the subjective and objective parts of the examination.

THE SUBJECTIVE EXAMINATION

The easiest way to find out what is wrong with a patient is to ask him or her. This is the subjective part of the examination, which comes first. If you simply ask "what is wrong?" you will either get too brief a response, ("my arm hurts"), or you will get a life history. Neither response will help you reach a conclusion, so you need to structure the subjective examination by asking specific questions. There are six questions that you need answered, we will look at each question in turn to see exactly what information it will extract from your patient. I phrase each question in a form that could be put to the patient. You do not need to phrase it in exactly the same terms each time, but you should always make sure that the patient understands exactly what it is you are asking.

Question 1: The Onset

The question is: "How did this episode start?"

Note that you are asking about this episode, not the last six times they had something similar—that will come later. The patient may start off by saying something like "now I have to go back about 5 years." Do not try and stop him, as it is usually futile, but do make sure that when he has finished you have found out how the *present* episode started. In clinical practice you will find that all the possible responses to this question can be put into one of two categories. The symptoms either came on suddenly or gradually. These two categories can then be further clarified by establishing if there was a cause of onset. "Suddenly" means the patient woke up and the symptoms were there full-blown or fell down and the pain was immediate and has stayed with him since. Gradual onset might be that the patient felt a bit stiff for a few mornings on waking, and then over a period of time felt pain in the mornings, then pain all day and so on.

A cause for the condition, if there is one, comes down to two things. Either it is due to trauma (such as a fall) or to overuse (a sore shoulder developing after the first baseball practice of the season). Be careful, as you will often have patients say they hurt themselves when they fell, but that the pain came on 3 days later. I once had a 60-year-old lady with an acute back pain tell me that it was due to a fall at school when she was 15 years old—even though she had never had any back symptoms in the intervening 45 years. So be sure that the incident is directly connected to the condition. When you are clear on the history note down all the relevant information that the patient has given you. Then decide if the condition came on gradually or suddenly, if there was a cause, and if so, whether it was trauma or overuse.

Question 2: Duration

The question is: "When did this episode start?"

What you are trying to discern is the acuity of the condition. Make it clear to the patient that it is only this episode that you are asking about. He may have had knee problems for 20 years, but if this episode started a week ago then one week is the finding that you record. It is not uncommon to have a patient who was barely able to crawl into the clinic tell you that he has been like this for 2 years, but then you discover he only signed off work a week ago. On further questioning you will find he has had recurrent symptoms for a long period of time, but it is only in the last week or so that he has been suffering this kind of pain. The duration of the condition is then 1 to 2 weeks. Record the exact date of onset if there is one, as well as the causative factors; you never know when you may have to make a report on a patient for a lawyer or insurance company.

Question 3: Frequency

The question is: "How many similar episodes have you had before?"

Be specific, it is this episode that we are concerned with; previous episodes must therefore have consisted of essentially the same symptoms. While other symptoms occasionally can be important, in verifying the cause of symptoms the most effective sign is recurrence of the same symptoms, not just similar ones, in the same area. It is not necessary to record the dates of every occurrence—simply note if it happens frequently each year, or only once or twice a year, or once every year or two, etc. Where possible record the year during which symptoms first occurred. Sometimes a patient's symptoms will have varied over the years, but will still be relevant to your assessment. For example a patient may have started having pain in the left side of his low back 3 years ago. Then last year in addition to the back pain, he also had pain in his left buttock. Now this year the pain in the back is not as bad, but the buttock pain is worse, and there is also pain in the back of the thigh. This can be a fairly typical history as a bulging disc progresses to the point of herniation. In this type of case it is necessary to record the progression of symptoms. If you, or the patient, feel that differing symptoms relate to the same condition then record them here. If you feel they do not relate, then record them under "previous history" at the end of the subjective examination.

Question 4: Area of Symptoms

The question is: "Show me exactly where your symptoms are?"

Get the patient to show you by having him put his finger or hand on the place where the typical symptoms are felt. We are back to that "typical" thing again. Patients have an annoying, but understandable, habit of showing areas where pains used to be or of showing you where the last three things they had wrong would hurt if they had them now. Do not get sidetracked and do not be content with a description. Patients will say that they have pain in their hip joint if the pain is in the buttock, the lateral aspect of the upper thigh, or over the anterior of the hip (which incidentally is the site of true hip joint pain). Having them show you the area, is much less confusing in the long run.

The other point to note is that you should ask them to show you where they feel their symptoms, not their pain, as some patients do not have any pain as such, they may simply have stiffness or numbness. Get a precise description of where they are feeling their symptoms and then record it by shading the appropriate area on a body outline. If there is more than one area of symptoms then number them, recording the one that the patient feels is most important as number 1, the next most important as number 2, and so on.

Question 5: Type of Symptoms

The question is: "What are your typical symptoms?"

Again you use the word "symptom" instead of "pain," although pain is of course, the commonest complaint. When it comes to pain the majority of patients are fairly unimaginative; "it hurts" is the usual answer. Although no doubt true, this does not help you very much. Different structures in the body often produce different and sometime typical types of pain. The commonest pains are dull, sharp, shooting, stinging, aching, or burning. The other common symptoms are numbness or tingling. Combine the recording of these findings with those from the area of symptoms (question 4) by noting beside your shaded area on the body outline what type of symptoms the patient has at that site.

An additional point to note here is one that crosses over into the objective part of the assessment. Whenever a patient describes a symptom always ask them exactly where they feel it. This should become second nature to you, so that when a patient is bending forward for example and says, "I can feel that pulling a bit," you automatically ask "where?" If the patient says "I get tingling in my hand," you need to know if that is in the hand and fingers, or just the fingers or part of the fingers, or only some of the fingers and not others. Keep asking for clarification until you are sure you understand precisely what the patient is experiencing.

Question 6: Miscellaneous

The question is: "Is there anything else you can tell me about your condition?"

This section deals with possible symptoms that the patient might complain of that are significant when analyzing your assessment findings. For example, patients will often describe hearing "a pop" when they have torn a ligament in their knee. In each chapter that covers assessment findings you will find a list of these miscellaneous signs and symptoms, with each one related back to the possible causes.

Medical History

I have not included this as one of the specific questions as it does not usually help in the diagnosis of the common conditions covered in this book. Nonetheless it is an important area to cover in your charting.

The question is really in two parts:

1) "Are you currently suffering any other problems?"
2) "Do you have any other previous medical problems?"

These questions can sometimes open a floodgate, which may not necessarily help you make a diagnosis, but it is important to know about your patients' general health before you start treating them. It is not enough to ask about "their health in general." On more than one occasion I have had patients tell me that their general health is excellent, only to find the scar from recent heart surgery when conducting the physical examination. As far as they are concerned the surgeon has cured them, but from your point of view it is important to know that they have a history of heart disease before you plan their exercise program. So ask if they have ever had any medical problems and then give them examples, "such as heart disease, diabetes, or epilepsy." Concurrent conditions can also affect your treatment planning, for example, in planning speed of progression of exercise, or even knowing something as simple as not being able to lay a patient flat because he gets reflux from a hiatus hernia.

For a review of the body systems the patient should be asked to complete a general health questionnaire such as the one shown at the end of this chapter. Any positive findings should be followed up by the therapist during the assessment.

THE OBJECTIVE EXAMINATION

This is the point where you start to move and touch the patient; before you do so you need to have the patient undress enough to see all of the area you are going to be examining. Be very aware of the patient's dignity, there is nothing more humiliating than being scrutinized while your rear end is hanging out of a hospital gown. Only uncover those parts of the body that you need to see and give the patient some adequate means of covering the rest of his body.

For the sake of simplicity I am going to divide the objective part of the examination into six sections. Each section has a title that relates to the major activity that you or the patient will undertake. These are your "bread and butter" techniques of patient evaluation and will be augmented by many other varied tests. However, in many cases these techniques alone are enough to allow you to establish a working diagnosis on which to base your plan of treatment.

Observation

Note that the first thing you do is look at the patient, but not touch him. There is always a terrible temptation to start prodding the patient with thumb, finger, or hand as soon as he has finished telling you his problem. This is particularly true if he has just shown you the part that hurts or some area that he thinks is swollen. Avoid the temptation: literally the last thing we are going to do is touch the patient. There are two good reasons why you should look not touch. In the first place, if you do touch you may well leave a red mark. Since one of the signs you will be looking for is redness in or around the affected area, things can become confusing. Second, if you start prodding something that hurts, then it usually starts to hurt even more. This in turn can make it more difficult for the patient to move and you end up with an erroneous finding. So stand back and have a good look at the patient.

Your observation of the patient often begins before you have even started the subjective part of the assessment. This is because wherever possible you should observe the patient as he makes his way into the examination room. Check to see if he has a normal gait pattern or if he is limping. Is his posture upright, or does it deviate in any way. Are his arms swinging normally or is he holding one or both arms stiffly. You will also note if he is using any kind of assistive device such as crutches or a cane, or if he is wearing any form of protective or supportive device. You can learn a lot about patients before they even sit down, and it is a chance to observe them when they are not aware of your scrutiny. We all tend to stand just a little more upright when we know we are being watched.

The official observation of the patient begins immediately after the subjective examination and should include the whole patient, not just the affected area. Look at the patient's posture in general, and then at the way he holds the affected area in particular. If it is a leg or back problem, then is he taking weight evenly on both feet in standing and on both buttocks in sitting? Next look at the affected area. Note down anything out of the ordinary, such as redness, swelling, or loss of body contour. With the arms and legs this is easy, as most people have two and you can usually compare the "good" side with the affected side. When the patient has problems with either both arms or both legs, or if the condition affects the trunk, then you have to compare what you see with what you believe to be normal for the patient's age and sex. There are not a great variety of things to look for, but the likelihood of encountering any one finding, and the significance of that finding, does vary from area to area. Do not just gloss over this part of the assessment, as it can sometimes give a good indication of underlying pathology and it also allows you to formulate an impression of the patient's general physical condition.

Active Movements

This is possibly the most important part of the objective examination, as most patients presenting for treatment will have a problem with movement in one way or another. The first thing to do is to get the patient to do the moving and the first thing to move, if it is an arm or leg problem, is the un-affected arm or leg. This lets you establish the norm for that patient, against which you can compare the performance of the other side. If the problem is in the trunk then you do not have much choice about what you are going to move. In that case you have to compare what the patient achieves against what you would consider normal considering his age and sex.

When checking movements look for a pattern, noting down movements in order of restriction, with the most limited first, the next most limited second, and so on. This pattern of movement restriction is often more important in your analysis of findings than the actual degree of restriction for any single movement. However, be sure to note down the actual amount of restriction for each movement, either in degrees or as a percentage of expected normal. This will help you to determine the patient's progress with treatment, and is very important in terms of medico-legal reports. As the patient is carrying out each movement note if it appears normal in terms of quality of movement. A normal active movement is smooth, controlled, and purposeful. Pain will often make movements hesitant or jerky, and weakness can make them uncoordinated. Patients will also on occasion use accessory movements to try and enhance the range of weak, stiff, or painful body segments. The most common of these is probably the reversed scapu-lohumeral rhythm seen in many chronic shoulder conditions, in which the patient raises the shoulder girdle on the affected side to overcome lack of range of motion in the glenohumeral joint.

Also note the cause for any restriction against each movement. Do this by asking the patient what is stopping him from moving any further. The commonest answer to this is some variation on "it hurts." Always ask where it hurts and if possible get the patient to point to the area of pain or stiffness. I prefer my patients to give a running commentary on what they are feeling as they move, as symptoms can vary through range. You need to know the answers to questions such as: when does the pain occur? does it get worse if the patient tries to move further, or is the level of pain the same? and does the pain spread as the patient pushes further into movement? I always instruct patients not to push into ranges of movement that they are not comfortable with, so that if they are worried about hurting themselves they will feel empowered enough to limit the degree of examination. If the patient does say that there is pain during a movement, clarify if it is more than normal, as patients may answer that a certain movement is painful simply because the pain they are already feeling is still there when they do the movement. You need to know if the movement *changes* the pain in any way.

In the chapters in the book covering specific conditions, we will be looking at the different patterns of movement restriction related to common underlying causes. There can at times be variations in these patterns in different patients suffering from the same condition. In cases where this may be a significant factor it will be noted under the miscellaneous section for that body area.

Passive Movements

Having asked the patient what limits his movements, it is now time for you to test the feel of the movement for yourself. Moving the part passively allows you to do this. This means the patient should do nothing and just let you move him around. Unfortunately this is not always an easy feat to accomplish, as the patient often tries to assist you or sometimes simply does not trust you enough to relax completely. It is important to explain clearly to the patient what you are going to do and why. Assure him that you will be as gentle as possible. Do not tell him you are not going to hurt him, because there is a good chance that you will, as you will be taking the movement to the end of available range, which is usually where the pain occurs. Since you want the patient to trust you and relax as much as possible while you are carrying out the movements, it is important to fully support the body segment as you move it. Your grip should be firm but gentle, while the movements are made slowly and smoothly. Always be ready to stop the movement if the patient shows signs of discomfort. You may have to continue the movements beyond that point in certain circumstances, but if so then check that the patient is willing to let you continue the movement and tell him to let you know anytime he wants you to stop.

The passive movements for each body section will be described in the relevant chapters. In general the two most important considerations regarding passive movements are how they compare in range to the active movements, and what type of sensation you, the examiner, feel at the end of the movement. Dr. James Cyriax originally elucidated these points in *Textbook of Orthopaedic Medicine* and although some of his interpretations of the findings have been questioned by recent studies, the description of those findings are still useful in collating assessment data. The comparisons of active and passive movements will be covered in the relevant sections for each body segment for specific conditions. The *end feel* of movements will be covered here, as they are more generic in nature.

Bone-to-bone is described as an abrupt halt to movement when two hard surfaces meet. The end range of full passive extension of the normal elbow gives this type of feel.

Spasm of muscle coming actively into play (Cyriax described it as a "vibrant twang") gives a hard unforgiving end feel, but not as solid a feel as bone-to-bone.

Capsular end feel is like a piece of thick leather being stretched or two pieces of tough rubber being squeezed together. It is the feel that you get at the end of rotation in the normal shoulder or hip.

Springy block is a bouncy rebound at the end of available range.

Tissue approximation is when movement is halted by engagement of one body part with another, as happens at the end range of flexion in the normal elbow or knee.

Empty end feel is where the patient stops the movement, either by resisting it or by begging the examiner to stop, but the examiner can feel that further movement is possible and there does not appear to be any intrinsic resistance to movement in the joint itself.

For each movement you test note down the type of end feel and the range of motion, starting with the most limited and ending with the least limited. This will make it easier for you to compare the active and passive ranges.

Resisted Movements

There are two findings to be recorded after resisted testing: was the movement painful? was it weak? You have to test for these two things separately. The reason you want to know if a particular movement is painful is to determine if it is the muscle producing that movement that is the cause of the patients' symptoms. To do this you have to produce a gentle isometric contraction of that particular muscle. If you let any movement occur, then if pain is experienced it might be due to pathology in a joint structure and not the muscle. On the other hand, if you manage to get an isometric contraction but resist it very strongly then again, you may simply be stressing joint structures, or any pain produced could come from accessory muscles recruited to counteract the heavier resistance. So tell the patient to hold the position you put them in, which if at all possible should be painless to begin with, and then apply a gentle pressure in the opposite direction to the movement you want to test. Descriptions of how to resist particular movements are given in the chapters dealing with individual body segments.

To test muscle strength you can apply a lot more resistance, but it should only be enough to confirm if the muscle is as strong as would normally be expected. Again compare against the good side if there is one. Record the muscle strength as an estimate compared to expected normal, or use any other accepted method such as the Oxford Scale. The recording of the results can go beside the other movement recordings so that you end up with something like this: Abduction limited 60%, pain at end range, pain on isometric testing, muscle strength grade 4/5. Flexion limited 30%, stiff at end range, no pain on isometric testing, muscle strength grade 4+/5.

Palpation

Palpation is usually the thing you are most tempted to do during an assessment, particularly when you are not sure what is wrong with the patient. The idea is that if you poke around enough, you are going to find something that hurts. Palpation can occasionally prove very useful, but in the majority of common conditions it does not tell you anything that the previous 10 parts of the assessment have not. However, patients do tend to have a lot more faith in you if you are able to "put your finger right on it," and to a great extent that should be the purpose of your palpation—to confirm what you already suspect and identify the particular anatomical structure at fault. This is another good reason for leaving the palpation to last. In the chapters on particular body regions you will find photographs showing where you should palpate, with reference to the most probable underlying pathology. One point to note is that when you are checking for increased skin temperature it is best to use the back of the hand, as it is more sensitive.

Specific Tests

Whole books can be written on all the different tests that could be used in an orthopaedic examination. In this book I have tried to cover only those that are both simple to use and most singularly indicative of a particular condition. In clinical practice I use these tests as a means of confirming a diagnosis or as a final differentiation between two otherwise similar conditions. Under this heading, in the sections on specific conditions, I have also included any individual findings that are particularly characteristic for a given condition.

Posture

It sometimes seems that good posture is a thing of the past. A great many patients presenting with spinal problems have poor posture, which is probably the cause of the condition rather than caused by the condition. If time is taken to view the general population it is often hard to find any one individual who demonstrates what would be called "good posture." This section deals with some points regarding posture, mainly the postural abnormalities that can be encountered during physical assessment. It is not and cannot be a comprehensive review of postural analysis and the reader is advised to consult other texts that deal with the subject of posture in detail. The points covered here should be considered memory aids, and will help the informed reader to remember salient points relating to postural analysis of the patient during physical examination.

In the patient with good posture, an imaginary line passing through the patient from top to bottom when viewed from the side should fall in front of the upper part of the cervical spine and behind the ear roughly through the mastoid process. It should fall behind the clavicle, approximately through the point of the shoulder, in front of the thoracic spine, through the bodies of the lumbar vertebrae, through the hip joint, in front of the knee joint, and in front of the ankle joint.

If a person is able to sustain a correct posture then the muscles in the posterior cervical region only have to contract minimally to keep the head in balance. The same light degree of work is required in the erector spinae muscles to maintain the upright posture when the cervical, thoracic, and lumbar curves are balanced as described above. With the line of gravity passing through the hip, no muscle work is required to maintain the position of this segment of the body. When it falls in front of the knee, tension in the anterior cruciate ligaments, the hamstring muscles, and the gastrocnemius resists the tendency of the knee to fall into extension, so when the knee is fully extended it does not require any specific muscle action to maintain that position. With the line of gravity falling anterior to the ankle joint, a mild degree of contraction in the soleus muscle is usually sufficient to maintain the position of this joint relative to the erect posture.

Problems arise when the body segments fall out of line with the ideal situation described. The therapist should be aware of the following common postural faults. It is usually best to view the patient initially from the rear without telling them that their posture is being assessed. In that case the patient will stand more naturally, being less self-conscious than when being viewed from the side or the front. The therapist should look for the following possible abnormalities starting at the top and working down:

- One ear higher or lower than the other so that the head is held in a slight degree of side flexion.
- Lateral deviation of the cervical spine. This is usually associated with difference in ear height as noted above and suggests movement of the spine away from the midline. The deviation usually is away from the painful side and occurs in some neck conditions.
- The points of both shoulders should be at equal heights. Dropping of one shoulder can occur in some neck and upper back conditions or in some shoulder conditions. It should be remembered that the shoulder of the dominant arm tends to be slightly lower than the shoulder of the non-dominant side.
- Deviation of side flexion, rotation, or a combination of both in the thoracic spine may be seen in association with a scoliotic curve, where one scapula may seem to stand out more noticeably than the other; there may also be some protrusion of the ribs.
- Skin creases at the level of the lower rib cage may be more marked or more numerous on one side, suggesting a lateral deviation of the spine to the opposite side and subsequent side flexion to the side where the creases are more marked.

- The iliac crests and the dimples marking the sites of the posterior superior iliac spines should be level.
- The gluteal folds at the upper part of the thigh just below the buttock should be level and symmetrical.
- Bowing of the knees may occur, either genu valgum ("knock knees") or genu varum ("bow legged").
- The heels should be straight and should not angle in or out.

When the patient is viewed from the front the therapist should look for the following possible abnormalities:

- The ears out of alignment, with the lobe of one ear higher than the other, and the chin tilted to one side.
- One clavicle may appear lower than the other when one shoulder is dropped excessively or when one shoulder is raised more than the other. Again, bear in mind the normal slight dropping of the shoulder on the dominant side.
- One acromioclavicular joint may seem higher than the other if there has been a separation of the shoulder.
- Any variation in the skin folds around the lower ribs and waist on one side could denote lateral deviation of the spine.
- One iliac crest or anterior superior iliac spine may be higher or lower than the other when there is rotation of the pelvis, lateral deviation of the spine, or a leg-length discrepancy.
- The knees are again checked for the presence of genu varum or genu valgum deformities.

When the patient is viewed from the side the following possible abnormalities might be observed:

- A line taken vertically down from the lobe of the ear falls in front of the clavicle. This is the typical forward head posture found quite commonly in the general public, as well as in patients with neck and back problems. If this is present the patient's chin tends to poke forward, hence the term head "forward head posture."
- Excessive curvature of the thoracic spine may be noted in conjunction with rounding of the shoulders if an excessive thoracic kyphosis exists, possibly in compensation for excessive lordosis in the cervical and/or lumbar spine, or if the patient's abdominal tone is poor. Excessive weight carried in the abdominal area can best be noted from the side view and may predispose the patient to an increased lumbar lordosis.
- Excessive curvature may be present in the lumbar spine. This should not be confused with a well-pronounced posterior, which may give an impression of an increased lumbar lordosis. The lumbar spine should be palpated to see if there is, in fact, increased curvature present.
- Excessive tilting of the pelvis may be present. This is again usually associated with either an increased or decreased lumbar lordosis.

- The knees may be curved back behind the normal line of gravity in genu recurvatum, or the patient may stand with their knees slightly flexed to relieve pressure on a nerve root. In chronic knee conditions this can be due to tight or painful hamstring muscles.

The above postural points can be reviewed quite quickly when examining the patient, although care must be taken not to miss any minor deviation, which can on occasion have a significant impact on the patient's functional capabilities.

GAIT

The reader is encouraged to refer to other texts that deal in detail with normal and abnormal gait patterns to be able to effectively assess the patient's gait pattern the therapist needs to understand normal gait, a subject far too detailed to deal with comprehensively in this text. During physical assessment the following points of gait disturbance should be kept in mind when observing the patient, both when he enters the clinic or examination room, and specifically when checking the gait during the physical assessment. As in review of posture the patient should be viewed from the front, back, and side, and the therapist should be aware of the following possible gait abnormalities that might be present:

- Antalgic gait: This type of gait is quite often seen in patients with back and lower extremity problems. It is due to pain, with decreased time being spent in the stance phase on the affected leg. It may be combined with such signs as facial grimacing and gripping or holding of the affected region of the back or leg while walking.
- Trendelenburg gait: This is most commonly seen in patients with hip problems and is due to weakness in the hip abductor muscle so that when the patient takes weight on the affected leg the pelvis on the opposite side drops. This pronounced dropping of the pelvis was made famous by Marilyn Monroe (although in her case the condition appeared to be bilateral), and the accentuated swinging of the pelvis that results is sometimes known as the chorus girl's swing.
- Stiff leg gait: This is seen in patients who have a stiff hip or knee who go higher onto their toes on the unaffected leg to give themselves room to swing the stiff leg out as well as forward. This type of gait may also be associated with a shorter stance phase on the affected leg and a shorter step taken with the affected leg.
- Leg length discrepancy: If a patient has one leg shorter than the other he will have a tendency to shift the spine laterally, onto the affected side, with dropping of the pelvis on that side. The patient appears to tilt over to one side on every other step, giving a slight rocking appearance to the gait.

A further and important part of gait analysis is observation of the patient's footwear, in particular checking for uneven wear (as described in Chapter 5).

POSSIBLE CAUSES OF CONCERN

Throughout the assessment and treatment of a patient the physical therapist should be aware of certain warning signs that may suggest more serious pathology and that could necessitate referral of the patient to a general
practitioner or a specialist. There are countless signs and symptoms of
medical disease. While it is not the role of the physical therapist to make a
diagnosis of a medical condition, the therapist must have a basic grasp of
signs and symptoms related to the various body systems. A routine scan
for symptoms should be included in any physiotherapy assessment. One
simple means of acquiring necessary information from the patient is to use
a questionnaire such as the one shown at the end of this chapter. This will
allow the therapist to tell at a glance if the patient has any underlying, possibly undiagnosed, problems; suitable questioning can then clarify the patient's medical condition. There are several signs and symptoms that may
be considered "red flags"; some of these are given.

Patient Not Improving With Treatment

If a definitive orthopaedic diagnosis has been reached, but a patient does
not show response to treatment as expected, then consultation should take
place between the therapist and the referring physician, even in the absence
of any other findings of concern. This is particularly true of patients who
show no change in their condition despite physical intervention as compared to patients who get either better or worse.

No Variation in Symptoms with Activities or Rest

When a patient's symptoms do not change despite exercise or specific activities, or on resting, either in a weight bearing or non-weight bearing position, then there is a possibility that their condition is not mechanical in
origin and there may be some underlying pathology. There may be some
change in symptoms from time to time, most probably a steady increase in
discomfort and a decrease in function that the patient is unable to relate to
any specific cause.

Gradual Onset with No Cause

This is a quite common form of onset for several of the conditions discussed within this book. However, this form of insidious onset can also be
the first sign of serious underlying pathology. When it is coupled with the
absence of any other mechanical findings it should make the therapist more
cautious in his approach to treatment. Consultation with the referring physician may be necessary.

Unexplained Weight Loss

When a patient complains of loss of weight with no change in diet or
level of physical activity, then their physical condition needs to be fully

investigated. This is a common finding in conditions such as malignancy, gastrointestinal disorders, diabetes, systemic infections, hyperthyroidism, and adrenal insufficiency.

Fatigue and General Loss of Energy (Malaise)

This is a common complaint in chronic pain states, but is also found in patients suffering from systemic infections, diabetes, hypothyroidism, rheumatoid arthritis, cancer, or nutritional problems.

Fever

Presence of a fever may indicate something as simple as the flu; however, ongoing fever is also a sign of occult infections and cancer, and its cause should be fully investigated.

Nausea and Vomiting

Feelings of nausea and vomiting are two of the commonest side effects of some of the medications that patients with orthopaedic conditions may be taking. However, they can also be signs of gastrointestinal problems or some forms of cancer. They can also occur commonly in pregnancy, particularly in the early stages.

Temporary Loss of Consciousness (Syncope)

Patients may suffer brief loss of consciousness associated with hypoglycemia or the side effects of some medications. Any patient who reports regular occurrences of syncope should be referred to his general practitioner for a full investigation, if this has not already been done.

Shortness of Breath

During exercise patients may commonly display shortness of breath; the degree of exercise required to produce this state will vary with the patient's overall physical condition. Shortness of breath on relatively light exercise or following any form of mild exertion may indicate cardiovascular or pulmonary disease.

Changes of Bladder Function

Painful or difficult urination (dysuria) and change in urinary frequency could indicate problems with the urogenital system.

Difficulty Passing Urine/Mild Bowel Incontinence

These two signs, found either separately or together, are possible signs of spinal cord compression and may occur in patients who are only suffering mild, or possibly no, back symptoms whatsoever.

Increased Urination With Excessive Thirst

When a patient complains of ongoing thirst with increased frequency of urination, despite increasing their fluid intake, the possibility of diabetes should be considered. The patient may not necessarily complain of these problems, but may simply be seen to drink excessively during treatment sessions.

Skin Lesions

Because of the necessity of undressing a patient to view the relevant areas during an examination, the therapist has a unique opportunity to observe the patient's skin condition, particularly in areas where the patient may not be able to observe it himself, such as the middle of the back. Particular signs to note when observing a skin lesion are variation of skin color within the area, an irregular border, a raised irregular surface, and crusting or ulceration. All of these signs are indications of possibly serious pathology.

General Changes in Skin

If areas of redness or roughness of the skin are noted the patient should be questioned about the length of time that these conditions have been present and if the problem has been viewed by a doctor. Many conditions that produce these types of signs may be benign, and respond well to medical treatment.

Skin Color

A bluish discoloration of the skin (cyanosis), which may be particularly noticeable in the area of the tongue, the lips, or the skin and nails of the hands and feet, may indicate cardiovascular or pulmonary problems or problems with the local circulation. A yellowish discolouration of the skin (jaundice) may indicate a liver or blood disorder.

Clubbing of the Nails

When this occurs the nail base is swollen and soft and the nail bed can be seen to lie at an angle to the skin (i.e., the nail points downward when the finger is laid flat, where normally it would be in horizontal alignment with the skin).

Pain in Chest on Exertion

Complaints of tightness or pressure in the chest, particularly when associated with breathlessness, may indicate the presence of myocardioischemia. Any patient complaining of these symptoms should be taken off exercises and the condition reviewed by the therapist and a doctor.

Severe Incessant Pain

The presence of constant excruciating discomfort is one of the signs of skeletal metastases. Any such complaints should be thoroughly investigated, particularly if the patient complains of unchanging or worsening symptoms with treatment. This kind of symptom can also produce a hysterical reaction in a patient, which may incline some health professionals to discount to some degree the patient's description of his discomfort.

Rebound Tenderness

If, during palpation of the abdomen, pain experienced by the patient is worse on sudden release of the palpatory pressure, compared to the pain elicited when pressure was first applied, there may be peritoneal irritation present and possibly serious pathology. Any patient demonstrating this particular sign should be sent immediately to his general practitioner.

Decreased Tenderness with Abdominal Contraction

If tenderness is found on palpation of the abdomen with the patient supine, which decreases if the patient contracts the abdominal muscles by raising their head and neck off the bed, but the pain returns when the abdominal muscles are allowed to relax, there is the possibility that the discomfort is produced by the deeper visceral structures lying within the abdominal cavity.

Neurological Findings

Various tests of the neurological system are included within the text related to various specific conditions. One finding not covered is the Babinski sign. This is elicited by stroking the plantar surface of the patient's foot with either the thumb nail or the end of a reflex hammer. A stroke is taken from the heel along the lateral aspect of the foot to the heads of the metatarsals and then medially across the foot to the base of the great toe. A positive result is one of extension of the great toe and fanning out of the other four toes. A normal response is flexion of all the toes. This response is reversed in the neonate for the first few weeks. A positive Babinski sign is suggestive of an upper motor neuron lesion.

ASSESSMENT FINDINGS

In subsequent chapters of the book you will find individual findings grouped according to the most likely pathologies that produce them. I believe that this is the method we use when conducting the assessment of a patient. We build up a picture piece-by-piece as we receive a series of impressions from the patient's history and the physical findings. I think this is a suitable point at which to give a word of warning—do not jump to conclusions. Make your final decision regarding the patient's condition only at the end of the full assessment procedure. It is easy to fall into the trap of making your diagnosis on some piece of information that the patient gives you in the history, and then using the rest of the assessment to prove that you were right. If you have a patient with back pain and his history is typical of a disc protrusion, then you should be trying to prove in your physical examination that it is not a disc protrusion. Then, at the end of the examination when everything does point to a disc protrusion, you can bask in the happy knowledge that you were right all along. Another word of warning—the more experienced you become in patient examination, the more prone you are to this particular failing.

The tables of findings related to specific conditions should not be looked upon as an easy way to make a diagnosis. In fact, in the majority of cases the likeliest scenario is that a differential diagnosis will be made consisting of two or three possibilities for the ultimate cause of the patient's problem. There is no simple formula to use in these tables (for example, if three or four of the signs or symptoms suggest one particular condition, then it must be that condition). In fact, half of the patient's signs and symptoms may suggest one condition, and three or four may suggest another condition, yet the lesser number may prove to be true as regards final diagnosis. I think the value of these tables lies rather in the enhancement of a logical approach to viewing and reviewing the signs and symptoms in terms of the conditions that may be causing them. Always keep in mind two possibilities: being wrong and the patient having more than one problem at one time.

TABLE 1.1 Health History—Please place a check next to all current and past conditions:

Muscles / Joints / Nerves	Heart / Circulation	Digestion
tension or migraine headaches	high or low blood pressure	nausea or vomiting
whiplash / motor vehicle accident	chronic congestive heart failure	constipation
neck pain / stiffness / injury	heart attack or stoke	rapid weight loss
arm pain / weakness / tingling	chest pain / angina	appetite changes
back pain / stiffness / injury	varicose veins or phlebitis	diarrhea
hip or thigh pain / stiffness / injury	cold hands & feet	bad taste in mouth
leg pain / weakness / tingling	swelling in legs or hands	conditions of the colon
head trauma / concussion	diabetes	ulcers
loss of co-ordination / dizziness	light-headedness / fatigue	gall bladder problems
sleep or personality changes	poor healing / bruising	cancer
epilepsy / seizures		

TABLE 1.1 (Continued)

Muscles / Joints / Nerves	Heart / Circulation	Digestion
tooth / jaw / ear pain	**Lungs / Respiration**	**Genitourinary**
vision or hearing difficulty	asthma or bronchitis	painful urination
multiple sclerosis	emphysema	unusual color /
degenerating discs	shortness of breath	odor
osteo / rheumatoid	frequent colds or	hip or flank pain
arthritis	sinus	gynecological
osteoporosis or bone	chronic cough /	concerns
disease	smoking	Are you pregnant?
spasm / strain or sprain		
tendonitis / fibrositis /	**Skin / Immunity**	**Life Questions**
bursitis	open sores / cuts /	I exercise regularly
fractures / pins, wires,	warts	I feel good about
plates	contagious skin	life
fibromyalgia	disease	I have good sleep-
sports or work-related	tuberculosis or	ing patterns
injury	hepatitis	I have poor energy
repetitive strain	HIV	level
injury (RSI)	allergies /	I suffer from too
carpal tunnel syndrome	anaphylaxis	much stress

Use this space to elaborate on any of the above questions checked or
other conditions not listed

_____

_____

_____

Please list any prominent diseases in your immediate family (eg: heart
disease, cancer, diabetes):

_____

_____

_____

That having been said, I believe that if the majority of the signs and
symptoms, when viewed in the tables, suggest one particular diagnosis,
then the thrust of treatment is best aimed towards the anatomical structures
typically involved in that condition. The material within the tables is based
on current thinking as shown in a selection of standard texts on the subject.
Where there is a lack of agreement between texts about the significance of
particular findings, I have gone with my own personal clinical experience
based wholeheartedly on trial and error. In difficult cases I have always
found it useful to make a written list of the assessment findings, writing
against each finding the possible conditions that could give rise to it. I have
found that this can yield surprising results in what can otherwise appear to
be very obscure or confusing examination findings.

BIBLIOGRAPHY

Agur A.M.R., Ming J.L.: Grant Atlas of Anatomy (9th ed). Williams and Wilkins, Baltimore, 1991

American Physical Therapy Association: Guide to Physical Therapist Practice. Amer. Phys. Ther. Assoc., Alexandria, Virginia, 1997

Apley G.A., Solomon L.: Apley's System of Orthopaedics and Fractures (6th ed). Butterworth, London, 1982

Corrigan B., Maitland G.D.: Practical Orthopaedic Medicine. Butterworth, London, 1983

Cyriax J.: Textbook of Orthopaedic Medicine, Vol. 1, Diagnosis of Soft Tissue Lesions (8th ed). Bailliere Tindall, Eastbourne, J.K. 1982

Dambro M.R.(ed): Griffith's 5-Minute Clinical Consult. Lippincott Williams and Wilkins, Baltimore, 1992

Donatelli R.A., Wooden M.J. (eds): Orthopaedic Physical Therapy (2nd ed). Churchill Livingston, New York, 1994

Field D.: Anatomy: Palpation and Surface Marking. Butterworth-Heinemann, Oxford, J.K. 1997

Goldie B.S.: Orthopaedic Diagnosis and Management: A Guide to the Care of Orthopaedic Patients (2nd ed). ISIS Medical Media, Oxford, U.K., 1998

Gross J, Feeto J., Rosen E.: Musculoskeletal Examination. Blackwell Science, Cambridge, MA, 1996

Magee D.J.: Orthopaedic Physical Assessment (2nd ed). Philadelphia P.A., W.B. Saunders, 1992

Malone T.R., McPoil T.G., Nitz A.J. (eds): Orthopaedic and Sports Physical Therapy (3rd ed), St. Louis 1997

Prentice W.E. (ed): Rehabilitation Techniques in Sports Medicine–New York W.C.B./McGraw Hill, 1999

Williams, P.L. et al (eds): Gray's Anatomy (37th ed). Churchill Livingston, Edinburgh, 1989

The following tables contain test movements for examination of the shoulder and upper arm. The starting positions and a description of each movement are given. These would be considered the optimal test positions in each case, but would have to be modified for individual patients who are unable to achieve or sustain a described position.

Active Movements at the Glenohumeral Joint

Name of Movement	Starting Position	Movement
Flexion	Most easily tested in either sitting or standing, it can be tested in supine or side lying. The patient's hand is held at their side with the palm of the hand facing towards the leg.	The patient is instructed to raise the arm forwards and above the head, keeping the elbow straight. Average range of motion: 180°
Extension	Movement most easily tested in standing or lying, it can be tested in side lying or prone lying. The arm is held at the side with the palm facing towards the leg.	The patient is instructed to take the arm backwards as far as possible with the elbow kept straight. The movement is then repeated with the elbow bent. Average range of motion: 50–60°
Abduction	Tested most easily in sitting, standing, or side lying. The arm is held at the side with the palm of the hand facing the body.	The patient is instructed to keep the elbow straight and raise the arm sideways away from the body and above the head. Movement is repeated with the thumb turned out away from the body (lateral rotation of the shoulder) and with the thumb facing in towards the body (medial rotation of the shoulder) Average range of motion: 180°
Lateral Rotation	Most easily tested in sitting or standing, can be tested in supine or side lying.	The patient is instructed to move his hand out and away from the body while contact is maintained between the elbow and body.

(continued)

Active Movements at the Glenohumeral Joint (*continued*)

Name of Movement	Starting Position	Movement
	Arm is held into the side with the elbow flexed at 90° and the thumb facing upwards (forearm in neutral position).	Average range of motion: 80–90°
Medial Rotation	Most easily tested in sitting or standing, can be tested in supine lying.	The patient is instructed to move his hand in towards the abdomen. If movement is stopped by contact with the abdomen a second test, in sitting or standing, is to have the patient reach their hand up behind their back, between the shoulder blades, as far as possible. (This combines medial rotation with extension).
	Arm is held into the side with the elbow flexed at 90° and the thumb facing upwards (forearm in neutral position).	Average range of motion: 70–90°
Adduction	Most easily tested in sitting or standing, can be tested in supine or side lying.	The patient is instructed to carry the arm across the chest with the elbow kept straight.
	Shoulder in approximately 90° of flexion.	The arm coming into contact with the chest wall normally limits movement.

Passive Movements of the Shoulder

Name of Movement	Starting Position	Movement
Flexion	Movement can be tested in sitting, standing, supine lying, or side lying. Grasp the patient's arm with one hand placed above the wrist and the other hand above the elbow with the shoulder held in a neutral position (between medial and lateral rotation).	The arm is carried upwards and forwards so that the hand is taken above the head while the elbow is kept straight.
Extension	The movement can be tested in sitting, standing, or side lying. Grasp the patient's arm at the anterior aspect of the elbow and upper forearm with one hand. The other hand is placed over the superior aspect of the shoulder, stabilizing the shoulder girdle.	The arm is drawn backwards while the elbow is kept straight. The movement is repeated and the elbow is allowed to bend.
Lateral Rotation	The movement can be tested in sitting, standing, supine lying, or side lying. The arm is held into the side with the elbow bent to 90°. Support the midforearm with one hand and hold the patient's elbow into the side with the other hand.	The patient's hand is carried out and away from the body.
Medial Rotation	The movement can be tested in sitting, standing, supine lying, or side lying. The arm is held into the side with the elbow bent to 90°. Support the midforearm with one hand and hold the patient's elbow into the side with the other hand.	The patient's hand is carried in across the body to bring it into contact with the abdomen.

(continued)

Passive Movements of the Shoulder (*continued*)

Name of Movement	Starting Position	Movement
Lateral Rotation in Abduction	The movement can be tested in sitting, standing, supine lying, or side lying. Take the patient's arm into 90° abduction (if comfortable) with the elbow flexed at 90° (forearm parallel to the floor if the patient is in sitting or standing). Support the upper arm with one hand and hold the patient's wrist with the other hand.	The patient's hand is carried upwards above the head while the shoulder is maintained in 90° of abduction and the elbow flexed at 90°.
Medial Rotation in Abduction	The movement can be tested in sitting, standing, supine lying, or side lying. Take the patient's arm into 90° abduction (if comfortable) with the elbow flexed at 90° (forearm parallel to the floor if the patient is in sitting or standing). Support the upper arm or forearm with one hand and hold the patient's wrist with the other hand.	The patient's hand is taken downwards towards the hip with the shoulder maintained in 90° of abduction and the elbow flexed to 90°.
Adduction	The movement can be tested in sitting, standing, supine lying, or side lying. Support the patient's upper arm or forearm with the shoulder held in 70–80° of flexion.	The arm is drawn across the patient's body to bring it into contact with the chest wall, if possible. The movement is first tested in the neutral position and then retested in full medial and full lateral rotation.

Resisted Movements of the Shoulder

Name of Movement	Starting Position	Movement
Flexion	The movement can be tested in sitting, standing, supine lying, or side lying. With the patient's arm held at his side with the elbow straight, apply pressure to the anterior aspect of the upper arm.	Either try to push the arm backwards with the patient resisting the movement or have the patient try to move the arm forwards and then resist the movement.
Extension	The movement can be tested in sitting, standing, or side lying. With the patient's arm held straight at his side, apply pressure to the posterior aspect of the upper arm.	Either try to push the arm forwards with the patient resisting the movement or have the patient push the arm backwards and then resist the movement.
Abduction	The movement can be tested in sitting, standing, supine lying, or side lying. Hold the patient's arm into his side with the elbow straight. Then apply pressure to the lateral aspect of the upper arm just above the elbow.	Resist the movement as the patient tries to raise his arm sideways away from his body.
Adduction	The movement can be tested in sitting, standing, supine lying, or side lying. Hold the patient's arm into his side with the elbow straight. Then apply pressure to the medial aspect of the upper arm just above the elbow.	Attempt to draw the arm out and away from the body while the patient resists the movement.

(continued)

Resisted Movements of the Shoulder (*continued*)

Name of Movement	Starting Position	Movement
Lateral Rotation	The movement can be tested in sitting, standing, supine lying, or side lying. Hold the patient's arm into his side with the elbow flexed to 90° and the forearm in the mid position. Then apply pressure to the posterior aspect of the forearm.	Attempt to push the forearm in towards the body while the patient resists the movement. The patient's elbow must remain in contact with his side during testing.
Medial Rotation	The movement can be tested in sitting, standing, supine lying, or side lying. Hold the patient's arm into his side with the elbow flexed to 90° and the forearm in the mid position. Then apply pressure to the anterior aspect of the forearm.	Attempt to push the forearm out away from the body while the patient resists the movement. The patient's elbow must remain in contact with his side during testing.

Resisted Movements of the Shoulder Girdle

Name of Movement	Starting Position	Movement
Elevation	The movement can be tested in sitting or half lying with the patient's arms resting at his sides.	1. Apply pressure over the superior aspect of both shoulders and instruct the patient to shrug his shoulders. 2. Have the patient shrug his shoulders fully, then apply pressure over the superior aspect of the shoulder while the patient tries to maintain the position.
Retraction	The movement can be tested in sitting or half lying. Place one hand on each of the patient's shoulders over the posterior acromial rims.	1. Instruct the patient to maintain position while trying to push the shoulders forward. 2. Have the patient fully retract his shoulders, apply pressure to try to push the shoulders forward while the patient resists the movement.
Protraction	The movement can be tested in sitting. Place one hand over the anterior of each of the patient's shoulders.	1. Attempt to push the shoulders backward while the patient resists the movement. 2. Have the patient round his shoulders (bring them into protraction) then try to push the shoulders backward while the patient resists the movement.

Examination Findings Related To Specific Conditions

	Onset				
Sudden Due to Overuse	Sudden Due to Trauma	Sudden No Cause	Gradual Due to Overuse	Gradual After Trauma	Gradual No Cause
Acute Rotator Cuff Tendonitis Pectoral Muscle Tear	Rotator Cuff Tear Acromioclavicular Joint Injury	Acute Rotator Cuff Tendonitis	Acute Rotator Cuff Tendonitis Bicipital Tendonitis Subacromial Bursitis Chronic Rotator Cuff Tendonitis Chronic Instability of the Shoulder Joint	Chronic Instability of the Shoulder Joint Acromioclavicular Joint Irritation Adhesive Capsulitis	Chronic Rotator Cuff Tendonitis Adhesive Capsulitis Acromioclavicular Joint Irritation (in the older patient)

Typical Age Ranges

20–40 Years	30–50 Years	35–70 + Years	40–65 Years
Chronic Instability of the Shoulder Joint Acromioclavicular Joint Irritation Acromioclavicular Joint Injury Pectoral Muscle Tear Acute Rotator Cuff Tendonitis	Acute Rotator Cuff Tendonitis Chronic Rotator Cuff Tendonitis Rotator Cuff Tear Biceps Tendonitis	Chronic Rotator Cuff Tendonitis Subacromial Bursitis Adhesive Capsulitis	Rotator Cuff Tear Adhesive Capsulitis

Duration

Less Than 3 Weeks	Less Than 6 Weeks	6 Weeks to 3 Months	3 to 6 Months	6 Months to Years
Rotator Cuff Tear	Acute Rotator Cuff Tendonitis	Chronic Rotator Cuff Tendonitis	Adhesive Capsulitis	Chronic Instability of the Shoulder Joint
Acromioclavicular Joint Injury	Biceps Tendonitis (in athletes)	Adhesive Capsulitis	Acromioclavicular Joint Irritation	
Pectoral Muscle Tear		Biceps Tendonitis		
		Subacromial Bursitis		

Frequency

First Occurrence	First Occurrence Of These Symptoms/Recurrent Episodes of Other Minor Shoulder Problems	Similar Episodes Occurring Once or Twice per Year for 1–3 Years	One Long Single Episode of Varying Intensity
Acromioclavicular Joint Injury	Rotator Cuff Tear	Acute Rotator Cuff Tendonitis	Acromioclavicular Joint Irritation
Pectoral Muscle Tear	Adhesive Capsulitis	Chronic Rotator Cuff Tendonitis	
		Bicipital Tendonitis	
		Chronic Instability of the Shoulder Joint	
		Subacromial Bursitis	

(continued)

Examination Findings Related To Specific Conditions (continued)

Area of Symptoms

Anterior Shoulder Region	Anterior and Lateral Shoulder Region	Anterior and Lateral Shoulder and Upper Arm	Posterior/Superior Shoulder to the Point of Deltoid Insertion	Poorly Localized around the Shoulder and Upper Arm	Point of the Shoulder
Bicipital Tendonitis	Acute Rotator Cuff Tendonitis	Chronic Rotator Cuff Tendonitis	Rotator Cuff Tear	Adhesive Capsulitis	Acromioclavicular Joint Injury
Pectoral Muscle Tear		Chronic Instability of the Shoulder Joint			Acromioclavicular Joint Irritation

Type of Symptoms

Sharp Pain on Movements of Shoulder	Dull Ache—Worse After Activity	Dull Ache At Rest/Sharp Pain on Sudden Movements	Sharp Pain on Movements Followed By Ache	Stiffness—No Particular Pain	Crepitation on Movement
Rotator Cuff Tear	Chronic Rotator Cuff Tendonitis	Acute Rotator Cuff Tendonitis	Bicipital Tendonitis	Adhesive Capsulitis	Chronic Instability of the Shoulder Joint
Acromioclavicular Joint Injury	Acromioclavicular Joint Irritation	Adhesive Capsulitis	Chronic Instability of the Shoulder Joint		Chronic Rotator Cuff Tendonitis
Acute Rotator Cuff Tendonitis		Subacromial Bursitis	Acromioclavicular Joint Injury		
			Pectoral Muscle Tear		

Observations

Nil of Note	Swelling Anterior Shoulder Region	Reverse Scapulo-Humeral Rhythm	Muscle Wasting—Scapular Area	Muscle Wasting—Shoulder Region	Step / Bump at Point of Shoulder
May (and often does) apply to any of these conditions	Acute Rotator Cuff Tendonitis / Bicipital Tendonitis / Pectoral Muscle Tear (early days)	Chronic Rotator Cuff Tendonitis / Adhesive Capsulitis	Chronic Rotator Cuff Tendonitis / Rotator Cuff Tear (later on)	Adhesive Capsulitis / Chronic Rotator Cuff Tendonitis	Acromioclavicular Joint Injury / Acromioclavicular Joint Irritation

Active Movements

Full and Pain Free	Mild Limitation of Abduction	Mild Limitation of Abduction and Flexion	All Movements Limited—Particularly Lateral Rotation and Abduction	Limitation of Lateral Rotation when Arm in 90° Abduction
Chronic Instability of Shoulder Joint	Acute Rotator Cuff Tendonitis / Rotator Cuff Tear / Acromioclavicular Joint Injury	Chronic Rotator Cuff Tendonitis	Adhesive Capsulitis / Acromioclavicular Joint Injury	Bicipital Tendonitis

(continued)

Examination Findings Related To Specific Conditions (continued)

Pain and Limitation on Abduction and Medial Rotation	Full Range but with Pain in Mid-Range Abduction or Flexion	Pain with Mild Limitation of Extension and Lateral Rotation	Pain with or without Restriction on Abduction and Lateral Rotation	Pain on Flexion from Full Extension
Subacromial Bursitis	Subacromial Bursitis	Pectoral Muscle Tear	Rotator Cuff Tear Acromioclavicular Joint Irritation Acromioclavicular Joint Injury	Bicipital Tendonitis

Passive Movements

Full and Pain Free	Mild Limitation of Abduction	Restriction of All Movements, Particularly Lateral Rotation and Abduction	Pain on Adduction	Pain and Mild Limitation on Combined Extension and Lateral Rotation
Rotator Cuff Tear Chronic Instability of the Shoulder Joint	Acute Rotator Cuff Tendonitis Acromioclavicular Joint Irritation	Adhesive Capsulitis	Acromioclavicular Joint Injury Acromioclavicular Joint Irritation	Pectoral Muscle Tear

Pain on Medial and Lateral Rotation at 90° Abduction	Pain on Medial Rotation at 90° Abduction	Pain Only in Mid-Range Abduction and Flexion	Pain on Combined Extension of Shoulder and Elbow
Chronic Rotator Cuff Tendonitis Acromioclavicular Joint Injury	Subacromial Bursitis	Subacromial Bursitis	Bicipital Tendonitis

Resisted Movement

Pain on Abduction	Pain on Lateral Rotation	Pain on Medial Rotation	Pain on Flexion	Pain on Adduction
Acute Rotator Cuff Tendonitis (Supraspinatus Tendon)	Acute Rotator Cuff Tendonitis (Infraspinatus Tendon)	Chronic Rotator Cuff Tendonitis	Acromioclavicular Joint Injury	Pectoral Muscle Tear
Chronic Rotator Cuff Tendonitis	Chronic Rotator Cuff Tendonitis	Pectoral Muscle Tear	Acromioclavicular Joint Irritation	
Rotator Cuff Tear	Rotator Cuff Tear		Pectoral Muscle Tear	
	Acromioclavicular Joint Injury			

Pain on Elbow Flexion (Shoulder in extension)	Mild Weakness— Most or All Movements	Weakness on Adduction and Medial Rotation	Weakness on Both Rotations	Shoulder Gives Way under Strong Resistance
Bicipital Tendonitis	Adhesive Capsulitis	Pectoral Muscle Tear	Chronic Instability of the Shoulder Joint	Chronic Instability of the Shoulder Joint
	Subacromial Bursitis (later stages)		Subacromial Bursitis	

Palpation

Pain—Anterior Shoulder Region	Pain below Anterior Acromial Rim	Pain below Anterolateral Acromial Rim	Tenderness over Bicipital Groove	Tenderness by Bicipital Groove and Anterior Wall of Axilla	Pain over Point of Shoulder	Soft Tissue Thickening at Point of Shoulder	Excessive Play in Joint Felt during Movement
Chronic Rotator Cuff Tendonitis	Acute Rotator Cuff Tendonitis	Rotator Cuff Tear	Bicipital Tendonitis	Pectoral Muscle Tear	Acromioclavicular Joint Injury	Acromioclavicular Joint Irritation	Chronic Instability of Shoulder Joint
	Chronic Rotator Cuff Tendonitis	Subacromial Bursitis			Acromioclavicular Joint Irritation		

PALPATION OF THE SHOULDER AND UPPER ARM

In this section a description is given of the method of palpating each structure referred to in relation to the following conditions:

- Acute Rotator Cuff Tendonitis
- Chronic Rotator Cuff Tendonitis
- Rotator Cuff Tear
- Adhesive Capsulitis
- Bicipital Tendonitis
- Impingement Syndrome
- Chronic Shoulder Joint Instability
- Acromioclavicular Joint Injury
- Acromioclavicular Joint Irritation
- Pectoralis Muscle Tear
- Subacromial Bursitis

Deep palpation at the anterior of the shoulder below the acromial rim will always produce pain (just try it on yourself) so palpate with even greater care than normal in this area. The following structures need to be identified.

The Acromial Rim (Fig. 2.1)

Pass a finger along the anterior border of the clavicle laterally and it will move onto the anterior border of the acromion. Follow this around as it

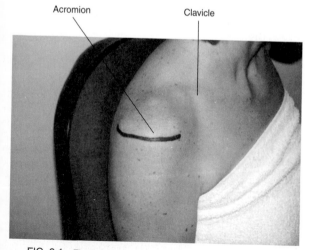

FIG. 2.1   The line marks the acromial rim of the right shoulder.

turns posteriorly and it then becomes the lateral border. This then passes medially to become the posterior border, which in turn forms the lower lip of the spine of the scapula (Fig. 2.2). Palpate under the rim of the acromion, all the way around from front to back, to see if it is possible to elicit any tenderness. Also check the same area with the back of the hand for increased warmth.

Supraspinatus Tendon

This is most easily palpated with the finger placed half an inch below the lateral acromial rim. The examining finger will be on the contour of the shoulder over the greater tubercle (Fig. 2.3). The arm is then placed in about 30 degrees of abduction and passively rotated—this will move the tendon under the examining finger.

Biceps Tendon (Fig. 2.4)

This structure lies about 1 inch medial to the greater tubercle in a groove that is usually quite easy to palpate. The tendon can be felt to move in its

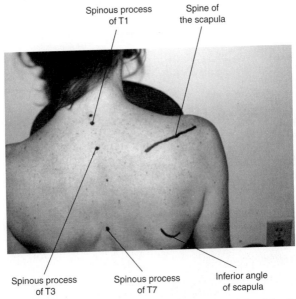

FIG. 2.2   The spine and inferior angle of the right scapula in relation to the thoracic spinous processes.

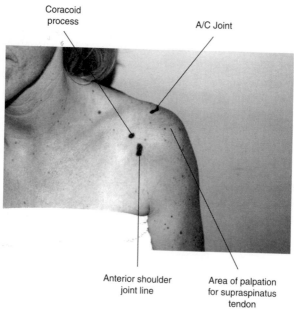

Coracoid process

A/C Joint

Anterior shoulder joint line

Area of palpation for supraspinatus tendon

FIG. 2.3 The area for palpation of the supraspinatus tendon at the left shoulder.

groove as the arm is rotated medially and laterally while in 90 degrees of abduction.

Acromioclavicular Joint

Follow the line of the clavicle as it flattens out on top of the acromion—at its lateral end there is a small tubercle. Just lateral to this landmark it is possible to palpate the acromioclavicular joint line (Fig. 2.5), which is easier to do when the joint is in motion. Downward pressure should be applied to the lateral end of the clavicle to determine if this produces any tenderness in the region of the acromioclavicular joint.

Crepitation

This phenomenon deserves a special mention in the shoulder region because it can be either very significant or totally irrelevant, depending on the patient's condition. In this author's experience, about one half of all

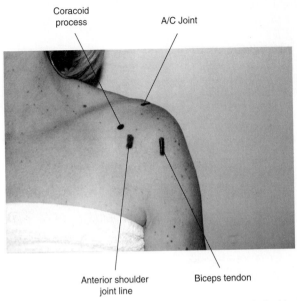

Coracoid process

A/C Joint

Anterior shoulder joint line

Biceps tendon

FIG. 2.4 The area for palpation of the biceps tendon at the left shoulder.

shoulders examined make cracking and grinding noises. These are felt particularly well when one hand is placed over the shoulder and the other hand is used to passively rotate the arm while it is held in 90 degrees of abduction. When this crepitation is found in both shoulders and is painless, it appears to have no diagnostic significance. If it is only present in the affected shoulder, and hurts, then it suggests that the rotator cuff tendons are being rubbed between the acromion and the greater tubercle of the humerus. The patient will often complain that his shoulder "joint" creaks, but this seldom occurs, except in a truly arthritic shoulder. In that case there will be clear x-ray findings. Once you have palpated an arthritic shoulder you will not forget the difference between bone grating and tendons rubbing.

SPECIFIC TESTS FOR THE SHOULDER AND ARM

Painful Arc of Movement

This is tested by raising the arm, both actively and passively, from the side while keeping it straight. If a painful arc is present the patient will expe-

Acromio-Clavicular
joint

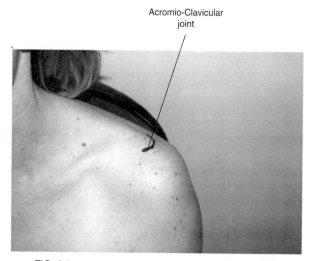

FIG. 2.5   The line marks the left acromioclavicular joint line.

rience discomfort between 60 and 120 degrees of abduction. In the classic painful arc of movement there is no discomfort below 60 degrees or above 120 degrees of abduction. However, in many cases, particularly in more chronic conditions, there will be less pain rather than no pain after approximately 120 degrees of abduction, compared to the discomfort felt in the 60 to 120 degree arc.

Yergason's Sign

The patient is tested in sitting with the arm held into the side with the elbow flexed to 90 degrees. The forearm is placed in the pronated position, then the movements of supination of the forearm and lateral rotation of the arm are resisted. Pain experienced in the region of the bicipital groove is indicative of bicipital tendonitis.

Speeds Test

The patient is tested in sitting or standing with the arm straight and the forearm supinated. The examiner then resists the movement of flexion of the shoulder. The test is considered positive if it produces increased tenderness in the bicipital groove on palpation during testing.

Shoulder Joint Instability

Many tests can be used to check for instability of the glenohumeral joint. Only three are given. These three are know as the Rowe tests for multi-directional instability. These tests are used to determine if there is a tendency towards subluxation of the joint. However, they can also indicate an increased degree of laxity compared to the expected normal. With the patient standing in a slightly forward flexed position with the arm relaxed and hanging, place one hand over the glenohumeral joint, with the thumb placed on the posterior aspect over the head of the humerus and the first two fingers over the anterior aspect of the humeral head. Apply light traction to the arm pulling it down towards the floor. Then carry the arm into approximately 25 degrees of extension and apply pressure to the posterior of the humeral head with the thumb, pushing it forwards. The patient's arm is then brought into approximately 25 degrees of flexion and pressure is applied to the anterior of the humeral head with the fingers to push it posteriorly. To test for inferior instability greater traction is applied to the arm; if truly significant instability is present, an indentation will be noted below the acromial rim laterally. This is known as the Sulcus sign.

Acromioclavicular Shear Test

The patient is tested in sitting and the examiner places the heels of the hands so that they cup the deltoid muscle anteriorly and posteriorly in such a way that the one hand is on the clavicle and the other hand over the spine of the scapula. The examiner then squeezes the hands together, applying a shearing stress to the acromioclavicular joint. Pain felt at the shoulder or an abnormal degree of movement present during testing suggests pathology of the acromioclavicular joint.

Impingement Tests

The patient is tested in sitting with the arm flexed to approximately 90 degrees. The arm is then passively internally rotated as far as possible. The sign is considered positive if during the maneuver pain is produced, which may be felt at the shoulder or upper arm.

Emptying Can

This is another impingement test. In this case the patient is instructed to sit with the arm elevated to approximately 90 degrees and positioned halfway between abduction and flexion, with the shoulder in a position of full lateral rotation. The patient is then instructed to turn the hand over as if they were emptying out a can. Pain produced towards the end of available range of medial rotation suggests impingement of either the supraspinatus or biceps tendons.

SHOULDER AND UPPER ARM CONDITIONS

Acute Rotator Cuff Tendonitis

This condition is usually found in the 25 to 40-year-old age range. The patient's history may have to be sifted through carefully because the symptoms will often be attributed to one particular injury. However, further specific questioning will usually reveal that the patient has had mild ongoing shoulder pain related to repetition of a particular activity, and this is just the worst episode so far. This could be called an acute on chronic condition, as the supraspinatus tendon can be subtly injured by compression between the acromion and the greater tubercle of the humerus when the arm is used repetitively at or about shoulder height. This leads to degeneration of the tendon, which in turn leads to bouts of acute inflammation. Given time and neglect this condition can become truly chronic; to avoid this care should be taken to remedy the cause, that is, the particular overhead activity that produces the recurrent symptoms, not just the present symptoms (1, 2, 5, 8, 25).

Subjective Findings

Onset This is usually gradual due to overuse, although any particular episode may be classified by the patient as sudden due to overuse. The commonest age range is 25 to 40 years, but can be younger if the patient participates in a sport with repetitive overhead activity, such as serving in tennis or pitching a baseball (2, 12, 16).

Duration To classify as an acute episode the time since onset should not be more than about 6 weeks, although it is the presentation of the condition that will define acuity. In general terms the longer the patient has suffered the problem, the more chronic in nature the underlying inflammatory process.

Frequency The condition typically reoccurs once or twice a year over a 2- or 3-year period, and can often be related to the start of a particular sports season or to working on a particular activity at home, such as "spring cleaning" (5, 8, 12, 16).

Area of Symptoms The patient usually complains of symptoms at the anterior of the shoulder joint region and over the anterolateral aspect of the acromial rim (Fig. 2.6) (3, 4).

Type of Symptoms Pain is often experienced as a dull ache following activity, with sharp anterior shoulder pain reported on sudden movements of the arm (12, 14, 15).

Miscellaneous The patient usually complains of pain on overhead activities and an inability to sleep on the affected side or pain on turning over in bed (14, 15).

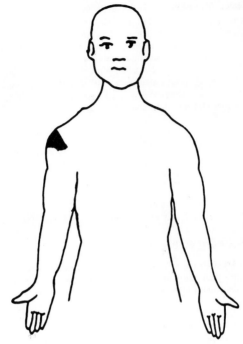

FIG. 2.6 The area of symptoms for acute rotator cuff tendonitis at the right shoulder.

Objective Findings

Observation Occasionally swelling can be seen at the anterior aspect of the shoulder below the acromial rim, particularly in the first few days following onset. Otherwise the joint will appear normal (14).

Active Movements In the truly acute condition, range of movement will be full, although in a severe case there may be limitation of abduction, medial rotation and flexion at mid-range due to pain. The patient will be unable to lift their arm past mid-range for a few days (1, 11, 15).

Passive Movements The findings on passive testing will be the same as on active movements in terms of both pain and any possible limitation of movement (1, 11, 13, 15).

Resisted Movements There should be near full strength on all movements, particularly if they are tested in an initially pain-free position, such as with the arm by the side. There may be weakness due to pain if abduction is tested at 90 degrees, and any strongly resisted movement is likely to produce some discomfort in the shoulder region due to stress placed on the rotator cuff as it stabilizes the shoulder joint. In very acute cases resisted abduction may be painful if the supraspinatus is the offending tendon, lateral rotation may be uncomfortable if the infraspinatus is at fault, and adduction can cause pain when the subscapularis muscle is affected (10, 11, 13).

Palpation A tender cord, the tendon of insertion of supraspinatus, can often be palpated below the anterior portion of the acromial rim (Figs. 2.1, 2.3). It is most easily palpated during passive medial and lateral rotation of the shoulder with the arm in approximately 30 degrees of abduction (2, 12, 21, 22).

Specific Tests It is not uncommon for the patient to present with a painful arc of movement somewhere between 60 and 120 degrees of abduction (13, 21, 23).

Treatment Ideas (1, 2–4, 7–9, 12, 15, 24, 26, 27)

Initial Treatment A trial of ice and rest is often beneficial in the early stages. It is particularly important to have the patient avoid any specific activity that appears to be an ongoing cause of recurrent bouts of symptoms. Rest *should not* exclude all movements of the shoulder, as sensible range-of-motion exercises within the available pain-free ranges will help to reduce the chance of the condition turning into a chronic problem.

The use of modalities that promote the body's repair processes can also prove beneficial. However, those that produce tissue heating are not indicated while ice is being employed as an anti-inflammatory agent. This stage of treatment should be continued for at least 2 days, and if the patient is making progress then there is no reason why it should not be pursued for a further 6 or 7 days. If the use of ice is not beneficial in the first 2 or 3 days, then continuing with this particular approach is likely to prove futile in the long run.

Whether the use of ice is effective or not, the progression of exercise remains the same. The application of heat can now be used prior to exercise, both to relax the patient and to make early exercise less uncomfortable. Continue active exercises for all shoulder movements with the patient carrying each movement to the end of pain-free range, but not into pain. Isometric-resisted exercises in pain-free ranges for flexion and extension will often prove beneficial with progression to resisted rotations, abduction, and then adduction as long as the patient is able to tolerate them. These exercises can be progressed to isotonic-resisted work through available range as symptoms subside. Continued use of modalities such as ultrasound, laser, and interferential therapy can help alleviate post-exercise discomfort.

The use of reciprocal pulleys can help patients both to maintain the range of motion that they have gained and to stretch out the soft tissues of the shoulder joint. Patients' usually find this exercise quite easy and relaxing, and it is a form of therapy that they can set up for themselves at home. Exercises using a cane held in both hands, done in both lying and standing, can provide a form of active-assisted exercises, with the unaffected arm helping the affected limb. Patients also often tolerate free-swinging exercises very well. Attempt these initially just using the weight of the arm and then, as the patient demonstrates an ability to tolerate the exercise, weights can be held in the hand or, preferably, wrapped around the wrist, as this allows for greater relaxation of the rotator cuff during the exercise. Patients may also benefit from a program of active shoulder girdle exercises as pain and muscle tension, or outright muscle spasm, can occur in the upper trapezius muscle on the affected side.

As treatment progresses strengthening of the rotator cuff becomes paramount. Use of a resistive exercise band is a simple and effective means of applying resistance to the movements of rotation of the shoulder. Initially only the rotations are strengthened, as this will allow for observation of the effects of the exercise and show if the patient is fully ready for the progression of their exercise program. Concentrating on the rotators impresses upon the patient the singular importance of this muscle group as the primary stabilizers of the shoulder joint.

Resisted exercises for all the other movements of the shoulder are initiated as soon as the patient is able to tolerate resisted rotation. One set of the resisted-rotation exercises can be carried out after every set of exercises for each of the other movements, as this once again impresses on the patient the importance of the rotator cuff. It will also help to improve stability of the joint at a crucial stage in the rehabilitation process.

A routine of stretching exercises for all movements of the shoulder will help to reduce the risk of soft tissue restrictions later on, and should be combined with the resisted exercises. Activities that have been identified by the patient as possible causative factors should be analyzed to determine which specific movements of the shoulder are involved. A progressive exercise program should then be designed that is geared to the patients' lifestyle, both work and leisure, and that can be continued at home or in a gym, depending on the degree of exercise required. The two most important considerations in this exercise program will be stretching of tight soft-tissue structures and strengthening of weak muscle groups, as identified during ongoing assessment of the patient.

Restrictions In the early stages of treatment the patient is advised to stop any activity that produces his typical symptoms. The patient may be able to sustain some activities for a short period of time before their symptoms start to appear, then after a rest they may be able to continue with the activity again, stopping once more as soon as any symptoms become apparent. The patient has to use a good deal of common sense in stopping and starting these activities and should be advised to err on the side of caution whenever they are unsure of the effect that a particular activity is having on their condition. If the therapist feels that the patient is likely to put himself at risk, more specific restrictions should be applied.

In the majority of cases, working with the arms held at or above 70 degrees of flexion or abduction for any period of time is likely to prove problematic. Typical activities of this type are dusting and cleaning walls or ceilings, cleaning windows, or hanging out washing. In sports, overhead shots with a racket or throwing activities should be strongly curtailed in the early stages of the condition. Symptoms may not appear until 1 to 2 hours after an activity; the patient must be made aware of this possibility. The activity should then be stopped, as the chances of accidental exacerbation of the condition will be high. If the patient is able to change the way that an activity is carried out so that it no longer produces symptoms, they can, of course, do so. On the other hand, this should not place any undue strain on another part of the body or it will produce more problems than it solves. Keen athletes and conscientious workers are two categories of patients who are prone to this type of ill-advised activity modification.

As the patient gains pain-free range of motion with exercises above shoulder level, he can begin to attempt activities that previously produced symptoms. Return to these activities must be graduated, using only low weights and short durations of activity initially. Duration of the activity should be progressed first. As the patient tolerates increased duration, then the degree of weight or force involved in the activity can also be increased. It is important to have the patient simulate work, sports, or leisure activities in the clinic before attempting them in those actual environments.

In truly acute rotator cuff tendonitis, complete recovery should be expected within 4 to 6 weeks of treatment. The important issue is prevention of further recurrent episodes through rectification of causative factors and good muscle conditioning.

Chronic Rotator Cuff Tendonitis

Overview

Most rotator cuff problems have a chronic history (see acute rotator cuff tendonitis); the main factors that produce chronicity are simply time and neglect. The neglect is on the part of the patient who, having suffered mild recurrent shoulder problems, that always cleared up with time and a little rest in the past, now continues with activities that produce the symptoms and ends up with a condition that refuses to improve. The pathological process is the same as that described for the acute form of this condition, but the tendon becomes chronically swollen or damaged with subsequent scarring and thickening of the tissues. Signs of impingement at the shoulder can often be found concurrently with this condition (3, 5, 28).

Subjective Findings

Onset This is usually gradual with no known cause, or possibly associated with recurrent overuse (3, 4).

Duration The present episode will have usually persisted for at least 2 months, and often longer, before the patient seeks treatment.

Frequency There should be a history of previous episodes of similar symptoms, but less prolonged and less restricting, going back over the previous 2 years or more (3, 8).

Area of Symptoms Presence of symptoms is indicated in the anterolateral aspect of the shoulder and upper arm by the patient demonstrating the area with the whole hand, as the symptoms are usually poorly localized (Fig. 2.7). There may also be complaints of discomfort in the upper trapezius on the affected side, possibly due to muscle spasm (2, 11, 14).

Type of Symptoms The pain is described as a dull ache that is worse with activity. The patient often complains of sharp pains on certain shoulder movements, usually those involving some degree of rotation of the joint (14, 15).

Objective Findings

Observation Upset in scapulohumeral rhythm may occur on shoulder abduction and there may also be a mild degree of muscle wasting around the shoulder and scapula regions (6, 19, 21).

Active Movements Mild limitation of active abduction and medial rotation is often found, with complaints of stiffness and discomfort, rather than pain, at end range of these movements (6, 8, 9).

Passive Movements Pain can be elicited through the mid range of medial and lateral rotation when the movements are tested with the arm abducted to 90 degrees. End feel to abduction and both rotations is usually one of tight soft-tissue resistance, which is like trying to stretch a thick piece of rubber (6, 8, 13, 15).

Resisted Movements Pain is usually elicited on isometric abduction. Either or both rotations may also produce discomfort, but to a lesser degree (2, 13).

Palpation There may be diffuse tenderness around the anterior aspect of the shoulder joint below the anterior rim of the acromion. In some cases localized tenderness may be elicited over the supraspinatus or subscapularis tendons (Figs. 2.1, 2.3) (3, 14, 22).

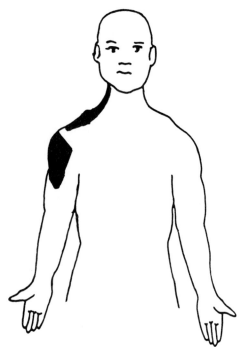

FIG. 2.7   The area of symptoms (usually poorly localized) for chronic rotator cuff tendonitis at the right shoulder.

Specific Tests   A painful arc of movement is often present on both passive and active abduction of the shoulder. Pain may also increase towards the end of available range of abduction as the movement becomes stiff; however, there should still be comparatively greater pain between 60 and 120 degrees of abduction (13, 21, 23).

Treatment Ideas (2, 4, 5, 7, 10, 12, 15, 16, 26, 27)

Modalities and physical agents can be used to heat the area of the affected joint and are combined with active exercises in order to regain lost mobility. The use of assisted movements and auto-assisted exercises performed by the patient are often most effective in regaining lost range of movement, without producing undue discomfort, in the early stages of treatment. The patient will benefit from advice on how to set up a reciprocal pulley system at home. Modalities such as interferential therapy and transcutaneous electrical nerve stimulation can help to alleviate post-exercise discomfort.

Pendular free-swinging exercises can be started with the patient standing erect, rather than leaning forward, because when the patient leans forward the swinging arm is already in the painful arc range of 60+ degrees of flexion. With the patient standing erect instruct him to swing the arm reasonably vigorously, initially with no weight and then with steadily increasing weight as he shows an ability to tolerate the exercise. The exercise should be done with a certain amount of vigor so that the momentum built up by the weight of the arm will provide a mobilizing force for tight, stiff, soft tissue around the affected joint.

As pain decreases and range of motion increases the patient can be progressed onto a full set of active exercises for the shoulder, shoulder girdle, and elbow. At the same time general resisted exercises can be started, initially in early ranges, which should be pain-free. The exercises are then progressed through range and with increasing resistance. Use of a resistive exercise band is an effective way of providing resisted exercises in a format that the patient can continue to use easily at home. Initially exercises with the resistance band can be done in a lying position. Patients usually find it easy enough to do straight arm flexion to approximately 90 or 100 degrees, alternating arms. This can be followed by working from a position with the arms held in 90 degrees of flexion of the shoulder, and drawing the arm back down to the side for resisted extension. Then again, with the arms in the same 90 degree of shoulder flexion starting position, the arms can be drawn away from each other into horizontal abduction. Lateral rotation can be carried out simultaneously for both arms, with both elbows tucked into the sides and bent to 90 degrees. Get the patient to draw his hands apart to produce the movement of lateral rotation at the shoulders. To resist medial rotation the resistance band needs to be tied to some immovable object, such as a door knob or railing, and the movement is carried out with the elbow flexed at 90 degrees and the hand carried in towards the body.

The resisted exercises for flexion, extension, and abduction, which were previously done in a lying position, can now be done sitting or standing. In the standing position resisted abduction can be added to the exercises with the patient instructed to draw the arm away from the side into approximately 90 degrees of abduction at the shoulder. Once the patient is able to do these exercises without any discomfort he can increase the range to go past the 90-degree point for flexion and abduction. The use of thermal agents and other modalities can be continued at this stage, although their value diminishes once the patient gains a reasonable range of motion (70–80%). As soon as resisted rotations are painless, emphasis can be placed on progressive strengthening of the rotator cuff, as this will help to decrease the likelihood of future recurrence of symptoms.

In many cases gains in range of motion are erratic; at those times when the patient appears to have reached a plateau, further gains can be made by the use of different passive movements. The simplest form of this treatment approach is the use of the same passive movements that were used in assessing the patient. With the patient supine, grip the upper arm and support the arm fully. Each movement is then carried to the end of available range where a gentle overpressure is applied. This overpressure can be applied in two ways, either in the form of small amplitude movements repeated many times, or in the form of sustained pressure applied at the point of resistance to movement, which is then held for 15 to 20 seconds at a time. These movements should not be particularly uncomfortable because if they are, the patients' voluntary resistance to the movement will prevent any effective gains in range.

Latter Stages   The patient can be progressed to a gym-type exercise program suitable to their lifestyle and rehabilitation goals. Full range of motion should be present by this time and the aim of treatment should be to restore full functional muscle strength with the emphasis on rotator cuff strengthening in order to stabilize the joint. This can be accomplished by having the patient repeat resisted rotation exercises, particularly lateral rotation, between sets of general strengthening exercises for the upper extremities. Strengthening of the biceps muscle can also be very helpful, as the action of the long head of the biceps as it passes over the top of the humerus and through the shoulder joint is to draw the humerus down away from the acromium, thus providing more space for the inflamed tendons of the rotator cuff. It is important for the patient to have a home-exercise program of general upper extremity stretches; these should be employed at regular intervals throughout the weight-training program to promote flexibility of the soft tissues of the shoulder girdle and upper extremities.

Restrictions   These are the same as those suggested for acute rotator cuff tendonitis with avoidance of overhead activities in the early stages. Return to those types of activities should commence only as and when the patient demonstrates the ability to perform the movements without any undue discomfort. Return to activities identified as producing the patients' symptoms should be gradual and monitored by the therapist, with correction of technique as required.

Chronic rotator cuff tendonitis can clear quite quickly, but usually does not. It tends to be less responsive to treatment and the patient cannot be progressed as quickly as one who is suffering from the acute form of this condition. However, in the long run the result should be the same and the patient is expected to gain full recovery in about 8 to 12 weeks.

Rotator Cuff Tear

Overview

In the majority of cases rotator cuff tear is now suspected to be an acute injury occurring in an already degenerate tendon, despite the fact that the patient often does not give a history of previous problems with the shoulder. The mechanism of injury is usually a fall onto the outstretched arm, or it may follow a sudden and unaccustomed degree of strain applied to the shoulder during pushing or pulling activities. Tears can be partial or complete; if diagnosed as complete, referral for an orthopaedic consult is warranted. Often only the deep surface of the tendon is torn or, more rarely, just the superficial surface (5, 17, 19, 25).

Subjective Findings

Onset The patient is usually between 45 and 65 years of age. Onset is sudden and due to trauma, although in the older patient the degree of force required to disrupt the tendon might be quite trivial (5, 11, 15).

Duration Patients are usually referred quite quickly because of the degree of incapacity that the condition can produce, so most patients are seen within a month of onset of their symptoms.

Frequency The patient often reports this as being the first such episode of these particular symptoms, although a history of recurrent minor shoulder problems might be given.

Area of Symptoms Symptoms should be well localized to the posterior and upper aspect of the shoulder or in the area of the deltoid insertion (Fig. 2.8) (2, 4, 11, 14).

Type of Symptoms Pain is sharp in nature, particularly on movement. There can also be a persistent deep ache even at rest.

Miscellaneous The patient often reports being unable to sleep on his back or on the affected side, and is woken by turning over in bed. The patient will also report being unable to lift or carry weight with the affected arm.

Objective Findings

Observation There is usual nothing out of the ordinary to observe, although in the early days following injury mild swelling may be seen around the area of the acromial rim. In longstanding cases muscle wasting may be noted in the area of the belly of the supraspinatus muscle, in the supraspinous fossa, or generally around the shoulder region (2, 4, 14).

Active Movements Abduction and lateral rotation of the shoulder are painful during movement and abduction will be slightly limited. Medial rotation may also be slightly limited and painful at the end of available range. In cases where the movement of abduction is grossly limited, but without any great degree of discomfort reported by the patient during testing, a complete tear should be suspected (13, 18, 19).

Passive Movements Passive movements are usually full and substantially pain-free, although some discomfort may be produced at the end of range on medial rotation. End feel will be normal for all movements of the shoulder (1, 2, 13, 19).

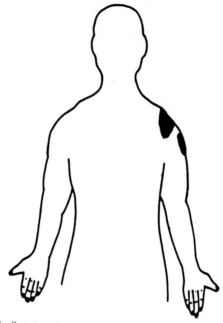

FIG. 2.8   Symptoms (usually well localized) for a rotator cuff tear at the right shoulder.

Resisted Movements Pain and weakness will be exhibited on resisted abduction and possibly also on lateral rotation. Marked painless weakness of a movement should alert the therapist to the possibility of a complete rupture of the tendon (1, 2, 13, 19).

Palpation Tenderness can often be elicited under the anterior and lateral aspects of the acromial rim (Fig. 2.1) (1, 19, 22).

Treatment Ideas (1, 2, 4–6, 9, 11, 14–17, 19, 30)

Initial Treatment If onset is recent then the RICE (rest, ice, compression and elevation) principles should be applied for the first 2 to 3 days. The patient is advised to ice the shoulder region for a period of 10–15 minutes every 2 hours, while avoiding as far as possible any movement that produces symptoms and also avoiding any sudden movements of the arm, as this is the way in which the patient most commonly exacerbates the condition. Compression and elevation of the shoulder are impractical, if not impossible.

To fully rest the arm the patient will often need to make sure that it is well supported when sleeping. One method of achieving this is to have the patient sleep in the supine position with a pillow placed behind the shoulder and along the length of the arm on the affected side. This both helps to support the arm, preventing the humerus translating posteriorly at the glenoid, and also tends to turn the patient slightly towards the other side so that he is less likely to roll onto the affected shoulder.

Active and assisted exercises should be commenced in lying initially and then progressed to sitting or standing. After the first few days the use of superficial heat therapy before exercise and ice after exercise can help to minimize discomfort, while other modalities such as laser and ultrasound can be used to enhance the body's response to injury.

Active exercise should be progressed by the use of assisted stretches at the end range of each movement. Mobilizing force can be applied to the joint by either the therapist or the patient. Passive mobilizations are done in the same way as that described for rotator cuff tendonitis. The patient can also carry out exercises using a cane held in both hands so that the unaffected arm is used to help mobilize the affected shoulder joint. It is best to start these exercises in a lying position and progress to standing. They can be combined with free-swinging exercises using the weight of the arm as a mobilizing force. Once this is tolerated by the patient a weight can be held in the hand or wrapped around the wrist.

Light resisted exercises to maintain general condition can be used for all non-affected, and therefore pain-free, muscles such as biceps, triceps, pectoral muscles, trapezius, and latissimus dorsi. Care should be taken to limit the degree of resistance so that the rotator cuff is not overtaxed in its role as a stabilizer of the shoulder.

At about 6 weeks post-injury resisted exercises can be started for the affected rotator cuff muscles, while general strengthening of the rest of the arm can be progressed steadily. More forceful passive mobilizations of the shoulder can also be used at this time if the patient is experiencing difficulty in regaining range of motion. Mobilization is best achieved by gentle but prolonged overpressure at the point of resistance to movement.

The patient should finally be progressed to a gym-type exercise program tailored to individual goals and the use of physical agents or electrical modalities should no longer be required. A program of general upper extremity stretches is given to the patient at this time to help maintain soft-tissue extensibility.

Restrictions In the initial stages following injury, activity at or above 70 degrees of either abduction or flexion of the shoulder should be avoided by using the other arm for daily tasks whenever possible and by using steps to reach objects at or above shoulder height, rather than reaching with the affected arm. If sports or recreational activities require movements into painful ranges, they should be curtailed for approximately 2 to 3 weeks.

Work activities should be modified to avoid work at or above shoulder height for the affected arm. The patient will have to exercise caution in activities such as climbing ladders or crawling on all fours.

As shoulder pain decreases and range of motion increases, then light work can be carried out at shoulder height; however, the frequency and duration of this kind of activity should be graduated to avoid recurrence of symptoms. When full pain-free range of movement is restored and shoulder stability has been established, then the patient can make a graduated return to all their pre-injury activities. Review of sports or work techniques is essential at this time to avoid recurrent shoulder problems.

Rotator cuff tears can be expected to clear completely with treatment. Prevention of further injury is important and requires a detailed understanding of the patient's lifestyle requirements. Return to full function can take 3 months, particularly if the patient's work or other daily activities tend to put a great deal of strain on the rotator cuff.

Adhesive Capsulitis

Overview

This condition is often referred to as "frozen shoulder," however, this term has come to be used to describe any shoulder condition that is painful and limits movement. It is far better to restrict the use of the term adhesive capsulitis to a chronic limitation of shoulder movement related to adherence of the capsule of the shoulder joint both to itself and to underlying bony structures. Primary adhesive capsulitis usually has no known cause of onset, however, the condition can also be secondary to virtually any other shoulder condition. It is usually described as having three overlapping phases (11, 12, 14, 15):

Phase 1: Pain is experienced in and around the shoulder joint and is made worse by movement, but there is minimal loss of range of motion.
Phase 2: Increasing pain that starts to seriously restrict movements and leads to loss of range of motion and the start of joint stiffness.
Phase 3: Steadily lessening pain but increasing stiffness and loss of range of motion.

This condition usually resolves spontaneously in 12 to 18 months with the third phase of the condition slowly easing so that movement in the affected joint returns gradually. The aim of therapy is to speed up the natural progression of the condition. It should be noted that although the majority of cases clear completely, a small percentage of patients do end up with permanent restriction of motion in the affected joint (12, 14, 18).

Subjective Findings

Onset The patient is usually between 40 and 60 years of age. Commonly, onset is gradual with no cause, although it can develop gradually after trauma (1, 5, 11, 17).

Duration Patients are rarely seen within the first 2 or 3 months following onset of the condition. Patients being referred 6 to 9 months after onset are not uncommon.

Frequency The patient usually reports this as being the first time he has experienced this type of symptoms; however, some patients may have a history of an old shoulder injury or other previous shoulder problems (5, 11, 17).

Area of Symptoms Symptoms are usually poorly localized in an area around the shoulder region and are often also referred into the anterolateral aspect of the upper arm (Fig. 2.9) (11, 15, 18, 19).

Type of Symptoms The typical pain is a poorly defined ache with occasional sharp pains on movement. Stiffness is a common feature after about the second month following onset. The degree of either pain or stiffness that the patient experiences will vary throughout the course of the condition.

Miscellaneous The patient usually cannot lie on his affected side and women will also complain of having great difficulty doing their hair or hooking their bra. Reaching back behind their body to pick up objects also presents major problems.

Objective Findings

Observation There is often general wasting of the musculature around the shoulder region with loss of the smooth shoulder contour on

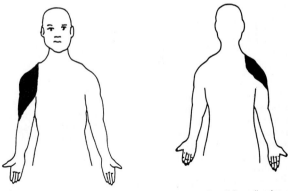

FIG. 2.9 The area of symptoms (usually poorly defined) for adhesive capsulitis at the right shoulder.

the affected side. This will become more marked in longer-standing cases (5, 17, 20).

Active Movements Restriction of all movements is usually present and progresses with time, with abduction and lateral rotation being particularly limited. Upset in scapulohumeral rhythm will be present on elevation of the arm (11, 12, 15, 21).

Passive Movements The pattern of restriction will be the same as that found on active movements. End feel will be stiff for most movements although adduction and extension may feel normal. Pain is often experienced on overpressure at end range of motion particularly on abduction and lateral rotation (12, 15, 21).

Resisted Movements In the initial stages movements are quite strong, but usually by the time the therapist sees the patient, there is some weakness of abduction, both rotations and, to a lesser extent, flexion of the shoulder joint (12, 13, 15, 16).

Palpation In most cases there are no findings of increased temperature or swelling, and no tenderness is elicited on palpation.

Treatment Ideas (1, 4, 6–8, 10, 12, 15–18, 29, 31)

Initial Treatment The use of physical agents and electrical modalities (for their thermal effects) can be useful in promoting early gains in range of motion. Active, passive, and assisted range-of-motion exercises are essential in the early stages of treatment. Any pain-relieving modalities are also appropriate when discomfort prevents attempted range-of-motion exercises. Passive distraction of the shoulder joint can be an effective way to stimulate gains in range of motion. When pain is still a major symptom care must be taken to work the arm only in available range, while pain-relieving modalities remain the treatment of choice.

Initial mobilizing exercises are done by the patient in supine and side lying. If the patient is able to elevate the arm past the point of 90 degrees, either in flexion or in abduction, then the weight of the arm will act as a mobilizing force while the exercise is carried out in the lying position. Instruct the patient to use either short oscillatory movements at end of available range or slow, steady, sustained pressure at the point of resistance to movement. The less painful the restriction of motion the more vigorously the stretch can be applied to the affected joint. When applying stretch at end of available range regulate the degree of force applied by observing the patient's reaction. Reciprocal pulleys allow the patient to mobilize the joint at his own pace, and are a very effective form of home exercise. Free-swinging exercises can be carried out by the patient in a slightly forward flexed position supporting the body weight with the hand of the unaffected arm on a chair or similar support. The aim of this exercise is to use the momentum of the arm to provide the mobilizing force.

Progression to resisted exercises is made as range of motion increases so that the patient's own musculature can start to provide a greater mobilizing force. If muscle wasting is a noticeable feature, then the use of neuromuscular electrical stimulation can hasten recovery of muscle function. The stimulation can be used in conjunction with either active or resisted movements. As movements become less painful and stiff, the passive mobilizations can become more aggressive in nature. Slow prolonged stretches of 1 to 2 minutes' duration at the end of available range are the authors' preferred method of mobilization, combined with longitudinal distraction of the glenohumeral joint.

Progression of resisted exercises into a gym setting can begin as soon as the patient can control movements with minor weights (4 to 6 pounds). Double arm work is particularly useful as the patient can use the unaffected arm to control the weights, while using the force generated to both help mobilize and strengthen the affected joint. Weights, repetitions, and range of motion for the resisted exercises are progressed as the patient demonstrates an ability to control use of the affected joint. Once pain has ceased to be a major symptom, progression of resisted gym exercises can be approached in as aggressive a manner as would be used for the healthy individual.

Restrictions Restrictions on activity during the painful stage of this condition should include restricting any activities that require stretching into painful ranges of motion. Activities in the early ranges of motion are usually fairly unrestricted, even if they require lifting or carrying relatively heavy weights. As long as the patient is not required to lift weight out and away from the body, he should not experience any pain and should be able to lift safely using his legs and torso.

Most activities that would be detrimental to the patient are self-limited by a mechanical inability to move the joint through the required range of motion. The patient should therefore be advised to show simple common sense in his approach to daily activities. Return to normal activities of daily living will occur spontaneously as range of motion and muscle strength return. The majority of patients will recover in 10 to 12 weeks with treatment. Patients who have not shown definite signs of improvement in about half that time need to be referred to a specialist for evaluation of other treatment options.

Bicipital Tendonitis

Overview

The tendon of the long head of biceps can become inflamed in the bicipital groove of the humerus. This does not necessarily relate to use of the biceps muscle, as the bony groove obviously moves every time the arm does, and it is this movement of the bone against the tendon that can produce pain and inflammation. The usual cause is repetitive or unaccustomed lifting the symptoms are often recurrent (4, 8, 14).

Subjective Findings

Onset   The patient is commonly between 30 and 50 years of age and will describe a gradual onset of symptoms following overuse of the arm (8, 18–19).

Duration   Normally the patient will have been suffering the condition for several weeks or even months before seeking treatment; however, in athletes, where performance is affected, the patient may be seen relatively early in an episode.

Frequency   The condition is often chronic and the patient will complain of previous episodes of the same type of symptoms over a period of months or years usually worsening with time (8, 12, 15).

Area of Symptoms   These are well localized over the bicipital groove at the anterior aspect of the shoulder. As the condition worsens with time symptoms may also spread down the anterior aspect of the upper arm as far as the elbow (Fig. 2.10) (11–14, 18).

Type of Symptoms   The patient's main complaint is of pain that is sharp in nature and occurs on movements of the arm. A general ache may be felt following use of the arm for any prolonged period.

Objective Findings

Observation   Appearance of the shoulder is usually unremarkable, although in the early days of a very acute episode there can be mild swelling and increased temperature over the area of the bicipital groove (4, 5, 17).

Active Movements   Lateral rotation of the shoulder is painful and will be limited when the movement is tested with the arm in 90 degrees of abduction. Pain may also be experienced on active flexion of the shoulder from the extended position (5, 11, 15, 17, 20).

Passive Movements   Pain will occur on passive extension of the shoulder when it is combined with extension of the elbow and pronation of the forearm. Passive lateral rotation of the shoulder with the arm abducted to 90 degrees will also be painful (11, 15, 17).

Resisted Movements   Pain can be reproduced by isometric flexion of the elbow and supination of the forearm when tested with both the shoulder and elbow joints extended (9, 20, 21).

Palpation   Tenderness will be elicited over the bicipital groove (Fig. 2.4). This is most easily detected by placing a finger over the groove while passively laterally rotating the shoulder in about 80 degrees of abduction (2, 15, 21, 22).

Specific Tests   In certain cases any contraction of the biceps muscle will produce some discomfort. Yergason's sign, pain felt at the anterior

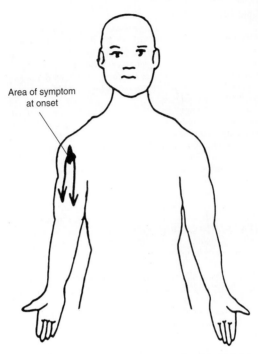

Area of symptom
at onset

FIG. 2.10 Area of symptoms (usually well localized) for bicipital tendonitis at the right shoulder.

of the shoulder on isometric resisted supination of the forearm, is definite corroboration of this diagnosis (1, 9, 21, 23).

Treatment Ideas (2–4, 5, 7–11, 14, 15, 17, 27)

Initial Treatment Ice and rest can be very effective in the initial stages of treatment but must be combined with avoidance of lifting and overhead activities. Active exercises focus initially on maintenance of range of motion in the shoulder, while modalities used to stimulate tissue healing can help to speed recovery and may reduce discomfort. The active exercises should not be carried into any range of motion that produces symptoms.

Isometric resisted shoulder exercises can be introduced as soon as the patient's level of discomfort starts to decrease. These exercises are best performed against a door jam. The patient is instructed to keep the arm straight at the elbow while placing the lateral aspect of the forearm against the door jam and pushing forward to resist flexion of the shoulder. The patient then stands sideways to the door and pushes the posterior aspect of the forearm against the door jam to resist abduction of the shoulder. Finally the patients puts his back to the door, and the anterior aspect of the forearm on the door jam, then pushes backwards to isometrically resist extension of the shoulder.

If these exercises are tolerated well, then isotonic resisted shoulder exercises can be combined with isometric elbow and forearm movements. Resisted elbow exercises can be carried out with the patient applying resistance to the movement using the opposite hand. Both flexion and extension are resisted with the elbow held in 90 degrees of flexion and the forearm supinated. Instruct the patient to apply enough pressure to make the muscle work strongly, but not so much resistance that discomfort is produced at the shoulder. Active stretches should be employed for the biceps muscle to prevent the formation of scar tissue adhesions. These can be combined with active shoulder stretches as all shoulder movements affect the biceps tendon in its groove. Thermal modalities can prove useful prior to stretching, and to stretch the biceps tendon effectively the shoulder has to be taken into extension with the elbow extended and the forearm pronated.

The patient is finally progressed to general upper extremity resisted work suitable to daily activities, while stretching of the upper extremities in general, and the biceps brachii in particular, remains an integral part of any treatment session. Advice and correction of techniques is required for any activity that appears to have been a causative factor for the condition.

Restrictions In the early stage, lifting with the affected arm should be avoided if possible, as should any repetitive or sustained work with the arm elevated more than 50 to 60 degrees. Forceful use of the arm, such as in throwing or pulling activities, is also unadvisable. The amount of weight allowed in lifting can be increased slowly as the patient shows improvement with treatment. Pulling a load from behind while facing forward (i.e., when the shoulder is extended) should not be attempted until the condition has fully subsided.

Complete recovery can be expected in cases of bicipital tendonitis but failure to control recurrent bouts of symptoms may lead to complete rupture of the tendon through attrition. This is particularly true in patients who are over 50 years of age.

Chronic Instability of the Shoulder Joint

Overview

This condition is also referred to as recurrent subluxation of the shoulder. It may occur following dislocation of the shoulder or as a sequel to a tear of the joint capsule. There is not always a history of previous trauma, particularly in athletes or people involved in heavy manual labor who also suffer from a natural joint laxity (double jointed). There will, however, always be a history of shoulder problems to one degree or another. To allow subluxation to occur there has to be a degree of laxity in the shoulder joint capsule, almost invariably in the anterior portion. Compared to other joints of the body, the shoulder joint has a propensity to laxity because of the uncommon degree of freedom of movement that the joint possesses (6, 12, 33, 36).

Subjective Findings

Onset Patients are commonly 20 to 40 years of age and give a history of gradual onset of symptoms following injury or overuse (4, 12, 18).

Duration The condition is chronic by definition, and patients will have usually been suffering symptoms for several months, if not years, before they are seen for treatment.

Frequency The patient will usually complain of recurrent symptoms over a period of 1 to 2 years, occurring particularly after specific shoulder movements such as throwing, pushing, or pulling activities (12, 14, 16).

Area of Symptoms Pain is often demonstrated by the patient putting their hand over the anterolateral aspect of the shoulder and the deltoid muscle (Fig. 2.11) (12, 14, 15, 18).

Type of Symptoms Pain after activity can often be so intense that the patient states that he was unable to move the affected arm. However, in milder cases there may only be a transient sharp pain followed by a general ache. Complaints of "popping and grating" on movements of the shoulder are common, and the patient may also experience weakness, or complain that he feels the joint is going to give way (14, 16).

Miscellaneous In some cases the patient may state that he is unable to lift or carry weights because he can feel the joint "slipping".

Objective Findings

Observation The area of the shoulder usually appears normal on inspection.

Active Movements All movements of the shoulder joint are of full range and will be pain free (3, 4, 12).

Passive Movements These are also full and pain free, but combined movements can produce discomfort or apprehension (see Specific Tests) (3, 12, 21, 35).

Resisted Movements Muscle strength is commonly within normal limits but in certain cases weakness of the shoulder muscles, in particular

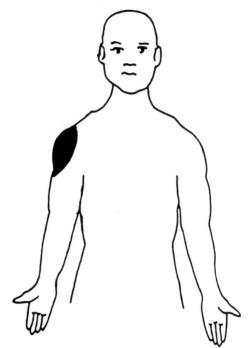

FIG. 2.11   Area of symptoms for chronic instability at the right shoulder.

the rotator cuff, can be part of the causative mechanism. Isometric resisted testing should be pain-free, but strongly resisted movements may bring complaints of giving-way at the affected joint (4, 16, 20).

Palpation   Joint laxity can often be felt while palpating the upper end of the humerus during passive movements. There should be no tenderness elicited or increase in skin temperature found during the examination (7, 16, 21, 22).

Specific Tests   The patient may display apprehension on passive lateral rotation of the shoulder joint when tested with the arm abducted to 80 or 90 degrees, as this puts pressure on the anterior portion of the capsule, the commonest site of the lesion. Passive distraction of the shoulder inferiorly may produce a distinct gapping between the upper humerus and the acromion (12, 21, 23, 35).

Treatment Ideas (3, 4, 6, 7, 12, 14–16, 18)

General isometric strengthening of the shoulder musculature is carried out with the arm at the side with the patient pushing against a wall or door jam, as described in the previous section on treatment suggestions for bicipital tendonitis. The movements of medial and lateral rotation can be resisted with the patient standing sideways by a wall with the elbow flexed at 90 degrees and the posterior of the forearm placed against the wall to resist lateral rotation. The patient then stands in a doorway so that he can rest the anterior aspect of the forearm against the wall, outside the door, in order to resist medial rotation. Progression of these exercises can be made by using a resistance band. The patient wraps the band around both hands and holds the affected shoulder in varying degrees of flexion, extension, abduction, or rotation. The unaffected arm is then drawn away from the affected arm in the direction that is opposite to the direction of the movement to be resisted, while the affected arm is held rigidly in position. The patient should be instructed to sustain as strong a muscle contraction as possible, but not so strong as to produce any sense of "giving way" in the shoulder joint.

The resisted exercises can be progressed by the use of neuromuscular stimulation that is applied to the supraspinous and infraspinous fossas bilaterally. The patient is instructed to maintain a strong isometric lateral rotation of the shoulders against a resistance band during stimulation. When the patient is comfortable with the isometric exercises, he can attempt isotonic strengthening, initially taking the movements through the first 25 to 35 % of range and increasing by increments of 10 to 15% of range. The first movements to be resisted in this way should be adduction and medial rotation; followed by flexion, extension, and abduction; and lastly lateral rotation. When the patient is able to complete full-range isotonic resisted exercises against significant resistance, he can be progressed onto combination movements such as lateral rotation with abduction. At this time proprioceptive neuromuscular facilitation techniques can be very effective, particularly when incorporating hold at different points through range.

As the patient's symptoms subside, neuromuscular exercises such as PNF and rhythmic stabilizations are essential in preventing reoccurrence of symptoms. Exercises for work hardening, or sports-specific training, should be included in the final stages of the rehabilitation program and the patient must continue with a home exercise program indefinitely in order to sustain stability of the shoulder joint.

Restrictions The patient should be advised to avoid sudden shoulder movements or sustained heavy shoulder activities, particularly any that require a combined movement of abduction with lateral rotation, such as throwing a ball. As symptoms subside these restrictions can be removed.

Compliance with a progressive resisted functional exercise program will produce satisfactory results. Cases that do not show improvement after

4 or 5 weeks should be sent for an orthopaedic consultation, as surgery may be required. The patient will have to continue with the exercise program even when the symptoms have cleared, particularly if he wants to continue with certain sports or leisure activities. Time is on the patient's side, as with advancing age the natural process of soft-tissue shortening will help to stabilize the joint.

Acromioclavicular Joint Injury

Overview

These injuries are very common in contact sports (I know I have one), and are usually the result of a fall onto the point of the shoulder or onto the outstretched arm. Three grades of injury are commonly described (12, 15, 16, 37):

Grade 1: A tear of the ligamentous support of the joint with no joint displacement.

Grade 2: More extensive ligament damage that allows mild displacement of the joint.

Grade 3: Disruption of the ligaments occurs, allowing the joint to dislocate, with the clavicle moving upwards on the acromion.

Objective findings vary depending on the degree of injury, but the subjective findings are fairly consistent.

Subjective Findings

Onset This is always sudden after trauma and the patient is usually 20 to 40 years of age (12, 15, 16).

Duration Patients will normally present for treatment a few days or up to 3 weeks after injury. If the patient is seen several weeks after the injury he is more likely to be suffering joint irritation, rather than the effects of the initial injury (see later).

Frequency This will be the first time that the patient has suffered the injury in this particular arm—it does not happen twice. However, the same injury occurring in the other shoulder is common in those whose sport or pastime makes them susceptible to this type of injury.

Area of Symptoms The patient will usually localize the area of symptoms by indicating the point of the shoulder with one finger (Fig. 2.12) (11, 12, 22).

Type of Symptoms Pain is sharp, particularly on movement, and is then often followed by a dull ache.

Miscellaneous The patient may complain of grating or rubbing during arm movements, which is felt at the point of the shoulder (11, 14, 15).

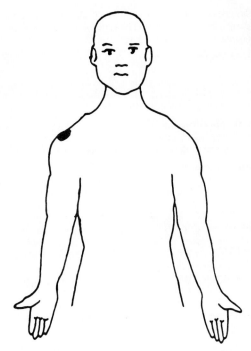

FIG. 2.12 Area of symptoms (usually well localized) for either acromioclavicular joint injury or acromioclavicular joint irritation at the right shoulder.

Objective Findings

Observation In grade 2 and 3 injuries a step may be noted between the medial end of the clavicle and the acromion. This may be concealed by swelling within a few hours following the injury, and for several days after (12, 15, 16).

Active Movements The available range of movements depends on the degree of injury and the time lapse since it occurred. In grade 1 injuries there is usually no loss of range of motion. Grade 2 injuries often produce minor loss of range of abduction and lateral rotation of the shoulder. Grade 3 injuries can produce in excess of 50% limitation of shoulder abduction and lateral rotation, with mild limitation of all other movements. However, even in grade 3 cases, range of motion should be near normal in a matter of 2 to 3 weeks post injury (9, 12, 15, 16, 19).

Passive Movements   In all grades of injury passive adduction of the arm across the chest will usually produce pain in the area of the affected joint. In grade 2 and 3 injuries pain is also produced during abduction of the shoulder and on rotations of the shoulder when tested with the arm abducted at 90 degrees (15, 16, 20).

Resisted Movements   Normal muscle strength is commonly present on isometric testing. Pain may be produced on strongly resisted abduction, flexion, or lateral rotation, particularly in more severe injuries (12, 15).

Palpation   Tenderness is elicited on palpation around the acromio-clavicular joint line (Fig. 2.1). Protrusion of the medial end of the clavicle can often be detected in grade 2 and 3 injuries (11, 12, 13, 22).

Treatment Ideas (2, 4, 12, 15–18, 37, 38)

Initial Treatment   For the first few days following injury the arm should be supported in a sling, and the patient should be advised to rest the arm and ice the shoulder regularly. The period of rest should be 48 to 72 hours, whatever the degree of injury, and active movements can be commenced immediately following that time period. Ultrasound and interferential therapy can also be started 2 to 3 days post injury. Heat packs often decrease discomfort on exercise if applied at the start of a treatment session, and ice packs can help eliminate post-exercise pain.

The rate of progression of active exercises into greater range will depend on the degree of injury, patients with less severe injuries being able to progress faster than those with more severe injuries. The active exercise program should also include shoulder girdle exercises for the movements of protraction, retraction, elevation, depression, and circumduction. Resisted exercises can be commenced for a particular movement when that movement is painless through range on active testing. Initial resistances should be low and the arm should not be carried into more than 60 degrees of flexion or abduction at that stage. The degree of resistance and range of motion are both progressed as tolerated by the patient.

Once the patient can cope with resisted exercises through all ranges of movement, he can progress into a gym exercise program and functional exercises involving lifting, carrying, pushing, and pulling, initially up to and then above shoulder level.

Restrictions   During the first few days following injury the patient should be advised to avoid activities requiring elevation of the arm beyond shoulder height. After this time the patient can attempt activities at increasing degrees of elevation of the arm, but only if not unduly uncomfortable. Forceful movements of the arm, such as in throwing activities or vigorous pushing or pulling, should be completely avoided at this time. Progression back to normal daily activities is usually quite rapid. However, work or sports activities that place heavy demands on the joint should only be attempted in a graduated manner, and only after the patient has demonstrated pain-free function of the joint against resistance throughout the required ranges. Prolonged activity at or above shoulder height should not be attempted until 5 to 6 weeks post injury, and then only when the patient has demonstrated tolerance to this type of activity in gym exercises.

Although patients with grade 2 and 3 injuries will be left with a possibly unsightly lump at the site of injury, they will still be able to regain full pain-free range of motion and function in the affected arm within 6 to 7 weeks of injury. Patients with grade 1 injuries can expect to achieve the same degree of recovery in about 3 or 4 weeks. Nevertheless, they will still have to avoid contact sports, or other activities that make them vulnerable to similar stresses and strains, until 6 weeks post injury, so as to allow for sufficient healing of the damaged soft tissues.

Acromioclavicular Joint Irritation

Overview

This condition can be found in younger people as a sequel to acromioclavicular joint injury or in the middle-aged patient as a primary condition, possibly part of a general osteoarthritic condition. The joint becomes chronically inflamed, with thickening and tightening of the periarticular structures. Repetitive stresses and strains lead to pain and occasionally loss of range of motion (1, 9, 15).

Onset

The age of the patient can vary between 20 and 50 years. Onset is usually gradual and following trauma, although in some cases, particularly in the older patient, no cause of onset can be established (1, 15).

Duration

This is, by nature, a chronic condition and the patient will often have suffered the symptoms for several months before seeking medical attention.

Frequency

There is usually a history of steadily increasing symptoms, but all considered as a single ongoing episode by the patient. A history of previous shoulder injury is common (1, 13).

Area of Symptoms

Patients can usually localize their symptoms to the point of the shoulder (Fig. 2.12) (1, 15, 22).

Type of Symptoms

The patient typically describes his symptoms as an aching pain that is worse following use of the affected arm (15, 16).

Miscellaneous

The patient may complain of difficulty sleeping on the affected side, and of feeling a grating sensation on movements of the shoulder.

Objective Findings

Observation Deformity may be observable if there was a previous injury, or swelling can be seen as a result of soft-tissue thickening around the joint. In many cases the joint appears normal on visual inspection (1, 16).

Active Movements There is usually no particular limitation of movement, although the last 50 to 60 degrees of abduction may produce some discomfort, felt at the point of the shoulder (13, 15, 16).

Passive Movements Adduction of the arm across the chest, end-range abduction, and end-range lateral rotation of the shoulder may all be painful and possibly limited. Crepitation can often be felt if the acromioclavicular joint is palpated during passive testing of movements (13, 15, 16).

Resisted Movements Resisted movements of the shoulder and shoulder girdle are usually strong and pain free. Occasionally the patient will complain of pain on strongly resisted flexion or abduction of the shoulder at or around 90 degrees of elevation (13, 15).

Palpation Soft-tissue thickening can often be palpated around the acromioclavicular joint line (Fig. 2.5) with varying degrees of tenderness present (13, 15, 22).

Treatment Ideas (1, 9, 13, 15, 16, 38)

Initially the most important element is to restrict the activities that produce the patient's typical symptoms. Thermal agents, such as hot packs and ultrasound, or the application of laser can help to alleviate pain and assist in mobilizing the affected joint. Active exercises should not be forced, but should be carried out within the patient's comfort zone of pain-free range of motion. Exercises should include all shoulder and shoulder girdle movements, starting as individual movements and progressing to combined movements for circumduction of both the shoulder and the shoulder girdle.

Resisted exercises can be started for the biceps and triceps initially, with progression to isometric resisted exercises for all shoulder movements. To begin, the movements should be carried out with the arm at the side and then progressed to 45 degrees, 90 degrees, and finally 135 degrees of arm elevation. When isometric exercises are carried out comfortably, progression can be made to isotonic resisted exercises, initially through 50% of range and then progressing to full range for each movement. Combined neuromuscular electrical stimulation of the upper trapezius and deltoid while the arm is abducted to 90 degrees, using a static arm hold against a resistance such as wrist weights, can help to promote stability in the affected area.

Patients should be able to progress to a gym exercise program 3 to 4 weeks after commencing treatment. All shoulder and shoulder girdle movements can be strengthened progressively, with the emphasis initially on endurance work and then a combination of endurance and power work with steadily increasing weights. Throughout the entire treatment program it is advisable to use ice at the end of each treatment session to help prevent any adverse reaction to the exercises.

Restrictions Whenever possible the patient should take strain or pressure off the joint. One problem that commonly occurs to further irritate the joint is that the patient lies on his affected side while sleeping. This can be avoided by putting a firm pillow under the affected arm, which will tend to stop the patient turning to that side during the night. Heavy lifting and carrying should be avoided in the early stages of treatment to allow the joint to settle down. Repetitive or prolonged use of the arm at or above shoulder height will also be likely to produce discomfort. The patient should be guided by his symptoms, and should stop activities before the point of onset of pain is reached. Work, sports, or recreational activities that have been shown to cause discomfort should all be limited until the joint irritation has cleared. A graduated return to these activities can then be coordinated with similar exercises in the clinic.

Acromioclavicular joint irritation can clear with conservative treatment, but all causative activities must be eliminated to allow this to occur. Maintenance of flexibility and strength in the shoulder girdle are also essential in preventing reoccurrence of symptoms, particularly in workers or athletes who place a large degree of strain on the shoulder girdle due to excessively heavy or exceptionally energetic use of the upper extremity.

Pectoral Muscle Tear

Overview

This is a relatively uncommon condition, and yet there is a good chance of seeing a patient suffering from a pectoral muscle tear every few months in a busy clinic. This is possibly due to the fact that more and more people are working out in gymnasiums, as weight training seems to be the cause of onset in the majority of cases (9, 17).

Subjective Findings

Onset Patients are usually between 20 and 40 years of age and give a history of sudden onset of symptoms following overuse, usually in the form of pushing a heavy weight.

Duration   Patients will normally present for treatment within one week of the injury, as they are unable to continue with their workouts.

Frequency   This will be the only time the patient has experienced these particular symptoms.

Area of Symptoms   Symptoms are felt at the anterior of the upper arm in the area of the bicipital groove over the attachment of the pectoralis tendon. They may also be felt in the area of the anterior chest wall over the muscle itself and at the anterior wall of the axilla (Fig. 2.13) (3, 14).

Type of Symptoms   A sharp pain is reported on movements, particularly when pushing or when lifting the arm forwards with a weight in the hand. There is also usually a more poorly defined ache following activity.

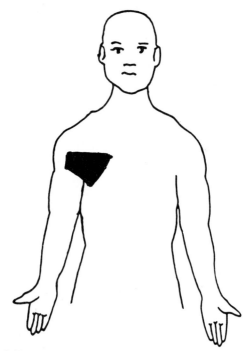

FIG. 2.13   Area of symptoms for pectoral muscle tear at right shoulder region.

Objective Findings

Observation There is normally nothing to see in the affected area, although there may be a small degree of swelling at the site of injury in the first few days following injury.

Active Movements Mild limitation of extension and lateral rotation of the shoulder is common, with pain reported at the end of available range (14).

Passive Movements Pain and possibly muscle spasm will be produced at end range of extension and lateral rotation with the same degree of limitation of movement as was found on active movement.

Resisted Movements The patient's typical pain is brought on during isometric resisted adduction, medial rotation, and flexion of the shoulder. Stronger resistance will also reveal weakness of these movements due to pain.

Palpation Tenderness will be elicited on palpation over the medial aspect of the bicipital groove and in the anterior wall of the axilla.

Treatment Ideas (17)

Ice and rest from any pushing activities for a few days help to alleviate discomfort and assist healing. Heat and increasing doses of ultrasound to the affected muscle can then be started, along with active arm exercises to maintain range of motion in the painless directions, with the patient instructed to stretch slowly and sensibly into extension and lateral rotation. Isometric resisted exercises can also be used to maintain strength in all pain-free directions. Ice should be advocated following exercise for the first 2 weeks in order to minimize any post-exercise discomfort.

Progression When full pain-free range of active movements has been restored, the patient can commence isometric resisted flexion, adduction, and medial rotation, with isotonic resisted extension, abduction, and lateral rotation. When the isometric exercises are painless when held at different points through range, then isotonic resisted exercises can commence for the pectoral muscles. Muscle stimulation can be applied to the pectoral muscles at this stage, with the patient supine and the arm of the affected side held against the contraction in a position of horizontal abduction combined with lateral rotation. This will provide a gentle end-range stretch to the muscle.

Latter Stages These patients will want to progress to a gym program quickly because they usually are involved in a weight-training program. They can continue with light endurance-type work with low weights and high repetitions for non-painful movements from about one week post injury. Progression to higher weights and to exercises that work the pectoral muscles should be made very gradually and in small incremental steps. The patient will need to show good common sense in their exercise progression; unfortunately, those involved in weight training often do not. The therapist should point out the very real dangers of chronic disability, as compared to a return to full pain-free function, if these rehabilitation guidelines are not followed sensibly.

Restrictions No pushing activities should be attempted in the first 2 to 3 weeks following injury. In weeks 3 to 6 these activities can be attempted again on a graduated basis. Lifting weights above shoulder height should also be avoided in the first few weeks following injury, and return to this type of activity should be made slowly as the patient demonstrates tolerance to similar activities in the clinic. Throwing is not advisable in the first 3 to 4 weeks following injury and should only be done at half pace for the next 1 to 2 weeks, with progression to full force made gradually over a further 2 to 3 weeks.

Complete recovery should be expected in cases of a pectoral muscle tear. Reoccurrence is rare if rehabilitation is carried out effectively and in a timely manner the first time around. Review of techniques in weight training is important when the cause of the injury is poor technique, or more probably the overestimation of ones abilities.

Subacromial Bursitis (Shoulder Impingement Syndrome)

Overview

The subacromial bursa lies between the supraspinatus tendon and the underside of the acromion, with the supraspinatus tendon forming most of the floor of the bursa. The bursa and tendon are therefore closely linked in both function and pathology. Inflammation of the bursa often occurs in connection with inflammation of the tendons of the rotator cuff within the subacromial space. However, occasionally the bursitis can occur as a separate and distinct pathological entity. The physical findings are often confusing because of an underlying mild tendonitis. This is a condition that often responds well to injection of corticosteroids; however, the patient may still require physical therapy interventions post injection (3, 12, 17, 33, 34).

Subjective Findings

Onset Onset is gradual either after overuse or with no known cause. Patients are typically over the age of 35 (2, 4, 17).

Duration In most cases the patient will have been suffering with symptoms for several weeks before seeking, medical intervention, as onset of symptoms is quite insidious. A typical time lapse from onset to initial assessment would be 6 to 12 weeks.

Frequency On most occasions this is the first time the patient will have experienced these symptoms, although in some cases there may be a history of one or two previous episodes occurring each year for 2 to 3 years (14, 17, 28).

Area of Symptoms Symptoms are usually localized to the antero-lateral aspect of the acromial rim with some referral into the anterolateral aspect of the upper arm (Fig. 2.14) (14, 16, 17).

Type of Symptoms The patient will complain of a deep ache at the shoulder and will often describe the shoulder and upper arm as being sore for most of the time, with increased pain occurring on certain movements (4, 14, 16, 28).

Miscellaneous The patient is often unable to work with his hands at or just above shoulder height, as in putting objects onto a shelf at head

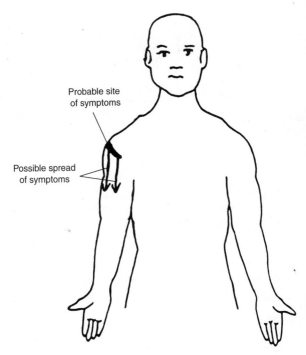

Probable site of symptoms

Possible spread of symptoms

FIG. 2.14 Area of symptoms for subacromial bursitis at the right shoulder.

height. With time the patient may also complain of pain in the area of the upper trapezius on the affected side, which appears to be due to protective spasm in the muscle (15, 28).

Objective Findings

Observation There is usually nothing to be observed at or in the region of the affected joint.

Active Movements In the early stages movements are full range, with pain experienced in mid-range of flexion and abduction. As the condition becomes more pronounced the patient may be unable to get the arm into full elevation. Medial rotation is limited when the arm is carried away from the side, as in trying to place the hand up the back and between the scapulae. If the course of the condition is prolonged there may be a general loss of range of motion due to disuse and the subsequent formation of soft-tissue adhesions (4, 12, 17, 19, 20).

Passive Movements Pain will be produced during mid-range abduction and flexion, as in testing for active movements. Stiffness may be felt towards end range of medial rotation when the movement is carried out with the arm in about 80 degrees of elevation midway between the positions of flexion and abduction (4, 15, 19, 20).

Resisted Movements In true acromial bursitis there is no pain on isometric testing of the muscles of the shoulder region. On the other hand, the effects of impingement on the rotator cuff tendons, with subsequent inflammation and swelling, can cloud the waters by producing signs of an underlying rotator cuff tendonitis. If bursitis is the primary lesion then these findings will not be particularly outstanding, so the pain on resisted testing will be relatively mild. On occasions there may be some general decrease in muscle strength due to disuse. There may also be a noticeable discrepancy between the strength of rotation compared to the strength of abduction and flexion. This weakness of the rotator cuff would be a possible contributing factor as regards onset of the condition (3, 4, 8, 16).

Palpation If the patient is able to relax the deltoid muscle sufficiently then tenderness may be elicited under the acromial rim at its lateral and anterolateral aspects (Fig. 2.1) (15 , 20, 22).

Specific Tests A painful arc of movement is often present and pain may be elicited on medial rotation when the arm is held in a position between abduction and flexion, with the arm elevated to 90 degrees (emptying a can) (12, 15, 21, 23).

Treatment Ideas (2–4, 10, 12, 14–18, 32, 34)

Initial treatment is aimed at increasing the space between the underside of the acromion and the upper end of the humerus. Ice and rest are often advisable, particularly in the acute case, and can produce good early results if combined with avoidance of activities that place the shoulder in the mid-range of flexion or abduction. After 2 or 3 days heat can be used prior to exercise, as this helps to relax the patient. The exercises should be carried out actively and through available pain-free range, as this may help to prevent an adhesive capsulitis developing secondary to the bursitis. The patient will usually be more comfortable doing these exercises and will gain more range if they are done in a lying position. Patients should also be able to use reciprocal pulleys to maintain range of motion without reproducing their symptoms. They can be taught how to set this up at home by using a rope or washing line run over a hook on the back of a door.

Progression of treatment can be made by initially introducing free-swinging exercises with no weight, and then using light weights, such as 3 to 5 pounds. These exercises should be done with the patient standing upright with his arm relaxed at his side. If the patient leans forward to do the exercise, then his arm will already be in some 60 to 70 degrees of flexion, which will place it in the impingement zone once the patient starts to swing the arm. The use of interferential therapy is often warranted prior to these exercises, as it can help to promote relaxation, thus allowing more effective motion of the affected joint. Once the patient's discomfort starts to subside, light resisted exercises for the rotator cuff and biceps muscles can be started. These muscles all help collectively to hold the head of the humerus down and into the glenoid, hence helping to prevent the mechanism of impingement.

In the final stages of treatment general strengthening of the upper extremity should be carried out, but with the emphasis on rotator cuff strengthening to make sure that there is no marked discrepancy in muscle strength between the deltoid and the rotator cuff muscles. To further promote distraction of the humerus, and so alleviate congestion between the greater tubercle and the acromium, the patient can be set up with neuro-muscular electrical stimulation applied to the upper trapezius on the affected side while sitting in a relaxed position in a hard-back chair with no arm rests. The affected arm is then allowed to hang dependent and a light weight (4 to 6 pounds) is attached to the wrist. Stimulation of the upper trapezius will produce elevation of the point of the shoulder, thus raising the acromium, while the weight around the wrist holds the arm down, thus effectively applying a distraction force to the glenohumeral joint. The degree of weight employed can be progressed as tolerated by the patient.

Manual distraction of the glenohumeral joint can also prove effective and should be carried out with the patient in lying with the arm comfortably supported. The distraction force is then maintained as either a long steady longitudinal pull or as a series of short longitudinal oscillations, in each case continued over a period of 30–60 seconds at a time. Resisted work for the biceps muscle can also help to decrease pressure under the acromium through the action of the tendon of the long head of the biceps. The tendon passes over the head of the humerus in its passage through the shoulder joint, therefore contraction of the muscle draws the humerus downwards away from the acromium. The patient can continue distraction at home using heat application to the shoulder with gentle swinging of a moderate to heavy weight, suitable to his physique. It is suggested that heat with stretch, followed immediately by icing with continued stretch, may help to conserve any gains in range achieved with the stretching.

Restrictions All activities requiring use of the arm with the shoulder held in a position between 60 and 120 degrees of elevation should be avoided. This will usually mean all activity carried out above 60 degrees, as working above 120 degrees usually involves repeated movements through the zone of impingement. Patients will also find that any sustained activity done with the arm held away from the body will bring on symptoms over time. This is probably due to tiring of the rotator cuff muscles, which then allow the humerus to move upwards under the acromion to produce excessive pressure on the bursa. This type of activity should either be avoided or the patient should be advised to take adequate rests, which in practice means stopping doing the activity at the first sign of onset of symptoms. It is unwise to advise a patient to rest the arm completely because adhesive capsulitis can develop as a secondary condition if active range of motion is not maintained at the shoulder complex.

REFERENCES

1. Dandy D.J., Edwards D.J.: Essential Orthopaedics and Trauma (3rd ed). Churchill Livingston, New York, 1998
2. Mercier, L.R.: Practical Orthopaedics (4th ed). Mosby Yearbook, St Louis, 1991
3. Braddom R.L. (ed): Physical Medicine and Rehabilitation. W.B. Saunders, Philadelphia, 1996
4. Crowther C.L.: Primary Orthopaedic Care. Mosby, St. Louis, 1999
5. Salter R.B.: Textbook of Disorders and Injuries of the Muscular Skeletal System (3rd ed). Williams and Wilkins, Baltimore, 1999
6. Donatelli R.A., Wooden M.J. (eds): Orthopaedic Physical Therapy (2nd ed). Churchill Livingston, New York, 1994
7. Payton O.D. (ed): Manual of Physical Therapy. Churchill Livingston, New York, 1989
8. Kasdan M.C. (ed): Occupational Hand and Upper Extremity Injuries and Disease (2nd ed). Hanley and Belfus, Philadelphia, 1998
9. Nicholas J.A., Hershman E.B.: Upper Extremity in Sports Medicine (2nd ed). Mosby, St. Louis, 1995
10. Kesson M. Atkins E.: Orthopaedic Medicine: A Practical Approach. Butterworth Heinemann, Oxford, U.K., 1998
11. Apley A.G., Solomon L.: Apley's System of Orthopaedics and Fractures (6th ed). Butterworth, London, 1983
12. Prentice W.E.: Rehabilitation Techniques in Sports Medicine. WCB/McGraw Hill, New York, 1999
13. Cyriax J.: Textbook of Orthopaedic Medicine: Vol.1, Diagnosis of Soft Tissue Lesions (8th ed). Bailliere Tindall, Eastbourne, U.K., 1982
14. Anderson B.C.: Office Orthopaedics for Primary Care: Diagnosis and Treatment (2nd ed). W.B. Saunders Co., Philadelphia, 1999

15. Corrigan B., Maitland G.D.: Practical Orthopaedic Medicine. Butterworth, London, U.K., 1983

16. Malone T.R., McPoil T.G., Nitz A.J. (eds): Orthopaedic and Sports Physical Therapy (3rd ed). Mosby, St. Louis, 1997

17. Skinner H.B. (ed): Current Diagnosis and Treatment in Orthopaedics. Appleton and Lange, Norwalk, CT, 1995

18. Snider R.K. (ed): Essential of Musculoskeletal Care. American Academy of Orthopaedic Surgeons, Rosemont, IL, 1997

19. Goldie B.S.: Orthopaedic Diagnosis and Management: A Guide to the Care of Orthopaedic Patients (2nd ed). ISIS Medical Media, Oxford, U.K., 1998

20. Gross J, Feeto J., Rosen E.: Musculoskeletal Examination. Blackwell Science, Cambridge, MA, 1996

21. Magee D.J.: Orthopaedic Physical Assessment (2nd ed). W.B. Saunders Co., Philadelphia, 1992

22. Field D.: Anatomy: Palpation and Surface Markings (2nd ed). Butterworth Heinemann, Oxford, U.K., 1997

23. Konin J.G., Wilksten D.L., Isear J.A.: Special Tests for Orthopaedic Examination. Slack, New Jersey, 1997

24. Wainner Maj. R.S., Hasz M.: Management of Acute Calcific Tendonitis of the Shoulder. J. Orthop. Sports Phys. Ther. 27 (3):231–237, 1998

25. Jobe F., Pink M.: Classification and Treatment of Shoulder Dysfunction in the Overhead Athlete. J. Orthop. Sports Phys. Ther., 8:427–432, 1993

26. Brewster C., Moynes Schwab D.R.: Rehabilitation of the Shoulder Following Rotator Cuff Injury or Surgery. J. Orthop. Sports Phys. Ther., 18:422–426, 1993

27. Nitz J.: Physical Therapy Management of the Shoulder. Phys. Ther., 66:1912, 1986

28. Cohen, R.B., Williams, G.R.: Impingement Syndrome and Rotator Cuff Disease as Repetitive Motion Disorders. Clin. Orthop., 351:95–101, 1998

29. Placzek J.D., et al. Long-Term Effectiveness of Translation Manipulation For Adhesive Capsulitis. Clin. Orthop., 356:181–191, 1998

30. Itoi E., Tabata S.: Conservative Treatment of Rotator Cuff Tears. Clin. Orthop. 275:165–173, 1992

31. Hanafin J.A., Chiaia T.A.: Adhesive Capsulitis: A Treatment Approach. Clin Orthop. 372:95–109, 2000

32. Conroy D.E., Hayes K.W.: The Effect of Joint Mobilization As a Component of Comprehensive Treatment for Primary Shoulder Impingement Syndrome. J. Orthop. Sports Phys. Ther. 28 (1):3–14, 1998

33. Warner J., et al. Patterns of Flexibility, Laxity and Strength in Normal Shoulders and Shoulders with Instability and Impingement. Am. J. Sport Med. (4):366–375, 1990

34. Neer C.S. Jr.: Impingement Lesions. Clin. Orthop. 173: 70–77, 1983

35. Levy A.S., et al. Intra and Interobserver Reproducibility of the Shoulder Laxity Examination. Am. J. Sports Med., 27 (4):460–463, 1999

36. Brown G.A., Tan J.L., Kirkley A.: The Lax Shoulder in Females: Issues, Answers but Many More Questions. Clin. Orthop., 372: 110–122, 2000

37. Philips A.M., Smart C., Groom A.F.G.: Acromial Clavicular Dislocation. Clin. Orthop., 353:10–17, 1998

38. Dias J.J., Gregg P.J.: Acromial Clavicular Joint Injuries in Sport: Recommendations for Treatment. Sports Med. 11:125–132, 1991

The following tables contain test movements for examination of the elbow, wrist, and hand. The starting positions and a description of each movement are given. These are considered the optimal test positions in each case, but should be modified for individual patients who are unable to achieve or sustain a described position.

Active Movements of the Elbow and Forearm

Name of Movement	Starting Position	Movement
Elbow Flexion	The movement can be tested in sitting, standing, supine lying, or side lying. The patient's arm is held loosely at the side with the palm facing in towards the body and the elbow straight.	The patient is instructed to bend his elbow, bringing his hand towards his shoulder as far as possible. Movement is normally limited by soft tissue approximation of the forearm to the upper arm. Average range of motion: 145–150°.
Elbow Extension	The movement can be tested in sitting, standing, side lying, or supine lying. The patient's shoulder is held in 90° of flexion with the elbow fully flexed and the forearm in the supinated position.	The patient is instructed to straighten his arm while maintaining 90° of flexion at the shoulder. Average range of motion: arm should be fully or nearly straight and movement of elbow is expressed as total movement from extension to flexion. (0–145°).
Supination of Forearm	The movement can be tested in sitting, standing, side lying, or supine lying. The patient's arm is flexed to 90° at the elbow with the forearm in the mid position (i.e., thumb facing up towards the head) with the elbow held in to the side of the body.	The patient is instructed to turn his hand over to bring his palm upwards, taking the thumb away from the body. Average range of motion: 80–90°.

Active Movements of the Elbow and Forearm (*continued*)

Name of Movement	Starting Position	Movement
Pronation of Forearm	The movement can be tested in sitting, standing, side lying, or supine lying. The patient's arm is flexed to 90° at the elbow with the forearm in the mid position (i.e., thumb facing up towards the head) with the elbow held in to the side of the body.	The patient is instructed to turn the hand over, bringing the palm downwards (thumb towards the body). Average range of motion: 80–90°.

Active Movements of the Wrist

Name of Movement	Starting Position	Movement
Wrist Extension	The patient's forearm is placed in the neutral position with the thumb facing upwards.	The patient is instructed to take his hand backwards, bringing the posterior aspect of the hand towards the posterior forearm. The fingers should remain relaxed and slightly flexed throughout the movement. Average range of motion: 80–85°
Wrist Flexion	The patient's forearm is in the neutral position with the thumb facing upwards.	The patient is instructed to bring his hand forward, approximating the palm to the anterior forearm. The fingers should remain relaxed and slightly flexed throughout the movement. Average range of motion: 80–85°
Radial Deviation	The patient's forearm is placed in pronation so that the palm of the hand faces towards the floor.	The patient is instructed to bring the thumb side of the hand towards the body. The elbow must not be allowed to flex during the test movement.

(*continued*)

Active Movements of the Wrist (*continued*)

Name of Movement	Starting Position	Movement
Ulnar Deviation	The patient's forearm is placed in pronation so that the palm of the hand faces towards the floor.	The patient is instructed to take his hand away from his body (i.e., to the little finger side). The elbow must not be allowed to extend during the test movement.

*Active movements of the wrist and hand are most easily checked with the arm resting on a small treatment table and the hand clear of the end of the table.

*The above four movements are repeated with the patient positioned so that the shoulder is flexed to 90° with the elbow held in full extension (i.e., with the arm straight) so as to stretch and test the muscles of the forearm that pass over the wrist and elbow. The movements of wrist flexion and extension can be combined with both ulnar and radial deviation to determine if this further provokes symptoms.

Active Movements of the Hand

Name of Movement	Starting Position	Movement
Combined Finger Flexion and Extension	The patient's forearm is placed in the neutral position midway between pronation and supination.	The patient is first instructed to make a fist and then to open the hand, straightening the fingers and thumb as far as possible. The movement is repeated several times.
Flexion and Extension of the Fingers at the MP Joints	The fingers are held straight with the forearm and wrist in the mid position.	The patient is instructed to bend his fingers at the proximal knuckle joint (metacarpal phalangeal joints), keeping the other joints of the fingers extended. All four fingers initially are tested simultaneously, then each finger separately if any discrepancy in movement is noted. Active range of motion: 0–80°

Active Movements of the Hand (*continued*)

Name of Movement	Starting Position	Movement
Flexion and Extension of the Fingers at the IP Joint	The fingers are held straight with the forearm and wrist in the mid position.	The patient is instructed to curl his fingers over to bring the tips of the fingers into contact with the palm of the hand at the level of the MP joints. The fingers are then straightened out completely. All four fingers are tested simultaneously, then each finger is tested independently if any discrepancy is noted.
Abduction / Adduction of Fingers	The patient's hand is placed flat on the table palm down.	The patient is instructed to spread his fingers as far apart as possible and then to draw them together to touch each other.
Flexion of the Thumb	The patient's hand rests on the table with the forearm in the mid position.	The patient is instructed to take the thumb across the hand to touch the base of the fifth finger (which is the average range of motion).
Extension of the Thumb	The patient's hand rests on the table with the forearm in the mid position and the thumb taken into the flexed position described above.	The patient is asked to draw the thumb out as far as possible directly away from the flexed position, stretching the web between the thumb and index finger. Average range of motion: 20°
Adduction of the Thumb	The patient's hand rests on the table with the forearm in the mid position.	The patient is instructed to bring the thumb in from the resting position so that the medial side of the thumb rests against the lateral side of the metacarpal of the index finger (which is the average range of motion).

(*continued*)

Active Movements of the Hand (*continued*)

Name of Movement	Starting Position	Movement
Abduction of the Thumb	The patient's hand rests on the table with the forearm in the mid position and the thumb in the fully adducted position as described above.	The patient is instructed to take the thumb directly away from the adducted position. This will carry it in a plane of movement at right angles to the plane of flexion and extension. Average range of motion: 70–80°
Opposition of the Thumb	The patient's hand rests on the table with the forearm in the mid position.	The patient is instructed to touch the tip of the thumb to the tip of the fifth finger or as close as he can reach. (Most patients are able to bring the two into contact)

*To check individual movements at the proximal interphalangeal joints grasp the proximal phalanx between finger and thumb and ask the patient to bend and straighten his finger. To test the distal interphalangeal joints hold the intermediate phalanx and ask the patient to bend and straighten the tip of the finger.

Passive Movements of the Elbow and Forearm

Name of Movement	Starting Position	Movement
Flexion of the Elbow	The movement can be tested in sitting, standing, side lying, or supine lying. Support the upper arm posteriorly just above the elbow and the forearm just above the wrist. The patient's shoulder is held in slight flexion.	Bend the patient's elbow to bring the forearm into approximation with the upper arm, if possible.
Extension of the Elbow	The movement can be tested in sitting, standing, side lying, or supine lying.	Take the patient's elbow from the fully flexed position described above until it straightens out completely. This requires posterior to anterior pressure on

Passive Movements of the Elbow and Forearm (*continued*)

Name of Movement	Starting Position	Movement
	The therapist supports the upper arm posteriorly just above the elbow and the forearm just above the wrist. The patient's shoulder is held in slight flexion.	the upper arm and anterior to posterior pressure on the forearm to ensure full range of motion.
Supination of the Forearm	The movement can be tested in sitting, standing, supine lying, or side lying. The patient's elbow is cupped in the examiner's hand with the elbow flexed to 90° and held into the patient's side. The examiner grasps the patient's hand (as in shaking hands).	The patient's hand is turned over so that the palm is facing upwards.
Pronation of the Forearm	The movement can be tested in sitting, standing, supine lying, or side lying. The patient's elbow is cupped in one hand with elbow bent at 90° and held into patient's side. Grasp the patient's hand (as in shaking hands).	Turn the patient's hand over so that the palm is facing downwards.

Passive Movements of the Wrist and Hand

Name of Movement	Starting Position	Movement
Wrist Flexion	With the patient's forearm pronated, grip the posterior forearm near the wrist to stabilize it, with the other hand placed over the dorsum of the patient's hand just proximal to the MP joints.	Apply pressure to the dorsum of the patient's hand to approximate the palm of the hand to the anterior aspect of the forearm (pushing the hand down towards the floor).
Wrist Extension	Place one hand on the posterior distal forearm to stabilize it. Place the other hand on the palm of the patient's hand.	Apply pressure to the palm of the hand to push the hand back, approximating the dorsal aspect of the hand to the posterior forearm.
Radial Deviation	With the patient's forearm pronated, grip the distal forearm to stabilize it. Hold the patient's hand between the fingers and thumb of the other hand.	The patient's hand is moved to the thumb side keeping the hand parallel to the floor (mid position between extension and flexion of the wrist)
Ulnar Deviation	With the patient's forearm pronated, grip the distal forearm to stabilize it. Hold the patient's hand between the fingers and thumb of the other hand.	The patient's hand is moved to the little finger side while maintaining the mid position of the wrist between flexion and extension.
Flexion of the Finger	With the patient's hand supported on the table and the forearm in the mid-prone position, place one hand over the dorsum of the patient's hand with the finger tips on the MP joints and the heel of the hand over the patient's fingernails.	Close your hand into a fist, pushing the patient's fingers into flexion at the MP and IP joints.
Finger Extension	With the patient's hand resting on the table and the forearm in the mid-prone position, place one hand over the dorsal aspect of the MP joint. The heel of the	Pressure is applied to the patient's fingertips to push the fingers out straight into extension while the other hand stabilizes the MP joints.

Passive Movements of the Wrist and Hand (*continued*)

Name of Movement	Starting Position	Movement
	other hand applies pressure to the palmar aspect of the patient's fingertips.	
MP Joint Movement	With the patient's hand resting on a table, grasp the metacarpal of the digit between finger and thumb of one hand and the proximal phalanx with the finger and thumb of the other hand.	The joint is carried into flexion and extension using the distal hand to produce movement while the proximal hand stabilizes the proximal bone.
Interphalangeal Joint Movements of Individual Fingers and Thumb	Use the index finger and thumb of each hand to grasp the phalanx on either side of an interphalangeal joint.	While the proximal hand stabilizes the proximal or intermediate phalanx, the distal hand moves the intermediate or distal phalanx to take the joint into flexion or extension.
Abduction / Adduction of Individual Fingers and Thumb	The patient's hand is placed flat on the table with the palm down. Grip the metacarpal joint with the index finger and thumb of one hand and the proximal phalanx with the index finger and thumb of the other hand.	The finger is moved side to side alternately away from and towards adjacent fingers or thumb.

*These movements are most easily tested with the patient in the sitting position with their arm resting on a small table with the hand clear of the end of the table. The therapist sits facing the patient.

Resisted Movements of the Elbow, Forearm, Wrist and Hand

Name of Movement	Starting Position	Movement
Elbow Flexion	The movement can be tested in sitting, standing, supine lying, or side lying with the elbow flexed at 90° with: 1. The forearm fully supinated 2. The forearm in the mid-prone position 3. The forearm in the fully pronated position	Place one hand on: 1. The anterior aspect of the forearm 2. The lateral aspect of the forearm 3. The posterior aspect of the forearm In each case pressure is applied to try and straighten the elbow as the patient resists the movement.
Elbow Extension	The movement can be tested in sitting, standing, side lying, or prone lying with the patient's elbow straight and the arm by their side. Grip the anterior of the patient's upper arm with one hand and the posterior forearm with the other hand.	Apply pressure to the posterior of the patient's forearm to try and bend the elbow while the patient resists the movement.
Wrist Extension	The patient's forearm is fully pronated. Grip the forearm with one hand and place the heel of the other hand over the dorsum of the patient's hand.	Apply pressure to the dorsum of the patient's hand pushing the hand down towards the floor (into wrist flexion) while the patient resists the movement.
Wrist Flexion	The patient's forearm is fully pronated. Place the heel of one hand on the palm of the patient's hand.	Apply pressure to the patient's palm to push the hand upwards (into wrist extension) while the patient resists the movement.
Radial Deviation of the Wrist	With the patient's forearm fully pronated, grip the lateral aspect of the hand (not the thumb) with your fingertips.	Pressure is applied to the lateral aspect of the hand to push it medially while the patient resists the movement.
Ulnar Deviation of the Wrist	With the patient's forearm fully pronated, grip the medial aspect of the patient's hand with your fingertips.	Apply pressure to the medial aspect of the hand to push it laterally while the patient resists the movement.

Resisted Movements of the Elbow and Forearm (*continued*)

Name of Movement	Starting Position	Movement
Finger Extension	The patient's forearm is placed in the mid-prone position with the fingers relaxed and slightly flexed. Place the palm of one hand over the posterior aspect of the fingers with the fingertips over the MP joints and the heel of the hand on the patient's fingernails.	Close the fist bringing the patient's fingers into flexion while the patient resists the movement.
Finger Flexion (Grip is best tested using specific equipment such as an isometric dynamometer)	Place your index finger in the palm of the patient's hand from the thumb (radial) side. The test is repeated with the finger inserted into the grip from the little finger (medial) side.	The patient is instructed to grip the finger tightly as you try to withdraw it from their hand.
Abduction / Adduction of the Fingers	The patient's hand is placed flat on the table with the fingers spread apart and the forearm fully pronated. Apply a fingertip to alternating sides of each of the patient's fingers.	Pressure is applied to alternating sides of the finger pushing it towards and then away from adjacent fingers, while the patient resists the movement.
Pinch Grip	Place your index finger between the tips of the patient's index finger and thumb.	The patient is instructed to grip the finger while you try to extract it from their grip.

Movements of the wrist and hand are best tested with the patient's arm supported on a small table and the hand clear of the end of the table.

Examination Findings Related To Specific Conditions

| | Onset | | | |
Gradual Due to Overuse	Gradual Due to Trauma	Gradual Due to No Cause	Sudden Due to Overuse	Sudden Due to Trauma
Lateral Epicondylitis	Olecranon Bursitis	Median Nerve Entrapment	de Quervains Tenosynovitis	MCP Joint Injury of Thumb
Medial Epicondylitis	Ulnar Nerve Entrapment	Carpal Tunnel Syndrome	MCP Joint Injury of Thumb	Strained Wrist
Olecranon Bursitis	Wrist Extensor Tendonitis	OA of CMC Joint of Thumb		
Ulnar Nerve Entrapment	Wrist Flexor Tendonitis	Trigger Finger		
Median Nerve Entrapment				
Carpal Tunnel Syndrome				
Wrist Extensor Tendonitis				
de Quervains Tenosynovitis				
Wrist Flexor Tendonitis				

Typical Age Ranges

20–40 Years	20–50 Years	35–55 Years	40–60 Years	50 + Years
Median Nerve Entrapment	Olecranon Bursitis	Lateral Epicondylitis	OA of CMC Joint of Thumb	Trigger Finger
MCP Joint Injury of Thumb	Ulnar Nerve Entrapment	Medial Epicondylitis		Duputryens Contracture
Sprained Wrist	Wrist Extensor Tendonitis	Carpal Tunnel Syndrome		
	Wrist Flexor Tendonitis			

Duration

0–3 Weeks	3–6 Weeks	6–12 Weeks	3–6 Months	6 Months–Years
Medial Epicondylitis	Wrist Extensor Tendonitis	Lateral Epicondylitis	Ulnar Nerve Entrapment	Carpal Tunnel Syndrome
de Quervains Tenosynovitis	de Quervains Tenosynovitis	Medial Epicondylitis	Median Nerve Entrapment	OA of CMC Joint of Thumb
MCP Joint Injury of Thumb (Trauma)	Wrist Flexor Tendonitis	Olecranon Bursitis	Carpal Tunnel Syndrome	Trigger Finger
Wrist Sprain			MCP Joint Injury of Thumb (Overuse)	Duputyrens Contracture

Frequency

First Time with These Symptoms	Recurrent Episodes Months Apart Over 1–2 Years	One Episode of Varying Intensity	One Episode of Steadily Worsening Symptoms	Episodes 1–2 Years Apart
Lateral Epicondylitis	Lateral Epicondylitis	Olecranon Bursitis	Trigger Finger	de Quervains Tenosynovitis
Wrist Extensor Tendonitis	Medial Epicondylitis	Ulnar Nerve Entrapment	Duputyrens Contracture	
de Quervains Tenosynovitis	Median Nerve Entrapment	Median Nerve Entrapment		
MCP Joint Injury of Thumb	Carpal Tunnel Syndrome			
Wrist Tendonitis	OA of CMC Joint of Thumb			
Wrist Sprain				

(continued)

Examination Findings Related To Specific Conditions (continued)

Area of Symptoms

Lateral Aspect of Elbow	Anteromedial Aspect of Elbow	Posterior Aspect of Elbow	Posterior Wrist and Hand	Medial 1½ Fingers/ Medial Hand and Forearm	Lateral 3½ Fingers Lateral Hand and Anterior Forearm
Lateral Epicondylitis	Medial Epicondylitis	Olecranon Bursitis	Wrist Extensor Tendonitis Wrist Sprain	Ulnar Nerve Entrapment	Median Nerve Entrapment

Lateral 3½ Fingers Lateral Aspect of Hand	Palm of Hand	Lateral Aspect of the Wrist and Thumb	Anatomical Snuffbox	Anterior Wrist	Medial Wrist
Carpal Tunnel Syndrome	Trigger Finger Duputryens Contracture Wrist Flexor Tendonitis	de Quervains Tenosynovitis Wrist Sprain	OA of CMC Joint of Thumb	Wrist Flexor Tendonitis	Wrist Sprain

Type of Symptoms

Sharp Pain on Activities	Ache following Activities	Ache at Rest	Stiffness in Morning or after Rest	Pain and Paraesthesia in Forearm	Motor Weakness in Forearm or Hand
Lateral Epicondylitis	Lateral Epicondylitis	de Quervains Tenosynovitis	OA of CMC Joint of Thumb	Lateral Epicondylitis	Ulnar Nerve Entrapment (later stages)

Medial Epicondylitis Wrist Extensor Tendonitis de Quervains Tenosynovitis Wrist Flexor Tendonitis	Medial Epicondylitis Wrist Extensor Tendonitis OA of CMC Joint of Thumb	OA of CMC Joint of Thumb	Ulnar Nerve Entrapment Median Nerve Entrapment	Median Nerve Entrapment (later stages) Carpal Tunnel Syndrome (later stages)
Pain on Elbow Contact with Surface	**Pain and Swelling at Wrist**	**Pain and Paraesthesia in the Hand**	**Stiffness with Deformity of Fingers**	**Pain on Taking Weight through Hand**
Olecranon Bursitis Ulnar Nerve Entrapment	MCP Joint Injury of Thumb Wrist Sprain	Median Nerve Entrapment Ulnar Nerve Entrapment Carpal Tunnel Syndrome	Trigger Finger Duputryens Contracture	Wrist Sprain

Observations

Swelling Lateral Elbow	**Swelling Posterior Elbow**	**Swelling Lateral Wrist/Thumb**	**Swelling at Base of Thumb**	**Swelling around Wrist Joint**	**Soft Tissue Thickening at Base of Thumb**
Lateral Epicondylitis	Olecranon Bursitis	de Quervains Tenosynovitis	MCP Joint Injury of Thumb	Wrist Sprain	OA of CMC Joint of Thumb

(continued)

Examination Findings Related To Specific Conditions (continued)

Thickening/Puckering of Skin in Palm	Wasting of Muscles Anterior Forearm/Hand	Wasting of Hand Muscles	Wasting of Muscles of Thumb	Nil of Note
Duputryens Contracture, Trigger Finger	Median Nerve Entrapment (later stages)	Ulnar Nerve Entrapment (later stages)	Carpal Tunnel Syndrome (later stages)	Wrist Flexor Tendonitis

Active Movements

Full and Pain Free at Wrist, Elbow and Hand	Pain on Forearm Pronation	Pain on Wrist Extension	Pain on Extension and Abduction of Thumb	Wrist Movements Near Full Range but All Movements Painful or Stiff	Decreased Range of Ulnar Deviation of Wrist
Early Lateral Epicondylitis, Medial Epicondylitis, Olecranon Bursitis	Median Nerve Entrapment	Medial Epicondylitis, Wrist Flexor Tendonitis	MCP Joint Injury of Thumb	Wrist Sprain	de Quervains Tenosynovitis

Decreased Range of Flexion of Thumb	Mild Limitation of All Movements of Thumb	Loss of Extension of Fingers	Normal Active Movements of Fingers but with Clicking or Jerking during Movements	Inability to Close Fist Fully
de Quervains Tenosynovitis	OA of CMC Joint of Thumb	Trigger Finger, Duputryens Contracture	Trigger Finger	Ulnar Nerve Entrapment

Passive Movements

Pain on Combined Wrist Flexion and Elbow Extension	Pain with Combined Wrist Extension and Elbow Extension	Pain on Full Elbow Flexion	Pain in Wrist on Ulnar or Radial Deviation	Pain in Wrist on Finger Flexion Combined with Ulnar/Radial Deviations	Pain on Posterior/Anterior Glides of the Wrist Joint
Lateral Epicondylitis	Medial Epicondylitis Wrist Flexor Tendonitis	Olecranon Bursitis	Wrist Sprain	Wrist Extensor Tendonitis	Wrist Sprain

Pain on Flexion of the Thumb Combined with Ulnar Deviation of Wrist	Pain on Rotation of Thumb	Pain on Extension and Adduction of Thumb	Soft Tissue Resistance to Finger Extension	Movements Full and Pain Free
de Quervains Tenosynovitis	MCP Joint Injury of Thumb OA of CMC Joint of Thumb	MCP Joint Injury of Thumb OA of CMC Joint of Thumb	Dupuytrens Contracture Trigger Finger	Ulnar Nerve Entrapment Olecranon Bursitis Carpal Tunnel Syndrome Median Nerve Entrapment Trigger Finger

Resisted Movements

Pain on Finger Extension	Pain on Wrist Extension	Pain on Wrist Flexion	Pain on Pronation	Pain on Abduction and Extension of Thumb	Pain on Adduction of Thumb
Lateral Epicondylitis	Lateral Epicondylitis Wrist Extensor Tendonitis	Medial Epicondylitis Wrist Flexor Tendonitis	Medial Epicondylitis	de Quervains Teno-synovitis MCP Joint Injury of Thumb	MCP Joint Injury of Thumb
Lateral Epicon-dylitis					

(continued)

Examination Findings Related To Specific Conditions (continued)

Weakness of Grip Radial Side of Hand	Weakness on Pronation, Wrist Flexion and Opposition of Thumb	All Movements Strong and Pain Free	Weakness of Grip Generally	All Wrist Movement Produce Pain on Strong Resistance
Carpal Tunnel Syndrome (Later Stages) OA of CMC Joint of Thumb	Median Nerve Entrapment	Olecranon Bursitis Carpal Tunnel Syndrome Trigger Finger Duputryens Contracture	Ulnar Nerve Entrapment	Wrist Sprain

Palpation

Tender Over Lateral Elbow	Tender Over Anteromedial Elbow	Poorly Localized Tenderness Posterior Elbow	Palpation over Carpus Produces Hand Symptoms	Pain over Anterior Carpus	Tender over Pisiform
Lateral Epicondylitis	Medial Epicondylitis Ulnar Nerve Entrapment	Olecranon Bursitis	Carpal Tunnel Syndrome	Wrist Extensor Tendonitis	Wrist Flexor Tendonitis

Pain At Medial or Lateral Wrist Joint Line	Pain Lateral Wrist and Thumb	Pain in the Anatomical Snuffbox	Pain in Palm over Base of Second Metacarpal	Snapping of Flexor Tendons Felt in Palm on Finger Extension	Thickening of Soft Tissue in Palm
Wrist Sprain	de Quervains Tenosynovitis	OA of CMC Joint of Thumb MCP Joint Injury of Thumb	Wrist Flexor Tendonitis	Trigger Finger	Duputryens Contracture

PALPATION OF THE ELBOW, WRIST, AND HAND

In this section a description is given of the method of palpating each structure referred to in relation to the following conditions:

- Lateral epicondylitis of the elbow
- Medial epicondylitis of the elbow
- Olecranon bursitis
- Ulnar nerve entrapment (cubital tunnel syndrome)
- Median nerve entrapment
- Carpal tunnel syndrome
- Wrist extensor tendonitis
- de Quervains tenosynovitis
- Metacarpophalangeal joint injury of the thumb
- Osteoarthritis of the carpometacarpal Joint of the thumb
- Trigger finger
- Wrist flexor tendonitis
- Dupytrens contracture
- Wrist sprain

The following structures discussed in the following sections must be identified.

Elbow Region

Lateral Epicondyle

With the patient's elbow flexed at 90 degrees, the most prominent point that can be seen and palpated at the lateral aspect of the elbow is the tip of the lateral epicondyle. If radial deviation of the wrist is resisted then the common extensor tendon can be palpated from its attachment to the lateral epicondyle distally into the forearm (Fig. 3.1).

Head of the Radius

Just distal to the lateral epicondyle is the rounded head of the radius. This is most easily palpated with the elbow extended and it can be felt to rotate during pronation and supination of the forearm when the elbow is flexed to 90 degrees (Fig. 3.2).

Medial Epicondyle

This is the most prominent bony point at the medial side of the elbow and it is most easily palpated with the elbow flexed to 90 degrees (Fig. 3.3). Just anterior to the tip of the epicondyle it is possible to palpate the attachment of the common flexor tendon. If flexion of the wrist is resisted with the patient gripping a pencil, it is then possible to palpate the tendons and muscle bellies of the flexor muscles of the forearm and the pronator teres muscle.

Lateral epicondyle

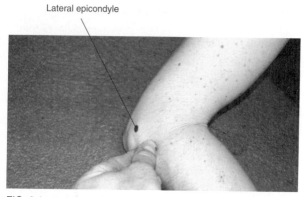

FIG. 3.1 Surface marking of the lateral epicondyle of the right humerus. The examiner's finger is placed on the common extensor tendon.

Lateral epicondyle

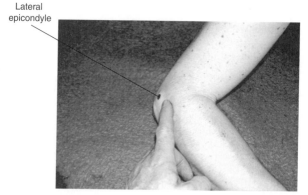

FIG. 3.2 Surface marking of the lateral epicondyle of the right humerus, the examiner's thumb and finger are holding the head of the right radius.

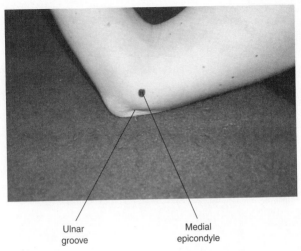

FIG. 3.3 The medial epicondyle of the right humerus and the ulnar groove at the right elbow.

Ulnar Groove

It is possible to palpate the ulnar nerve in its groove at the posterior aspect of the medial epicondyle, at which point the nerve can be rolled under a finger as it lies in the cubital tunnel (Fig. 3.3).

Olecranon

The olecranon is easily palpated as a bony lump at the posterior of the elbow and is most prominent when the elbow is flexed to 90 degrees (Fig. 3.4). If you pick up the skin and subcutaneous tissue over that area, you are then palpating the olecranon bursa.

Triceps Tendon

The tendon of the triceps muscle can be palpated at its attachment into the superior part of the olecranon (Fig. 3.5). This is most easily done when the elbow is flexed to approximately 45 degrees.

Biceps Tendon

This thick cordlike tendon is easily palpated at the anterior of the elbow on isometric resisted flexion of the elbow joint (Fig. 3.6).

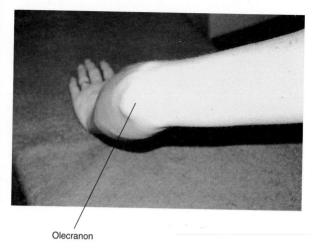

Olecranon

FIG. 3.4 The olecranon of the left humerus which is also the site of the olecranon bursa.

Wrist Region

Head of the Ulnar

When the forearm is pronated, the head of the ulna is easily palpated as a small bony protruberance at the medial aspect of the wrist (Fig. 3.7)

Wrist Joint Line

Dropping your finger off the head of the ulnar laterally and distally will take it onto the lower end of the radius, at which point it is easy to palpate the posterior wrist joint line and the concavity formed by the proximal row of carpal bones (Fig. 3.7).

Pisiform

Just distal to the head of the ulnar it is possible to feel the surface of a bone, the triquetrum. If the examining finger is brought around to the anterior aspect of the triquetrum, a small pealike bone, the pisiform, can be palpated at the anterior of the wrist joint. The tendon of the flexor carpi ulnaris muscle is easily palpated at its attachment to the proximal side of the pisiform on active or resisted ulnar deviation of the wrist (Fig. 3.8).

Triceps
muscle bulk

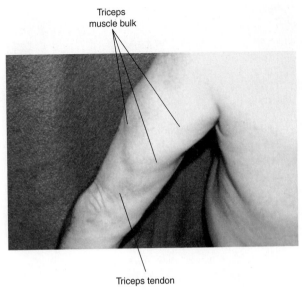

Triceps tendon

FIG. 3.5   The left triceps muscle and triceps tendon.

Radial Styloid

Follow the distal end of the radius on the posterior aspect of the wrist around to the lateral side and the radial styloid is palpable as a point of bone within the anatomical snuff box, which is an easily identifiable hollow at the lateral aspect of the base of the thumb, produced by the extensor and abductor tendons of the thumb when the thumb is held in extension and abduction (Fig. 3.9).

Flexor Carpi Radialis

The tendon of the flexor carpi radialis muscle can be palpated just lateral to the lateral border of the anatomical snuff box as it passes on its way to its attachment at the base of the second metacarpal (Fig. 3.10).

Carpometacarpal Joint of the Thumb

The joint line of the carpometacarpal joint of the thumb is palpable just distal to the radial styloid within the anatomical snuff box (Fig. 3.9). The tip of a finger or thumb placed in the base of the anatomical snuff box

Biceps muscle

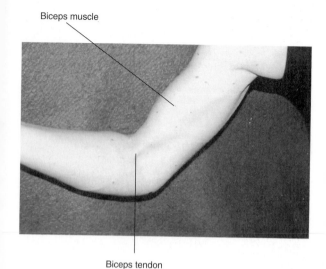

Biceps tendon

FIG. 3.6 The right biceps muscle and biceps tendon.

Head of ulna

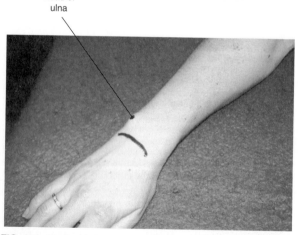

FIG. 3.7 The head of the right ulnar with a line marking the posterior wrist joint line.

Pisiform

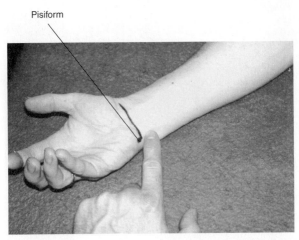

FIG. 3.8 Surface marking of the pisiform with a line marking the position of the anterior wrist joint line. The examiner's finger is placed on the tendon of the flexor capi ulnaris muscle.

C.M.C. Joint of thumb   Radial Styloid

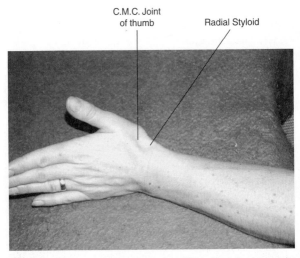

FIG. 3.9 The position of the anatomical snuff box at the left wrist containing the radial styloid proximally and the CMC joint of the thumb distally.

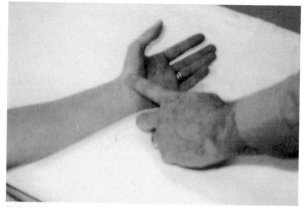

FIG. 3.10   The examiner's finger is placed on the tendon of the flexor carpi radialis muscle lying laterally to the lateral border of the anatomical snuff box.

will automatically fall on this joint line which is most easily identified when the thumb is moved either actively or passively.

Carpal Bones

It is very difficult to palpate the wrist joint line anteriorly, but there is a skin crease just proximal to the thenar and hypothenar eminences that is easily observed when the wrist is slightly flexed (Fig. 3.8). The bones of the carpus lie distal to this crease and mark the area of the carpal tunnel (Fig. 3.11). On the posterior aspect of the wrist just medial and distal to the radial styloid it is possible to palpate the bones of the carpus. The wrist extensor tendons run over this area.

SPECIFIC TESTS FOR THE ELBOW, WRIST, AND HAND

Lateral Epicondylitis

There are several tests for lateral epicondylitis. The simplest is to hold the patient's elbow fully extended with the forearm pronated and then passively flex the wrist. If pain is then experienced in the area of the lateral epicondyle it is considered positive for epicondylitis. Pain felt at the lateral epicondyle on isometric resisted radial deviation and extension of the wrist, while the hand is held in a fist and the forearm pronated, is a further confirmation of the presence of this condition. Isometric resisted extension of the fingers with pressure applied over the intermediate phalangese, while

Soft-tissue crease marking
anterior wrist joint line

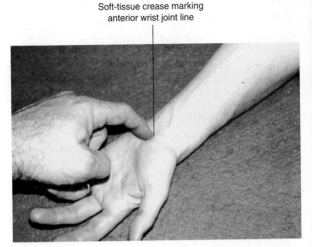

FIG. 3.11 The examiner's finger is in position over the carpal tunnel at the left wrist.

the forearm is pronated and the wrist held in a neutral position, will give further evidence of this condition if the test produces pain at the lateral aspect of the elbow.

Medial Epicondylitis

Only one test is commonly used to screen for this condition. The patient's elbow is held in a fully extended position with the forearm supinated. The wrist is then fully extended passively and pain felt over the area of the medial epicondyle will help to confirm diagnosis.

Cubital Tunnel Syndrome

The patient is asked to flex the elbow fully and hold it in this position for several minutes. Signs of paraesthesia in the distribution of the ulnar nerve in the forearm and hand are indications of a possible cubital tunnel syndrome.

de Quervains Syndrome

Have the patient hold his thumb inside his fingers while forming a fist, then passively ulnar deviate the wrist. This maneuver is positive if it produces pain in the affected tendons at the lateral aspect of the anatomical snuff box (Finkelstein's Test).

Thumb Carpometacarpal Joint

Hold the patient's thumb by grasping the first metacarpal. Apply compression force to the carpometacarpal joint by approximating the thumb to the forearm while rotating the joint. If pain is produced in the base of the thumb it is indicative of a carpometacarpal joint lesion.

Carpal Tunnel Syndrome

There are two commonly described tests for this condition. The first is to hold the patient's wrist in full flexion for one minute, if paraesthesia is produced in the thumb and lateral two and a half fingers, it is indicative of a carpal tunnel syndrome (Phalen's sign). Percussion over the anterior carpus using the tip of a finger or a reflex hammer will also produce paraesthesia in the thumb and the lateral two and a half fingers when the median nerve is compressed in the carpal tunnel.

ELBOW, WRIST, AND HAND CONDITIONS

Lateral Epicondylitis of the Elbow

This is a very common condition and is becoming more so due to an increase in the occurrence of repetitive strain injuries and a growing awareness of repetitive strain (1–3). The symptoms of this condition are often ignored by the patient for weeks, months, or even years, and the physician or therapist is not contacted until their symptoms are functionally limiting. The condition is believed to arise because of an excessive degree of pulling on the common extensor tendon, particularly at its attachment into the lateral epicondyle of the humerus. There appears to be a pathology of repeated microtrauma, where small areas of tendon tissue are torn away from the periosteum producing an associated inflammatory reaction that is initially minor but progresses to become recurrent, acute on chronic, and a major problem (3, 6, 10, 14, 25, 26, 31).

Subjective Findings

Onset   Onset is gradual due to overuse and is most commonly found in middle-aged patients. The condition can present in patients in their teens, and is particularly associated with the playing of musical instruments, but it is rare in the 60+ age group (2, 3, 6, 13).

Duration   The current episode may present as an acute problem of only a few weeks duration, but the condition usually presents as a chronic problem of between 6 weeks and 6 months duration, with regular recurrence of acute symptoms. Rarely the patient presents as a first-time acute case with the symptoms present for only a few days or one to two weeks.

Frequency Most commonly the patient will give a history of some previous episodes of similar symptoms that have been increasing in both duration and frequency. Recurrence of symptoms is often associated with a particular activity either at work, in the home, or related to a recreational pastime (1, 2, 15, 25).

Area of Symptoms The patient can usually localize the majority of his symptoms to the lateral aspect of the elbow over the anterior aspect of the lateral epicondyle. With repeated recurrence the pain will often radiate along the posterior aspect of the forearm to the wrist, and occasionally into the posterior aspect of the hand. (Fig. 3.12) (2–4, 14).

Type of Symptoms The patient complains of sharp pain at the lateral aspect of the elbow on certain activities. There will also be pain following activity, which is more of an ache and is located in the extensor muscle bulk at the posterior forearm. In more chronic cases the patient will also complain of paraesthesia affecting the forearm and hand (2, 3, 12, 15).

Miscellaneous Patients with lateral epicondylitis often report difficulty picking up an object while the forearm is pronated. This can be something as simple as picking up a cup of coffee. They also have difficulty using tools, such as a screwdriver or torque driver, particularly where a strong grip is required to control the tool (25, 28, 31).

Objective Findings

Observation In most cases there are no observable changes in the elbow or forearm. In very acute cases there may be a small swelling at the lateral epicondyle; in very chronic cases a degree of soft tissue thickening may be observed in the same area (3, 11, 12).

Active Movements In the initial stages of this condition, movement of the elbow, wrist, and hand are usually full range and painless. In more chronic cases there is loss of the last few degrees of elbow extension and pain may be reported on full flexion of the elbow, which is often described as a feeling of pressure at the lateral aspect of the elbow (4, 5, 11, 12).

Passive Movements Pain can often be produced at the lateral aspect of the elbow and along the course of the common extensor tendon when passive wrist flexion is combined with full elbow extension (2, 7, 21).

Resisted Movements Pain will be felt at the lateral aspect of the elbow and occasionally in the posterior aspect of the forearm on isometric resisted extension of the fingers and on extension or radial deviation of the wrist. Pain may be felt on only one or two of these movements or on all three, depending upon the severity of the condition during that particular episode. In either very acute or very chronic cases the same pain will also be produced on a strong full-hand grip or pinch grip (5, 7, 12, 15).

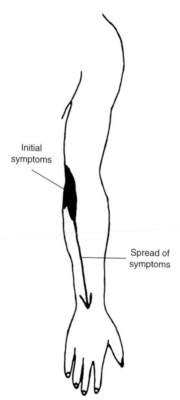

Initial
symptoms

Spread of
symptoms

FIG. 3.12   Area of symptoms for lateral epicondylitis at the right elbow.

Palpation Tenderness will be elicited over the lateral epicondyle of
the elbow (Fig. 3.1) in all cases; in chronic cases pain is also elicited along
the proximal part of the extensor muscle mass and over the common
extensor tendon. In the most pronounced cases the muscles of the forearm
will often feel full and tense on palpation, although this will not
necessarily be uncomfortable for the patient (10, 12, 18, 23).

Treatment Ideas (2–4, 8, 9, 11–13, 16, 26, 29, 30)

During any acute episode the patient is first advised to rest the arm, avoiding all activities that produce typical symptoms. This is the most singu-

larly important part of treatment at this stage, and must be thoroughly explained to the patient, as well as to the patient's employer, if necessary. The patient should be told that avoidance of pain-producing activities does not apply only to work, but also to any other activities, no matter how pleasurable. They should also be advised to use ice on the elbow and forearm for 15 minutes at least every 2 hours, both at work and at home.

Non-thermal doses of ultrasound are often useful in reducing symptoms and the sonation of anti-inflammatory preparations may also help. The use of a brace in this condition is a subject that produces a degree of discussion. For many years patients with lateral epicondylitis were instructed to use a wrist brace, as the condition is a problem of the wrist extensor muscles, not an elbow problem. However, since the condition is called "tennis elbow," and the symptoms appear at the elbow, it is virtually impossible to convince a patient that it is not an elbow problem. Therefore, the patient will tend to buy an elbow brace. I have found that the simple sleeve-type of elastic elbow brace does seem to help reduce symptoms, particularly if the rest and ice policy is followed effectively. The use of a strap-type forearm band, which in effect changes the origin of the muscle to take the strain off the common extensor origin, has, in my experience, reasonable short-term results, particularly in sports activities. In the long term and in the workplace, this type of brace tends to hide the symptoms for a period of time, but produces further discomfort more distally in the forearm later. My brace of choice in this condition is a wrist splint, which holds the wrist in mild extension and releases tension on the common extensor tendon.

In the early stages of treatment, active exercises should be aimed at maintenance of normal muscle length to prevent stiffness from occurring. The patient is taught gentle active finger flexion and extension, wrist extension, flexion, ulnar and radial deviation, and elbow extension and flexion. They must also be taught to take long rest breaks, even though the exercises are very light. These exercises should not be attempted at a level that produces any typical symptoms; if symptoms are produced the patient must rest until they disappear.

When the initial acute symptoms start to subside, muscle stretches can be introduced for the wrist extensors. These should not be carried out to the point of pain. The patient is taught to apply a gentle pressure, with the opposite hand on the knuckles of the affected side, holding the stretch for a minimum of 15 seconds and resting for 30 seconds between each stretch. These stretches should be progressed to include ulnar deviation combined with wrist flexion, as the extensor carpi radialis brevis muscle is usually one of the major structures involved in the pathological process.

Interferential therapy to the muscles of the forearm and transcutaneous electrical nerve stimulation to the common extensor tendon are helpful in reducing symptoms, particularly when combined with heat before exercise and ice after exercise. Once the patient can cope with simple active exercises and passive stretching of the affected muscles, without discomfort and through full range, then a useful treatment technique is the use of neuromuscular electrical stimulation to the extensor muscles of the forearm to produce a mild contraction. The patient then grips the edge of the table or pillow that he is resting on in order to hold against the contraction, to produce a simple, effective stretch of the extensor muscles.

Further progression of treatment is achieved through light resisted gripping exercises for the hand and isometric exercises for all four movements of the wrist joint. Light resisted elbow exercises using dumbbells are an effective way of working the forearm muscles. The patient has to be instructed to continue with the resting techniques he has been using, so that as the exercises progress, the symptoms do not. Progression of exercise can be achieved by gradually reducing rest periods as tolerated by the patient.

Neuromuscular electrical stimulation can now be used to recreate, in slow motion, the injury process. This is done by producing a stronger contraction in the extensor muscles. The patient is instructed to wait until a contraction is produced and then to push down against the contraction, bringing the wrist into flexion. Typically, in daily use of the arm, patients who suffer from these symptoms have had to carry out activities where they grip tools or objects and at the same time are required to flex their wrist. This produces a contraction of the extensor muscles of the wrist while the muscle is being forced to lengthen. The use of muscle stimulation can recreate this type of activity, but in a controlled manner that will help to condition the patient to similar work without producing injury.

The patient should be progressed to gripping and handling activities such as holding different sizes and weights of cans in the hand while flexing and extending the wrist, particularly with the forearm pronated. A general upper-extremity workout is also necessary to condition the whole arm; once again the patient must be instructed to take regular rest and stretch breaks to prevent any onset of symptoms. Return to work or sports activities should be carried out in a graduated manner, with reintroduction of the activities that produced the symptoms for a limited time period initially. As the patient copes with these activities without exacerbating their symptoms, the time spent on them can be increased.

Restrictions   In the early stages the patient should be advised to avoid all activities that produce their typical symptoms. I use the analogy of a finger being trapped in a door, and ask the patient to consider that if he was being treated for symptoms related to that type of injury he could not expect to get better if he continued to trap his finger in the door several times each day. Every activity the patient does that produces typical symptoms is no different than placing that finger in a door and closing it once again. If the patient is using a brace and can carry out some activities without producing those symptoms, that had occurred previously, either during or after the activity, then it is all right to continue with that activity.

The one thing that must be avoided at all costs is the use of a brace to simply decrease the symptoms, rather than abolish them, as this will inevitably lead to chronicity in the condition.

When lifting, the patient should be advised to have the arm supinated and the weights raised should never be heavy enough to produce symptoms. In sports, the patient cannot carry out any activities of a sudden explosive nature, such as throwing. The patient also has to be advised against prolonged or repetitive gripping, either with the whole hand or with a pinch grip. Increase in activities at work, in sports, or in the home should trail behind the patient's progression in the clinic. As the patient demonstrates ability to use the wrist and hand without symptoms, then he can attempt lighter activities at home, progressing to more strenuous activities when able. At any sign of a flare up in the condition, the patient should be advised to use ice on a regular basis and stop activities once again. Return to work and sports activities should be monitored by the therapist, with the patient advised against ignoring even minor symptoms. An aggressive approach to rest and a carefully graduated increase in activities is the only way to prevent this condition from becoming truly chronic and debilitating.

Medial Epicondylitis of the Elbow

This is a less common condition compared to lateral epicondylitis, but is still found in a large number of patients. It is a condition that is virtually chronic by nature, but occasionally can be found in acute cases. It is usually associated with a certain activity or activities either at work, in the home, or connected with sports or recreation (1, 8, 11, 12). Inflammation occurs in the common flexor tendon at its insertion into the medial epicondyle of the humerus. It is believed to be caused by repetitive microtrauma, in the form of minor periosteal tears, or through attrition of the tendon itself. It is often related to tight flexor muscles of the wrist and fingers, and occurs on more prolonged or more vigorous activities, such as gripping the handle of a tool, particularly if this is associated with vibration of the tool (for example, when using a jackhammer). It can also be produced by hard forearm shots in racquet sports or by throwing a ball. The condition is often ignored by the patient until not just the causative activities, but all daily activities, are affected by the symptoms (3, 7, 16, 25, 26, 28).

Subjective Findings

Onset This is usually gradual after overuse in patients commonly 35 to 55 years of age. It can be found in patients as early as in their teens or twenties, but is rarely seen in the over sixties. It is very seldom associated with a single incident (4–6, 11).

Duration Any one episode may present as an acute case and the patient is seen one to three weeks after onset. On the other hand, any one episode could last two to three months before the patient is referred for treatment.

Frequency   There is usually a pattern of recurrent episodes over a 1- to 2-year period, although with the higher profile that repetitive strain injuries enjoy today, you can occasionally find cases that are only a few days old, but this is rare (11, 13, 17).

Area of Symptoms   The patient will usually be able to localize symptoms to the anteromedial aspect of the elbow, with spread of symptoms along the anterior aspect of the forearm, occasionally as far as the wrist (Fig. 3.13) (5, 10–12).

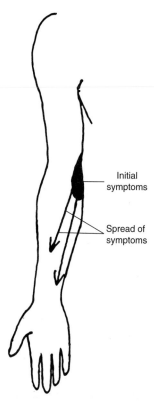

Initial symptoms

Spread of symptoms

FIG. 3.13   Area of symptoms for medial epicondylitis at the right elbow.

Type of Symptoms Patients will usually complain of a nagging ache at the elbow and in the anterior forearm, which is worse after activity. Occasionally on certain activities the patient will complain of a sharp pain more clearly localized to the anteromedial aspect of the elbow (10–12).

Miscellaneous Patients will often be able to continue with the activities that produce discomfort as the symptoms are not as disabling as those produced by lateral epicondylitis.

Objective Findings

Observation There is seldom anything to be seen in either the elbow or the forearm on examination. In very rare cases a small degree of swelling may be visible over the medial epicondyle itself (3, 6, 18).

Active Movements Movements of the elbow are usually pain free and of full range. Some discomfort may be felt on active extension of the wrist, particularly when the elbow is extended. All movements of the wrist will be of full range, although there might be pain and slight restriction on extension of the wrist when the elbow is fully extended (3, 10, 11, 16, 19).

Passive Movements Range of motion will be the same as in active testing. Pain will often be felt in the anterior aspect of the forearm on full passive extension of the wrist while the elbow is held in extension. In very acute or very persistent cases pain may be felt at the medial epicondyle on this same maneuver (12, 18, 19, 21).

Resisted Movements Pain will be experienced on isometric resisted wrist flexion and occasionally on flexion of the fingers. In some cases isometric pronation of the forearm may produce more pain than wrist flexion, but commonly both movements are uncomfortable. The pain will usually be felt at the anterior aspect of the medial epicondyle rather than in the forearm itself (7, 11, 13, 18).

Palpation Tenderness is often found on palpation over the anterior surface of the medial epicondyle of the humerus (Fig 3.3); occasionally tenderness will also be elicited along the forearm for 1 to 2 inches distal to that point. During acute exacerbations the forearm muscles often feel tight and tense, even with the arm relaxed and fully supported. This is most noticeable in comparison to the non-affected side 7, 13, 23).

Treatment Ideas (2, 3, 5, 6, 8, 12, 13, 16, 18, 29, 30)

The most essential part of early treatment is avoidance of all pain-producing activities, be that at work, at home, or in sports and recreational activities. This should be accompanied in the early stages by frequent icing at a minimum of 15 minutes every 2 hours. The use of splints is not particularly helpful in this condition. A wrist splint will often produce more discomfort as the patient is required to work against it while using the hand; rather than resting the affected muscles this will actually require them to do more work. Some patients' benefit from the use of a simple sleeve-type elastic support over the elbow itself. The main reason for this may be that they are made more aware of their condition and therefore less likely to do activities that produce ongoing symptoms. Active movements of the hand, wrist, forearm, and elbow should be continued within pain-free ranges to prevent onset of stiffness because, as noted earlier, tightness of the flexor muscles of the forearm is a common contributing factor to the condition overall.

As the patient's symptoms start to subside, heat can be substituted for ice and gentle stretching of the flexor muscles of the wrist can commence. This should be done both with the elbow in flexion and in extension. Stretches should be held for a minimum of 15 seconds with at least 30 seconds rest between each stretch.

Light resisted hand exercises can be incorporated into the treatment program, but the patient must be clearly advised on the use of rest and stretch breaks to prevent increase in symptoms during or following the exercise. Exercises that are tolerated well and produce no symptoms will help to condition the arm to further work. Exercises that exacerbate the patient's symptoms will lead to further chronicity of the condition. When the patient can tolerate passive stretching of the flexor muscles of the wrist, then a muscle stimulator can be used to produce contraction of the muscle, with the patient holding the wrist and fingers in extension against the force of the contraction. The amount of stimulation is steadily increased as the patient demonstrates the ability to tolerate this particular modality. At this stage thermal doses of ultrasound can be used to facilitate stretching of the common flexor tendon, and interferential therapy can be useful in promoting relaxation of the forearm muscles. If the patient shows a propensity towards postexercise pain, the use of ice is indicated.

Further progression can be made through more vigorous strengthening of the forearm muscles, initially with isometric wrist exercises and moving on to isotonic wrist and hand exercises. Again, rest periods should be designed to prevent increased symptoms during or after exercise; as the patient's condition improves these rest periods can be steadily reduced. Stretching of the flexor muscles of the wrist by the patient standing and leaning forward on a table, with palms placed flat on top, can be considered a final-stage stretch.

If after several sessions of treatment the patient still has some nagging discomfort at the medial aspect of the elbow, deep friction massage can be employed as a means of loosening restricted tissue and producing a local hyperaemia. If this particular form of treatment is not effective in one or two sessions it should be discontinued, as patient's tend to become angry and apprehensive from being repeatedly hurt without seeing any results from such treatment.

The patient is progressed into a general upper extremity workout, continuing with rest and stretch breaks as required. This should be work or sports specific, with the use of functional exercises such as lifting and carrying weights, handling tools or materials, or practicing movements involved in specific sports such as throwing a ball. The patient should be instructed to ice the arm vigorously (15 minutes every hour for 3 to 4 hours) at any sign of exacerbation of symptoms as the exercises progress. The exercise program must then be reviewed and revised with a more graduated strengthening regime. The use of all modalities should be judiciously discontinued as the patient shows no need for them. The final treatment of this condition is prolonged exercise with sufficient rest to prevent any onset of symptoms. Rest periods are then steadily reduced to the point where they would be considered normal levels of rest for the patient's particular work, sport, or other daily activities.

Restrictions The patient must be instructed to avoid all pain-producing activities, in particular any prolonged or repetitive gripping using either the whole hand or a pinch grip. All activities that the patient can relate to as causative factors should be reviewed, particularly as regards the size of handles on tools (to determine if they are too large or too small) and holding or carrying objects with the forearms supinated. Use of the fingers to grip around objects, such as when handling large pieces of material (i.e., 4×8 feet plywood or gypsum boards) or heavy objects such as concrete blocks, must also be avoided until symptoms are no longer present in the elbow. In sports activities throwing or the use of a racquet should be restricted until symptoms abate.

Return to gripping and carrying activities is made gradually with slowly increasing weights and duration of tasks. In racquet sports, forehand work can be built up by hitting a ball against a wall, lightly initially, and then increasing the force used as the patient is able to cope with the activity. I also advise patients who are returning to racquet sports to pick easy partners to begin with so that they are not in a pressure situation during competition until they are fully fit for it. For throwing activities, particularly for pitchers in baseball, a warm-up program of increasing speeds of throws needs to be developed in consultation with coaching staff. Where vibration in tools is a problem, vibration-reducing gloves or material should be used to reduce the effects on the soft-tissue structures involved.

Olecranon Bursitis

Inflammation of the bursa that lies between the olecranon of the ulna and the overlying soft tissues can occur after prolonged or repetitive leaning on the elbow, as in studying for long periods, or following a blow to or a fall onto the elbow. Objective signs are often minimal and the patient usually presents with an elbow that simply continues to cause occasional sharp twinges of pain, mainly on contact with an object (2, 5, 11, 12).

Subjective Findings

Onset Onset is usually gradual in nature following overuse due to pressure at the posterior aspect of the elbow. Occasionally onset can be gradual after trauma, such as a blow to the elbow or a fall. It can occur at any age but the majority of patients present in the 20 to 50 year range (4, 5, 13).

Duration The condition presents as chronic in nature with a history of pain at the elbow of at least 2 to 3 months duration, and often longer.

Frequency It is rare to have repetitive episodes of this condition. It is usually one ongoing episode that appears to be intermittent because pressure has to be applied to the elbow before symptoms are experienced. Recurrence of symptoms after an episode has cleared is uncommon (5, 9, 11, 15).

Area of Symptoms The pain is felt at the posterior of the elbow joint, usually more to the lateral side (Fig. 3.14) (4, 5, 23).

Type of Symptoms Sharp pain is reported on resting the elbow on a hard surface. Often the pain is not present on every occasion that the elbow comes into contact with a hard surface, however, when the pain does occur it is initially very sharp in nature. It is then followed by a more general aching discomfort that can last anything from a few minutes to 1 or 2 hours (4–7).

Miscellaneous Typically patients will feel a sharp pain on resting the arm on a table or similar surface, but when attempting to discover an area of tenderness they are unable to do so.

Objective Findings

Observation Swelling may be observable around the area of the olecranon (Fig 3.4). On rare occasions redness of the skin will also be present. In the majority of cases there are no visible changes to be observed (11, 13, 15).

Active Movement There is usually no limitation of movement at the elbow, although on occasions full flexion can be limited which will be particularly noticeable if the patient is wearing a heavy coat or jacket or any clothing with tight sleeves (5, 6, 11, 24).

Passive Movement Range of motion will be the same as in active testing. There may be a tightness to the last few degrees of elbow flexion, but no complaints of discomfort (5, 6, 11, 24).

Resisted Movement Movements of the elbow, wrist, and hand are strong, with no discomfort on isometric testing (5, 11, 19, 24).

Palpation It is often difficult to elicit any tenderness, although if the condition has been present for several months it is occasionally possible to feel soft tissue thickening around the olecranon. Increased skin temperature may be discernible generally around the posterior aspect of the elbow (17, 23, 24).

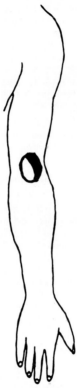

FIG. 3.14 Area of symptoms for olecranon bursitis at the right elbow. These are usually more pronounced on the lateral side.

Treatment Ideas (2, 3, 5, 6, 11, 13, 19)

A trial of intensive icing over a 3- to 4-/day period can sometimes produce good results. The patient should be instructed to ice the arm for 15 minutes every hour if possible, while at the same time avoiding putting any pressure on the elbow. A light elastic sleeve-type elbow support can be used as protection to prevent accidental knocking of the arm against objects. The support also helps to maintain the patient's focus on the condition, making him less inclined to put weight on the elbow. The use of interferential therapy or transcutaneous electrical nerve stimulation in conjunction with ice can often help to relieve discomfort, particularly the more chronic aching type of pain.

As the condition clears through rest and protection of the injured area, it is necessary to restore strength in the arm. This should be done gradually, initially using light free weights or exercise band for wrist, elbow, and shoulder exercises and then progressing the patient into a gym type program for general upper extremity strengthening. Any exacerbation of symptoms is treated immediately with the application of ice and the reintroduction of the use of a brace.

Restrictions Initially the patient has to be careful not to lean on or knock the affected elbow, otherwise most activities do not affect this condition to any great extent.

Ulnar Nerve Entrapment (Cubital Tunnel Syndrome)

The ulnar nerve lies in a groove behind the medial epicondyle of the humerus. The groove is covered by the cruciate ligament to form a fibrous tunnel. The nerve can become trapped in this tunnel by swelling or tissue thickening due to trauma or repetitive irritation following prolonged leaning on or constant use of the elbow (6, 9, 11, 15, 31, 33).

Subjective Findings

Onset This is typically gradual after overuse or on rare occasions following trauma. Even less commonly, onset is related to no particular cause. Patients are usually between 20 and 50 years of age (6, 11, 14).

Duration Initial symptoms are not severe so the patient often does not present for treatment until signs and symptoms have been present for at least 2 months, and often much longer.

Frequency Although the patient's history may suggest recurrent episodes, further questioning will reveal that it is, in fact, normally one long ongoing episode with exacerbations due to particular activities (9, 14, 16, 18).

Area of Symptoms Initial symptoms are felt in the medial one and a half fingers and the medial aspect of the forearm (the same distribution as when you strike your funny bone) Fig. 3.15. As the condition progresses symptoms are experienced at the medial aspect of the elbow and finally more symptoms may develop in the hand (4, 7, 10, 14, 18).

Type of Symptoms Initial symptoms are pain and paraesthesia in the forearm and fingers. Progression of the condition leads to pain being felt locally at the medial aspect of the elbow. If left untreated the condition can reach the point where the patient experiences motor weakness in the muscles of the hypothenar eminence and in the intrinsic muscles of the hand (4, 14, 15, 16, 18).

Miscellaneous Occasionally patients may complain of "something snapping" at the inside of the elbow on either flexion or extension of the joint or on both movements. The patient will often state that he tends to sleep with his elbows flexed and the forearms held into his chest. He then either wakes with, or is awakened by, the onset of symptoms.

Objective Findings

Observation In the early and intermediate stages of this condition nothing is observable at the elbow or arm. In the latter stages wasting of the

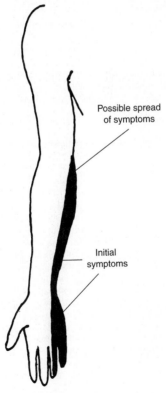

Possible spread
of symptoms

Initial
symptoms

FIG. 3.15 Area of symptoms for ulnar nerve entrapment at the right elbow.

muscles of the hand will be noted, in the form of hollows developing between the metacarpal bones and wasting of the muscles of the hypothenar eminence at the proximal and medial palmar aspect of the hand (14, 15, 18).

Active Movements   Normally the patient presents with full pain-free movements of the wrist, hand, and elbow. Although in the latter stages of the condition the patient may complain of difficulty in making a full fist (6–9, 18).

Passive Movements   All movements of the hand, wrist and elbow will be full and pain free (6, 7, 18).

Resisted Movements   As the condition progresses weakness can be noted on the patient attempting to grip small objects, such as a pencil, in a full-hand grip. This will be particularly noticeable if the patient attempts to hold onto the object while it is being pulled away from the medial side of the hand (5, 7, 10, 15).

Palpation   Occasionally it is possible to elicit tenderness at the medial aspect of the elbow over the ulnar groove (Fig. 3.3). It may be possible to feel the nerve subluxing in the groove while the elbow is palpated during active or passive flexion and extension of the elbow joint. In the later stages loss of muscle bulk and tone will be felt in the muscles of the hand (10, 18, 21, 22).

Specific Tests   Percussion with a reflex hammer over the area of the cubital tunnel may reproduce the patient's typical pain and paraesthesia (Tinnel's sign) (21, 22).

Treatment Ideas (3–8, 11, 15, 16, 18)

During the initial stages the use of padding around the elbow inside a light sleevelike brace can often help alleviate daytime symptoms. If the patient consistently wakes with the symptoms present and has a tendency to sleep with the elbows flexed and the arms held in tightly against the body, then extension night splints for the elbows can be prescribed to help to eliminate this particular cause of symptoms. Rest from any pain-producing activities will also allow the condition to settle more quickly.

Heat and active assisted exercises can be used to try and free the nerve from any adhesions that may have built up in the cubital tunnel due to trauma or inflammation. Full range-of-motion exercises are used, with a gentle prolonged passive stretch at end range of flexion of the elbow. A graduated resisted exercise program for strengthening of the muscles of the elbow, wrist, and forearm is often effective in speeding recovery of function as the patient's symptoms abate. Simple longitudinal distraction of the elbow in slight flexion may also help to mobilize the nerve in the cubital tunnel.

As the hand and forearm symptoms decrease in intensity, resisted exercises for the upper extremities should be introduced with the emphasis on hand function, particularly if the intrinsic muscles of the hand were involved, to help regain motor function. If these conservative methods fail, there are often good results following surgery.

Restrictions The patient should be advised against prolonged or repetitive elbow flexion, particularly towards the end range of movement. They should also avoid resting the elbow on any hard surfaces during daily activities. The patient should also be advised not to sleep with the elbows bent, although this usually requires some form of splintage, as sleeping habits are deeply embedded and extremely hard to alter.

Median Nerve Entrapment

The ligament of Struthers, when present, can produce compression of the median nerve at the elbow, or the nerve can get trapped in its course between the two heads of pronator teres. This can be associated with racquet sports or with work or leisure activities that require repetitive gripping with pronation of the forearm and extension of the elbow (i.e., a gripping, pushing, twisting motion) (3, 6, 11, 14).

Subjective Findings

Onset This is gradual, either after overuse or for no known reason. It occurs most commonly in the 20 to 40 year-old range (3, 6, 18).

Duration The patient invariably presents with a history of several months of recurrent symptoms, as the condition is never functionally limiting.

Frequency If the symptoms are associated with overuse then they are usually recurrent. If there is no known cause of onset the history is usually indicative of one long single episode (14, 16, 18).

Area of Symptoms Sensory symptoms are experienced in the lateral aspect of the hand and the lateral three and a half fingers. Motor symptoms may be found in the anterior forearm or the hand (Fig. 3.16) (7, 11, 14).

Type of Symptoms Initially paraesthesia is experienced in the lateral three and a half fingers and in the lateral aspect of the hand. As the condition progresses there will be decreased muscle strength on pronation of the forearm, flexion of the wrist, opposition of the thumb, and flexion of the second and third fingers (7, 11, 14).

Miscellaneous Patients quite commonly complain that they fatigue easily when using the hand or forearm musculature.

Objective Findings

Observations In most cases there is nil of note to be observed in the affected arm. In advanced stages of the condition there can be wasting of the affected muscles in the anterior forearm and hand (3, 8, 11).

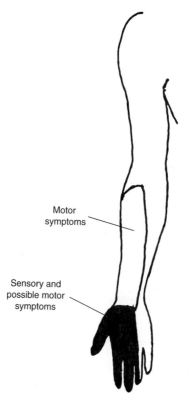

FIG. 3.16   Area of symptoms for medial nerve entrapment at the right elbow.

Active Movements These are usually full and pain free, although symptoms can sometimes be produced at end range of pronation of the forearm, particularly if this position is held for a period of time (6, 8, 14).

Passive Movements These are invariably of full range and pain free (6, 11).

Resisted Movements In the later stages of the condition weakness may be found on pronation of the forearm, flexion of the wrist, opposition of the thumb, and flexion of the second and third fingers. None of the resisted movements will produce any discomfort (7, 8, 14).

Palpation There is usually nothing out of the ordinary to be found on palpation.

Specific Tests Nerve conduction studies may be required to differentiate between this condition and carpal tunnel syndrome, as the two produce very similar symptoms. In the later stages, entrapment of the nerve at the elbow produces symptoms in the forearm which does not occur in carpal tunnel syndrome.

Treatment Ideas (3, 6–8, 11, 14, 16, 18)

This consists of rest and avoidance of activities that produce symptoms. At this time the application of heat in any form may be useful to ease muscle tension in the forearm and around the elbow.

If the patient's symptoms have been eased by rest, then stretching exercises can be started for all muscles of the forearm and wrist. Passive movements incorporating fascial-type stretches held for 1 to 2 minutes at the end of available range of motion are usually the most effective. Heat or thermal doses of ultrasound to the affected muscle can make the task of stretching easier.

Once the patient shows decreased symptoms consistently for a period of time he can be progressed into return to sports or work activities. These can be attempted in the clinic setting under controlled circumstances while the patient continues with stretching of the forearm, wrist, and hand muscles both before and after exercise. When the patient is able to cope with repetitions of exercises that would have previously produced symptoms, then he can attempt the same movements and stresses in daily life. This will usually involve activities of gripping while pushing, pulling, or twisting.

Restrictions In the initial stages the patient should avoid combining movements of pushing or pulling with pronation or supination of the forearm. A blanket restriction on all activities that provoke symptoms is the most effective way of controlling a patient's condition until the symptoms completely subside. A graduated return to these activities can then be started, as described earlier.

Carpal Tunnel Syndrome (CTS)

The median nerve is susceptible to compression as it passes over the carpal bones and under the transverse carpal ligament just distal to the anterior of the wrist joint. The nerve lies within the tunnel created between the bones and the ligament and is accompanied by eight tendons. Tightness of the overlying ligament and swelling of the tendons are two main factors in the pathology of this condition, and pressure on the nerve can be produced by either or both of them (6, 9, 11, 14, 16, 24, 31, 34, 36).

Subjective Findings

Onset Onset is gradual, often with no known cause, or it may be related to overuse. It is more common in women than men and the patient is usually between 35 and 55 years of age (4, 11, 15, 24).

Duration Symptoms may have been present for only a few weeks, but more commonly it will have been several months or even a year or two, since initial onset.

Frequency Episodes of symptoms are recurrent over months or years, and are often associated with a specific activity or activities involving particularly heavy or unaccustomed use of the hand (11, 14, 16, 24).

Area of Symptoms Symptoms are normally felt in the lateral three and a half fingers, but can also spread to the lateral two-thirds of the palm of the hand in chronic cases (Fig. 3.17) (7, 8, 11, 12).

Type of Symptoms Initial symptoms are paraesthesia and possibly numbness, which may eventually progress to loss of both muscle strength and muscle bulk in the thenar muscles of the thumb (7, 8, 12, 14, 16).

Miscellaneous The patient typically complains of waking in the night, sometime between 2 A.M. and 4 A.M. with tingling and numbness in the tips of the affected fingers. The patient often states that he is able to relieve these symptoms by hanging the arm over the side of the bed, putting the hand over his head or by working the hand by flexing and extending the fingers (5, 15, 18).

Objective Findings

Observation In most cases there is nil of note to be observed in the forearm, wrist, or hand. In the later chronic stages of the condition wasting of the thenar muscles of the thumb may be observed (5, 9, 12).

Active Movements Active movements are always full range and pain free in the wrist, hand, thumb, and fingers (4, 5, 9, 18).

Passive Movements These again are full and pain free, but over-pressure on flexion of the wrist may produce symptoms if sustained over a period of time (see "Specific Tests") (5, 7, 10, 12, 21, 35).

Resisted Movements In the early and intermediate stages of the condition movements of the fingers, thumb, and hand are strong and pain-less. In the latter stages of the condition weakness in the thumb may be noted, particularly on opposition. At no time are any of the movements of the thumb, wrist or hand painful (5, 10, 19, 24).

Palpation Occasionally tenderness may be elicited over the anterior aspect of the carpus of the hand, (Fig 3.11) particularly on deeper pressure. This may also produce onset of symptoms in the lateral 3 ½ fingers (5, 6, 17, 21, 23).

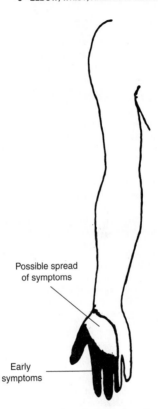

FIG. 3.17 Area of symptoms for carpal tunnel syndrome at the right wrist.

Specific Tests *Tinells Sign*: Repeated gentle tapping with the tip of a finger or a reflex hammer over the anterior carpus may reproduce the symptom of paraesthesia in the fingers (10, 12, 21, 22, 35).

Phalens Sign: If the wrists are held in flexion by pushing the backs of the hands together, and then held in this position for one minute, the patient's typical symptoms may be recreated in the fingers (10, 12, 21, 22, 35). Nerve conduction studies are often the most effective means of arriving at a definitive diagnosis of this condition.

Treatment Ideas (4, 5, 6, 8, 11, 15–19, 24, 36)

Complete rest for the wrist, with a splint to hold the wrist in a neutral position both during the day and at night, coupled with avoidance of any activities that produce symptoms, can be very effective in relieving the condition, particularly in the early stages. Initially the brace should be worn for 8 hours a day and 8 hours at night for 1 to 2 weeks, and then only at night for a further 3 to 4 weeks. Some patients also find benefit from repeated icing of the wrist, particularly if the condition is in its early stages.

Median nerve stretches (gliding) can be attempted by extending the elbow and wrist on the affected side with the arm abducted to 90 degrees and fully laterally rotated. The patient then side flexes the neck to the contralateral side. This should be done slowly and gently and stopped if any symptoms occur in the hand. Different types of glides can be attempted, either short oscillations or prolonged stretches over 15–30 seconds, with overpressure if no symptoms occur at the end of that time period. Claims are made for the effectiveness of both ultrasound and laser over the carpal tunnel. I have had some success using these modalities when combined with other treatment options, but I am unsure if they are truly effective in their own right.

If no progress is made with conservative means then surgery is indicated. However, if symptoms decrease with ice and stretching then strengthening of the muscles of the wrist, hand, and fingers can be attempted with regular rest breaks. The degree of activity is increased as the rest periods are decreased to steadily condition the patient back to their activities of daily living.

Restrictions   During initial treatment the patient should avoid any pain-producing activities. This usually has to be monitored closely by the patient, as the symptoms may often appear in the night following activities done during the day, so that identification of causative factors is often difficult. The patient should be instructed to stop all and any activities believed to produce symptoms and then reintroduce activities one by one and note any that do produce symptoms. These should then be excluded from the patient's daily routine until progress is made with treatment. All attempts to return to normal work, sports, or daily activities should only be attempted as those activities are simulated in the clinic and are shown to no longer produce symptoms.

Wrist Extensor Tendonitis

The extensor tendons of the wrists are prone to inflammatory reaction at or near their bony attachments. This is usually associated with trauma occurring when the wrist is extended and the hands in a fist, as in a fall onto the hand while holding a tennis racquet. Repetitive activity can produce similar symptoms when a strong full-hand grip is associated with repeated or sustained flexion of the wrist, as in gripping and carrying large paving slabs (11, 12).

Subjective Findings

Onset Onset is usually gradual following trauma or overuse and most commonly occurs in 20 to 50 year olds (11–13).

Duration The patient is normally seen some 3 to 4 weeks after onset, as initially the patient tends to either rest until the pain goes away or tries to "work it off." When either or both of these approaches fail, the patient then seek professional help.

Frequency This is usually the first time the patient will have experienced these symptoms (1, 3, 8).

Area of Symptoms The patient will normally indicate the area at the base of the hand posteriorly, just distal to the wrist joint (Fig. 3.18) (11, 13, 18, 23).

Type of Symptoms Pain is usually sharp on use of the hand with a persistent ache following activity.

Miscellaneous The patient will often complain of pain on gripping objects, particularly small-diameter objects. At times this condition can be found in association with lateral epicondylitis at the elbow in overuse syndromes (11, 12, 14).

Objective Findings

Observations There is usually nothing out of the ordinary to be observed in the forearm, wrist, or elbow.

Active Movements There is usually no restriction or discomfort on independent movements of the wrist or fingers. However, pain and restriction may be reported on active finger flexion when combined with wrist flexion. This will be particularly noticeable when gripping an object while flexing the wrist (11, 13, 18).

Passive Movements Ranges of motion will be the same as in active testing, although muscle guarding may be present at end range of movement of flexion of the wrist, flexion of the fingers, or both. Pain will also increase if ulnar or radial deviation is applied to a wrist and finger flexion stretch (11, 13, 18).

Resisted Movements Pain is often experienced on isometric wrist extension and is again worse if extension is combined with ulnar or radial deviation. Pain will be felt on either or both of the deviation movements depending upon the muscles affected (11–13).

Palpation Occasionally tenderness is elicited over the posterior carpus, particularly if the extensor tendons are palpated while on stretch (13, 18, 23).

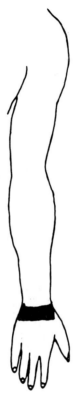

FIG. 3.18   Area of symptoms for extensor tendonitis of the right wrist (occurring just distal to the wrist joint line).

Special Tests   Resisted movements of extension with either radial or ulnar deviation will differentiate between lesions of the extensor carpi radialis longus or brevis and the extensor carpi ulnaris. The radial tendons are by far the more commonly affected (11, 18, 21).

Treatment Ideas (4, 11–14, 18)

The wrist is rested in extension in a splint and the patient is instructed to stop any pain-producing activities. Ice, pulsed ultrasound, interferential therapy, and transcutaneous electrical nerve stimulation can all help to ease discomfort. Active movements of the thumb, fingers, wrist, forearm, and elbow can all be continued within pain-free range to maintain flexibility of the soft tissues.

After a few days heat can be applied instead of ice, with thermal doses of ultrasound or the use of laser over the affected tendons. Active stretches into wrist flexion and finger flexion are started, with individual movements of the wrist or fingers initially, progressing to combined movements. If these stretches are tolerated, then light resisted wrist and hand exercises can be commenced, with rest and stretch breaks incorporated as required. Neuromuscular electrical stimulation of the extensor muscles with the patient holding the hand flat on a tabletop, against a gentle contraction of the muscle, will help to maintain mobility in the affected tissues.

Further progression is made by combining wrist and finger flexion stretches with ulnar and radial deviation of the wrist. Stretches are performed in two ways: relatively short stretches of 10 to 15 seconds repeated several times, and then longer stretches of 60 to 90 seconds with steadily increasing pressure applied either actively or passively. The use of neuromuscular electrical stimulation can be progressed by instructing the patient to actively flex his wrist against the extension contraction produced by the machine. This is, in turn, progressed by introducing ulnar or radial deviation in combination with the flexion movement. By this time the use of ice can be discontinued, but the continued use of thermal agents is often effective in aiding further stretch by both relaxing the patient and easing discomfort.

The patient should be progressed into a general upper-extremity workout and a hand and wrist exercise program using dead weights and resistance bands. Small hand equipment can be used for functional activities of gripping, lifting, pushing, and pulling, with rest and stretch breaks continued between each set of exercises. The amount of time that is allowed for rest is decreased slowly as the patient shows an ability to tolerate the exercise. The aim is to return the patient to repetitive and sustained exercises carried out over a significant time period that is relevant to their particular level of work, sports, or daily activities.

Restrictions Initial restriction is avoidance of all pain-producing activities. Most important precautions are in regards to strong gripping associated with movements of the wrist, particularly flexion with ulnar or radial deviation. Carrying weight in the hand is usually not as much of a problem as maneuvering weights, where torsion of the wrist and stress on the wrist through pushing and pulling activities can cause further symptoms to arise. Any sudden jerky movements applied to or by the hand should be avoided, as should rapid and repetitive finger movements such as keyboarding, particularly with the wrist flexed. Return to the use of tools or material handling should be done on a graduated basis and should lag behind similar activities simulated in the clinical setting.

Initially on attempting return to gripping activities the wrist must be maintained in a neutral or slightly extended position, so continued use of a wrist brace is normally required. Initial work should involve light weights and require minimal pressure to be applied through the wrist and hand. However, it should be noted that a prolonged static grip, even when applied lightly, is worse than active work of the wrist and hand when gripping is not required. The important factors for the patient (and his employer) to bear in mind are position, force, and repetition. Any task that combines awkward position of the hand with a strong force applied and a high rate of repetition will soon have the patient back in the clinic. It is essential to graduate each of these factors in an effective return to work program. Where this type of work is performed and cannot be modified then the patient must return to modified hours, only carrying out tasks for the time that he remains symptom free. Work time can be gradually increased as the patient shows no sign of exacerbation of symptoms.

de Quervains Tenosynovitis

The tendons of the abductor pollicis longus and extensor pollicis brevis muscles can become inflamed within the common sheath that they share at the lateral aspect of the wrist and thumb. This condition can be found under the various titles of de Quervains disease, de Quervains tenosynovitis, tendonitis, or stenosing tenovaginitis. Whatever the name, the pathology remains the same. It is associated with use of repetitive movements of the thumb, particularly a strong pinch grip, or with repetitive or sustained radial and ulnar deviation of the wrist. Friction of the tendons within the sheath while under pressure produce the inflammatory reaction, so the condition is almost always due to overuse. With the increased mechanization of tasks in light industry, which has removed the requirement to handle heavy weights, but has increased the repetition of activities to a marked degree, this condition is becoming more and more common (1, 2, 5, 9, 11, 14, 15, 18).

Subjective Findings

Onset Onset may be sudden or gradual and is due to overuse. Patients are usually 20 to 50 years of age (5, 11, 14, 17).

Duration The patient is most often seen quite early after onset of symptoms as the condition is often functionally very limiting. They therefore usually present within 1 to 2 weeks of onset and very seldom any longer than 6 weeks after onset.

Frequency Commonly this is the first time the patient will have experienced these symptoms, although recurrence of symptoms can occur as many as 1 to 2 years apart (4, 5, 9, 11).

Area of Symptoms The patient will be able to localize the symptoms to the lateral aspect of the wrist, particularly to the base of the thumb (Fig. 3.19). Usually the patient will run his finger over the lateral border of the anatomical snuff box when asked to show where the pain is felt (Fig. 3.10) (1, 15, 17, 23).

Type of Symptoms Pain is usually severe, sharp in nature, and occurs on movements of the wrist. There may also be complaints of a nagging ache present at rest (1, 4, 15, 17).

Miscellaneous The patient will report that a pinch grip is particularly painful. The history will also usually associate the symptoms with some form of repetitive activity of the hand, particularly involving unaccustomed use of the hand or thumb (11, 14, 15, 17).

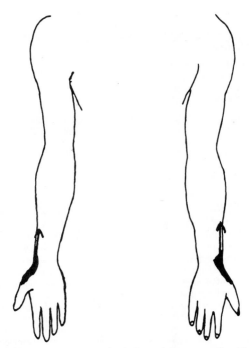

FIG. 3.19 Area of symptoms for de Quervains tenosynovitis at the tendons of the right thumb.

Objective Findings

Observation   In the majority of cases there will be a varying degree of swelling at the lateral aspect of the wrist over the offending tendon sheath (3, 7, 17).

Active Movements   There is usually no particular loss of range of motion either in the wrist or the thumb; however, there may be some decrease in range of motion of ulnar deviation of the wrist when it is combined with full flexion and adduction of the thumb. On the other hand this movement may be of completely full range, but it will almost invariably be painful (1, 2, 7, 10, 16, 22).

Passive Movements   As in active movements range should be within normal limits, however, passive ulnar deviation of the wrist with the thumb held inside the lightly clenched fist (i.e., adduction and flexion of the thumb) will reproduce the patient's typical symptoms (1, 2, 7, 16).

Resisted Movements   Pain is often experienced on resisted abduction or extension of the thumb, particularly when this is tested with the thumb in the adducted and flexed position. Strength of movements of the thumb and wrist will be within normal limits (1, 2, 16, 18, 19).

Palpation   Fine crepitation will often be felt on palpation of the tendon sheath at the lateral aspect of the wrist during either passive or active movements of the wrist (Fig. 3.9). Pain is also commonly produced on palpation of the tendon sheath (2, 5, 7, 21, 23).

Specific Tests   Production of typical symptoms with active or passive ulnar deviation of the wrist while the thumb is held inside a lightly clenched fist is known as Finklestein's test, and is diagnostic for this condition. However, it should always be compared with the unaffected hand, if there is one, as this movement does produce a degree of discomfort in the normal subject (10, 16, 18, 21, 22).

Treatment Suggestions (2–6, 9, 11, 13, 15, 16, 18, 19, 39)

The patient should be advised to rest the wrist and hand in a splint specifically designed for this type of condition, which includes support for the base of the thumb. In some cases, particularly where there is a marked degree of swelling present at the wrist, the patient may find that the pressure produced by the splint increases the symptoms. In these cases the use of a elasticized 2-inch bandage could be sufficient to protect the affected area. During this stage of treatment, ice, pulsed ultrasound, interferential therapy, and transcutaneous nerve stimulation help to decrease discomfort in the affected area. The patient must also be advised to stop all pain-producing activities at the first sign of symptoms. The patient must not attempt activities while using the brace simply because the brace makes the symptoms less apparent, as this will lead to increased irritation of the affected tendons and tendon sheaths, with subsequent increased chances of developing a chronic condition.

Once the patient starts to experience decreased symptoms, he can be progressed onto active exercises for the wrist, hand, and thumb within pain-free ranges and incorporating frequent rest breaks. The golden rule is that the patient should not exacerbate his symptoms, so he is instructed to rest from the exercise if any symptoms occur in the affected area until they are resolved, and before attempting further exercises. When active exercises are well tolerated, then stretching of the affected tendons can commence, initially using ulnar deviation of the wrist with the thumb in the neutral position. This is followed by active flexion and adduction of the thumb separately from the wrist movements, if both are well tolerated then the patient is progressed to a combined stretch of ulnar deviation of the wrist with flexion and adduction of the thumb.

Further progression can be made by the use of heat to the affected area followed by isometric resisted radial deviation of the wrist. This is best achieved by wrapping a piece of exercise band around the lateral aspect of the hand, excluding the thumb, and then flexing and extending the elbow joint with the hand held in the mid prone position (i.e., thumb upwards). When the patient is able to do this exercise with no problems, it is progressed by having the thumb inside the resistance band but resting on the index finger. Thermal doses of ultrasound or the use of laser along the affected tendon sheaths are indicated at this time. Ice is often still useful after exercise sessions and can help to prevent postexercise pain.

When the patient has achieved full pain-free adduction and flexion of the thumb, in combination with ulnar deviation of the wrist, then he should be progressed to graduated resisted gripping exercises for both whole-hand grip and pinch grip. Again, the use of rest and stretch breaks is important to prevent exacerbation of any underlying symptoms. Exercise can then be further progressed by decreasing the amount of rest, although it is often best to continue with stretching for as long as the exercise program is continued. At this time the use of modalities should stop and the patient is advised to control any sign of onset of symptoms by rest, and will have to do this while at work or in daily activities.

Exercises in the clinic should at this time be designed to mimic activities at home, at work, or in a recreational setting. The length of time for which the patient can continue with a specific hand and wrist exercise, particularly involving gripping, should be recorded and the length of time steadily extended to at least 20 to 30 minutes. The patient must learn to use rest periods as required to prevent onset of symptoms, rather than to rest the arm after symptoms occur. Once the patient has mastered this technique and is coping with up to 30 minutes of continuous exercise, he should be ready for most work, home, or leisure activities. Return to work or sports activities that specifically require forceful use of the thumb should be graduated and considered a continuation of the rehabilitation process.

Restrictions Initially all movements of the thumb should be restricted by the use of a brace or bandage. No gripping involving the thumb should be attempted in the early stages of treatment, particularly heavy lifting or carrying where the thumb is involved in the grip. The patient should also be rested from any activity that requires him to apply pressure with the end of the thumb.

As the condition improves the patient should be allowed to use grips in the mid range, that is, not holding small- or large-diameter objects. At this time a pinch grip should still be avoided. It is also important to avoid vibration while gripping, which can be done by wrapping the handles of vibrating tools in vibration-reducing material or by the use of gloves specifically made for this purpose. When the patient is able to cope with a reasonably strong grip in the semi-flexed position of the hand, he can progress to smaller and larger grips and can start to use the thumb in a pinch grip or to apply light pressure to objects. This progression of activity needs to be graduated carefully and the patient should be in a position that allows him to control the rate at which activities are carried out, so that he can rest as required to avoid exacerbation of symptoms.

Return to full use of the thumb for daily activities, whether at work, in sports, or at home, should only be attempted when the patient is coping with similar activities in the clinic without producing any symptoms. At this stage the patient should still be advised to rest at the first sign of exacerbation of symptoms, as this is the most effective form of prevention of recurrence of the condition.

Metacarpophalangeal Joint Injury of the Thumb (Ulnar Collateral Ligament Injury)

The ulnar collateral ligament of the thumb is easily injured by torsion or strain. In the days when every country estate had a game keeper, this used to be a repetitive injury for the game keeper, due to excessive pressure applied on the thumb when ringing the necks of fowl or other animals. In modern days the injury mainly occurs in sports, and is usually sudden and due to trauma.

The trauma is commonly produced by a fall while carrying something in the hand such as a ski pole or tennis racquet. If ligament instability is discovered on examination (which is shown by angulation of more than 15 degrees on passive testing as compared to the non-injured side), then referral to an orthopaedic surgeon is warranted, as this suggests a fullness thickness tear of the ligament. In cases of only partial disruption of the ligament it is reasonable to expect full recovery with conservative treatment. In the patient who is at risk from this type of injury, such as a regular sports participant, it is important to make sure that by the end of treatment the thumb is strong enough not only to take normal levels of strain, but also to withstand the sudden strain that a particular sport may cause (6, 7, 11, 16, 17, 37).

Subjective Findings

Onset Onset is sudden due to trauma or overuse and commonly occurs under the age of 40 (2, 7, 16).

Duration In acute cases, normally following trauma, the patient presents for treatment within 1 to 3 weeks of the injury. In more chronic cases, usually following overuse, the patient may not be seen for several months following original onset of symptoms.

Frequency This is almost always the first time the patient has experienced these particular symptoms as it often relates to a specific activity that the patient is then unable to continue because of their symptoms.

Area of Symptoms Initial symptoms are felt at the ulnar aspect of the thumb. In the later stages of the condition pain is felt around the metacarpophalangeal joint and radiates along the thumb (Fig. 3.20). The patient will often indicate the area at the apex of the anatomical snuff box as being the main source of symptoms (Fig. 3.9) (7, 11, 16, 17, 23).

Type of Symptoms Pain and swelling are found in the region of the base of the thumb in the early stages. Pain, weakness and instability of the joint may all appear in the later stages (6, 7, 16, 17, 37).

Objective Findings

Observation There may be swelling visible along the ulnar aspect of the thumb, particularly if the injury is due to trauma and if the patient is seen within one to two weeks of injury (2, 6, 7, 16).

Active Movements There is often no particular restriction of active movements of the thumb, fingers, or wrist; however, pain may be experienced on full extension and abduction of the thumb (stretching of the web between the thumb and index finger) (6, 7, 10, 16).

Passive Movements Pain will be produced by stretching the ulnar collateral ligament on both abduction of the thumb at the metacarpophalangeal joint and on rotation of the metacarpophalangeal joint (6, 7, 10, 16).

Resisted Movement Pain is usually reported on isometric adduction, particularly when tested at end range of abduction. Discomfort may also be present on flexion and opposition of the thumb if the movement is resisted strongly enough (6, 7, 16).

Palpation Tenderness will be elicited along the ulnar aspect of the metacarpophalangeal joint line of the thumb (2, 7, 10, 23).

Treatment Ideas (2, 6, 7, 11, 12, 16, 17, 24, 37, 38)

Ice and rest from activity should be instituted immediately following injury if possible and for the next 3 to 4 days. There are several varieties of

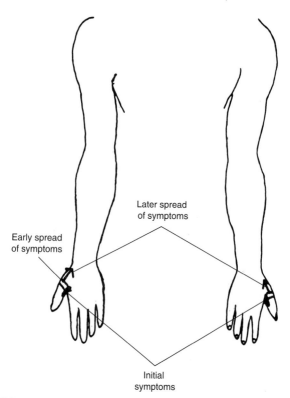

FIG. 3.20   Area of symptoms for injury of the MCP joint of the right thumb.

splints available for the thumb, and taping techniques are useful when done properly. Active movements of the thumb should be encouraged initially in individual ranges and then progressing to circumduction. In the athlete or heavy manual worker, strength of the wrist and fingers can be maintained with suitable resisted exercises without inclusion of the thumb.

At approximately 3 weeks following injury, passive stretching and gentle longitudinal distraction of the thumb can be employed to maintain range of motion in the soft tissues affected. At this time pain should be used as a guide by the therapist both listening to and watching the patient as the maneuvers are carried out. Progress is made to passive distraction of the thumb with valgus stretch applied to the metacarpophalangeal joint. This will start approximately 5 to 6 weeks postinjury. Light resisted exercises for the thumb, using a soft rubber ball for flexion and elastic bands for extension, can be started approximately 4 weeks after injury. The flexion activities are progressed to pinch grip, again using a ball or any other semisoft material. The exercises are progressed by increasing the density of the material used for exercising. Progression can also be made by the patient holding progressively larger and heavier cans in the hand while completing wrist exercises. A selection of different-sized cans containing sand or lead shot are useful pieces of hand-exercise equipment, which are both cheap and effective.

In the fourth or fifth week postinjury the patient can be progressed to upper extremity exercises in the gym using weights that can be handled without involving the thumb in gripping. By the sixth week the patient should be able to grip in a normal manner while dealing with weights suitable to their work, daily, or sports activities. In these later stages the patient should be tested for torsional forces on the thumb by the functional use of a screwdriver or hammer, or by using a twisting motion on the handle of resistance pulleys while working the shoulder and elbow.

Restrictions The patient should be advised against using a strong grip, particularly a pinch grip, for holding the shaft of any type of tool during the first 3 to 4 weeks postinjury. Once able to tolerate passive stretching of the thumb, it will be all right for the patient to handle tools and materials again, but torsional forces should be avoided until the sixth week. Return to repetitive or prolonged use of a pinch grip should be graduated, with suitable activities attempted in the clinic before they are attempted in work or leisure activities. A simple test of the patient's ability to handle torsional forces can be carried out by having the patient hold a light pole while the therapist tries to extract it from the hand by pushing, pulling, and twisting it. The degree of force involved is increased as the patient demonstrates the ability to tolerate the activity.

Osteoarthritis of the Carpometacarpal Joint of the Thumb

The carpometacarpal joint of the thumb possesses a high degree of freedom of movement and also sustains strong forces during a variety of gripping tasks. For these reasons osteoarthritis (OA) in this joint is quite a common occurrence, and will not necessarily be related to osteoarthritis anywhere else in the body. The pain that the patient experiences is produced by strain on tight periarticular soft tissues as the joint tends to sublux posteriorly or laterally. The aim of treatment is to gently stretch tight soft tissue while improving muscle condition to protect the joint (2, 5, 9).

Subjective Findings

Onset Onset is gradual with no specific cause. The patient is usually middle aged or older and it is more common in women than in men (2, 9, 13, 17).

Duration The patient will have been suffering symptoms for months or possibly years before seeking treatment, although some patients do present much earlier when there is a family history of arthritis, particularly if a close relative has rheumatoid arthritis, as the patient may be concerned that he is suffering from the same condition.

Frequency Patients usually report recurrent episodes of pain lasting for days or weeks, with each episode being separated from the others by weeks or even months. However, recurrence of symptoms will usually become more frequent and each episode more prolonged as the condition progresses (13, 17, 18).

Area of Symptoms The patient can usually localize their symptoms to the base of the thumb at the lateral aspect of the wrist (Fig. 3.21) (17–19, 23).

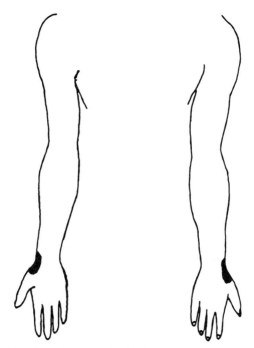

FIG. 3.21   Area of symptoms for OA of the CMC joint of the right thumb.

Type of Symptoms The patient complains of an aching pain that is worse with activities, particularly prolonged gripping, as in writing. The thumb may be stiff first thing in the morning or following rest after a period of activity (2, 9, 18).

Miscellaneous Applying pressure to the thumb when gripping, such as when opening the lid of jar, often produces the patient's typical discomfort.

Objective Findings

Observation There are commonly signs of soft-tissue thickening around the metacarpophalangeal joint of the thumb, which become more noticeable as the condition progresses (2, 5, 18).

Active Movements There is usually mild limitation of all movements of the thumb at the metacarpophalangeal joint, but particularly abduction and extension (2, 9, 13, 18).

Passive Movements Pain will be experienced at end range of motion of extension or abduction of the thumb at the carpometacarpal joint and on passive rotation of that joint. In some cases the pain will be noticeably increased when compression of the joint is combined with rotation (9, 13, 19).

Resisted Movements There may be mild weakness mainly due to pain and occurring particularly on extension and abduction of the thumb and on gripping either with a pinch grip or full-hand grip where the thumb encircles the object to be held. On testing of grip strength the radial side of the hand may be noticeably weaker than the ulnar side (9, 18, 19).

Palpation Soft-tissue thickening may be palpable around the carpo-metacarpal joint. There is often tenderness on palpation around the joint line (Fig. 3.9) (13, 17, 18, 23).

Specific Tests Pain on rotation of the thumb, particularly with compression of the joint, differentiates between this condition and de Quervain's tenosyovitis. X–rays can also help to confirm the diagnosis.

Treatment Ideas (2, 5, 9, 13, 17–19)

If the patient is suffering an episode of particular discomfort, rest is advisable, although the use of a splint may make the joints of the thumb stiff. The patient is therefore better advised to avoid using the hand, rather than to immobilize it. If it is thought that a thumb brace is not appropriate, then simple bandaging of the thumb and wrist using an elasticized bandage will often prevent the patient from using the hand while not particularly restricting motion. A warm hand bath with gentle unidirectional exercises for all movements of the thumb will help alleviate discomfort and maintain flexibility. Modalities such as ultrasound, laser, and transcutaneous electrical nerve stimulation help in some cases to alleviate discomfort, and ice can also be helpful postexercise.

As discomfort decreases in the affected joint hot packs can be applied and gentle passive distraction of the joint, with either small-amplitude repeated movements or gentle sustained traction, will help to maintain tissue length and reduce pain due to tight overstretched ligaments. Any modality that relieves the patient's discomfort should be continued and active exercises can be started using soft materials such as a foam ball to provide resistance. The patient should be advised to rest regularly and for relatively long periods between each set of exercises. Ice and transcutaneous electrical nerve stimulation combined at the end of treatment often help to reduce postexercise pain. The patient can be instructed to apply distraction to the joint while at home; again, this is usually more effective if attempted after the use of either a heating pad or a soak in hot water.

The patient will naturally pass through periods of remission, at these times strengthening exercises for the thumb and hand help to maintain correct muscle balance and hand function. The exercises should initially be attempted isometrically, then progressed to isotonic exercise as tolerated. Distraction of the joint can then be combined with rotations and abduction or adduction of the joint. Heat should still be continued both before and after exercise as required.

Restrictions   As stated earlier, to rest the affected joint the patient should be advised to avoid gripping activities involving use of the thumb for a period of 1 to 2 weeks, while using a brace or bandage if either is felt to be necessary. A gradual return to gripping movements should be made, with minimal force applied initially, using soft materials and low weights. Initially gripping should be attempted in the comfortable mid range position. Pressure on the thumb (such as in pushing on switches or buttons) must be avoided, and is an activity that the patient is unlikely to be able to tolerate at any time when suffering from this condition, so this restriction may become permanent. Gripping while rotational forces are applied to the hand produces strong torquing forces on the thumb, which the patient will be unable to tolerate on most occasions. The patient's ability to handle such forces can be tested by having him grip a pole or other similar object while the therapist twists it and the patient tries to hold it still. A particular problem will be experienced with machinery at work, such as air-driven torquing devices, that apply a strong twisting force to the hand and thumb. Again, strong consideration will have to be given to a patient permanently avoiding these types of activities when suffering from this condition.

Trigger Finger

Nodular thickening of the flexor tendons in the hand or fibrous thickening of the palmar tendon sheath can produce a stenosing tenosynovitis in the palm of the hand. This produces swelling and restricts movements of the flexor tendons in the hand. In the early stages of the condition physical therapy can be very helpful. In the later stages the patient is more likely to need injections or surgery, and may or may not require therapy after these procedures (5, 9, 14, 15, 17, 24).

Subjective Findings

Onset Onset is always gradual with no known cause. Patients are usually over 50 years of age (2, 9, 15, 17).

Duration The patient will have suffered from gradually increasing symptoms over a period of months or years (9, 15, 17).

Frequency The history the patient gives will be of one long ongoing episode, with symptoms worse on some days compared to others, but with no dramatic change in symptoms from day to day (6, 7, 15).

Area of Symptoms The problem is localized to the palmar aspect of the hand, usually over the area of the metacarpals most commonly affecting the third and fourth fingers (Fig. 3.22) (9, 15, 23).

Type of Symptoms The patient reports initially hearing a clicking in the area of the flexor tendons that progresses to difficulty in straightening the fingers from the flexed position. As the condition worsens the patient finds that he has to passively extend the finger after it has been flexed. This is often associated with a sharp click as the maneuver is carried out, hence the name of the condition. In extreme and chronic cases the patient cannot even flex the finger enough for it to become fixed (9, 10, 17, 19, 24).

Miscellaneous The patient may give a history of prolonged use of hand tools, but whether this is a direct contributing factor is debatable.

Objective Findings

Observation Thickening or puckering of the skin and subcutaneous tissues is usually observable over the affected tendons in the palm of the hand (5, 7, 15).

Active Movements Patients who are at a stage of the condition that is still amenable to therapy usually present with full active flexion and extension of the fingers, but with a jerk or click during the movement of extension from flexion. If the patient is already unable to extend the fingers fully, then the likelihood of physical therapy being effective is low. Sometimes active movements may be somewhat limited by pain if there is an underlying traumatic tenosynovitis associated with the condition, but in general restriction of motion is not associated with any particular discomfort (6, 7, 10, 19).

Passive Movements There is usually nil of note to be recorded on passive movements unless passive force is needed to straighten the flexed fingers.

Resisted Movements Muscle strength in the hand and fingers is usually within normal limits and there will be no discomfort felt on isometric testing of movements of the fingers and hand (7, 10, 19, 24).

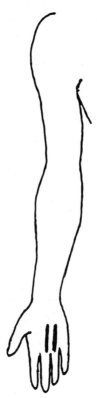

FIG. 3.22 Commonest distribution of symptoms for trigger finger in the right hand.

Palpation The therapist can usually feel a snap of the flexor tendons of the affected fingers when they are extended either actively or passively. This snapping will always be present on extension and may also be present on flexion. A thickened nodule or nodules may be palpable in the middle portion of the affected tendon (5, 17, 23, 24).

Treatment Ideas (1, 2, 5, 6, 7, 9, 13–15, 17, 19, 24)

In the early stages, particularly when clicking can be felt in the tendons during movement but the patient still has full active range of movement in the fingers, it is often beneficial to try a variety of modalities such as heat packs, laser, and ultrasound. These are followed by prolonged gentle stretches of the tendon, which may help to thin out the thickened part of the tendon and allow it easier access through the tendon sheath. The author has also found it beneficial in many cases to finish treatment with ice as the patient may experience some discomfort if the stretching is vigorous enough.

A further method of producing a good stretch of the flexor tendons is to apply muscle stimulation to the forearm flexor muscles. The patient then holds the fingers in full extension, either actively or passively, while the muscle stimulation contracts the affected muscles. Prolonged fascial-type stretches, where each stretch is held for 2 to 3 minutes or longer has occasionally proved useful in more severe or chronic cases. This protocol of heating and stretching of the affected tendons will normally produce results in six to eight sessions of treatment over a 2- to 3-week period. If definite results are not forthcoming in that time, then further treatment is unlikely to be effective. The patient seldom gains full recovery, but will plateau at a point where there is improved hand function and decreased restriction (or simply improved quality) of movement.

Restrictions   Patients suffering from this condition should be advised to avoid excessive use of a full-hand grip or repetitive movements of the fingers in order to reduce irritation of the tendon sheaths. Where a patient has to use a tool, that vibrates whether in a home or work activity, he should be advised to use vibration-absorbing material or gloves that are specifically manufactured to reduce the effects of vibration on the palm of the hand. Where extension of the fingers is particularly difficult then a custom-made splint can be supplied to maintain the fingers in the extended position. This can be worn for half the day, 1 hour on and 1 hour off, for 2 to 3 weeks while treatment is ongoing.

Wrist Flexor Tendonitis

Inflammation of the flexor tendons is less common than that of the extensor tendons, but is similar in nature in that it affects the tendons at or near their insertion into the bones of the wrist. It is commonly associated with a fall onto the anterior aspect of the hand while the fingers are held in a fist. It may also be associated with overuse, particularly where strong gripping combined with extension of the wrist is required, such as in the turning of a valve handle (11, 12, 14).

Subjective Findings

Onset   This is typically gradual after trauma or overuse and is usually found in patients 20 to 50 years of age (7, 12).

Duration The patient usually presents for treatment some 2 to 4 weeks following onset after either trying to rest following injury or attempting to work through the pain.

Frequency In virtually every case this will be the first time the patient has experienced these symptoms. On rare occasions it will present as recurrent episodes.

Area of Symptoms Symptoms are felt in the palmar aspect of the hand, just proximal to the wrist joint line (Fig. 3.23), either over the pisiform (Fig. 3.8) or at the base of the metacarpals (12, 14, 18, 23).

Type of Symptoms The patient usually reports suffering sharp pain on use of the hand with a persistent ache after activity. Patients will often complain of waking at night with the wrist aching (12, 14, 18).

Miscellaneous The patient may demonstrate or complain of particular pain on movement of the wrist from the position of radial deviation to the position of ulnar deviation while gripping an object, such as in hammering.

Objective Findings

Observation There is almost invariably nothing to be seen on examination of the affected area.

Active Movements Pain is reported on active extension of the wrist and is more intense if this movement is repeated with the hand held in a fist with the fingers fully flexed (7, 12, 14).

Passive Movements Pain may be reported at end range of wrist extension, but this is by no means present in all cases (14, 18).

Resisted Movements Pain is usually experienced on resisted flexion of the wrist. It will be worse if this movement is combined with either ulnar or radial deviation, depending on the specific muscle involved (7, 12, 18).

Palpation Occasionally tenderness is elicited over the distal insertion of the flexor carpi ulnaris into the pisiform or of the flexor carpi radialis into the base of the second metacarpal (Fig 3.10) (7, 12, 18, 23).

Specific Tests Pain experienced on resisted ulnar deviation from radial deviation tends to incriminate the flexor carpi ulnaris. Pain on resisted radial deviation from ulnar deviation suggests a problem with the flexor carpi radialis (7, 18, 21).

Treatment Ideas (1, 11, 12, 14, 18)

Initial treatment consists of rest from all pain-producing activities, with the wrist placed in a splint to hold it in a neutral position. In the first few days application of ice for 15 minutes every 2 hours can be helpful. After that time, pulsed ultrasound, and interferential and transcutaneous

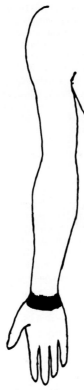

FIG. 3.23   Area of symptoms for flexor tendonitis of the right wrist (just distal to the wrist joint line).

nerve stimulation may all help to decrease discomfort. At that time active wrist and finger exercises should be started, but done separately and individually.

Patients are progressed onto the use of heat with active wrist stretches into the end range of extension. This is further progressed by introducing light resisted wrist and hand exercises. Neuromuscular stimulation may be applied to the flexor muscle of the wrist while the patient holds the hand statically against the contraction provided by the stimulator. As symptoms decrease and further stretching is attempted, then thermal doses of ultrasound or laser can be used. Laser appears to be particularly effective when areas of discomfort are easily palpable in the affected tendon. At this stage treatment sessions should still terminate with the use of ice.

Progression of treatment then involves stretches into wrist extension combined with hand grip. The objects held in the hand should be made steadily smaller in diameter. Muscle stimulation of the flexor muscles can now be combined with active extension of the wrist. Once an effective flexion contraction has been achieved with stimulation, it can also act as a test of the sensitivity of the tendons to stretch. At this time the use of ice can be discontinued.

The patient should finally be progressed onto a general workout for the wrist, hand, and upper extremities. The patient must be advised as regards the necessity of regular rest breaks and stretches, which should be long enough to prevent any increase in symptoms following exercise. As the patient demonstrates increased tolerance to exercise, the time allowed for rest and stretch breaks should be gradually decreased. Strengthening exercises should concentrate on hand grip and can be combined with wrist extension and deviation of the wrist to the side of the most affected muscle. The resisted exercise program should be related to the patient's particular work, sports, or leisure activities, particularly where these are incriminated in onset of the condition.

Restrictions   The patient should initially use the hand with the wrist kept in a neutral position and with no strong gripping or high rate of repetitions for any one movement. Carrying weight in the hand with the forearm supinated will be particularly problematic and should be avoided wherever possible. Progression of activities can be made with the patient dealing with heavier weights, but continuing to hold the wrist in a static neutral position, or by using light weights and increasing the amount of movement required at the wrist. The patient can return to activities requiring flexion and extension of the wrist before returning to activities that require ulnar or radial deviation. The patient can be weaned off the brace gradually by initially decreasing the time for which it is worn by 1 hour per day, then 2 hours, and so on as they find that they are able to cope with work or daily activities without exacerbation of symptoms.

Dupytren's Contracture

This is a fibrotic contracture of the palmar fascia with tissue thickening and adherence of underlying tissue to the skin of the palm of the hand. It appears to be an inherited condition, but is also associated with some disease states such as chronic alcoholism and epilepsy. Physical treatment only tends to retard progression of the condition and does not halt or reverse the disease process (4–7).

Subjective Findings

Onset Onset is gradual with no cause, and the disease is found in the 50 to 70-year-old age range. It is usually bilateral in nature with one hand often worse than the other (4, 7, 15).

Duration The patient will have been suffering from symptoms for many months or, more commonly, years before seeking or being referred to physical therapy.

Frequency This is a history of one long single episode.

Area of Symptoms Symptoms are localized to the palmar aspect of the hand commonly involving the fourth and fifth fingers and occasionally the third finger (Fig. 3.24) (2, 4, 14, 15).

Type of Symptoms The patient complains of contractures of the soft tissue with pain in the early stages of the condition followed by stiffness and then hand deformity (4, 14, 15, 18).

Miscellaneous In some cases this condition has been associated with recurrent and repetitive use of tools that require pressure on the palm of the hand, such as in the use of chisels when carving wood. However, the condition has been shown to be inherited by autosomal dominance (5, 6, 14, 18).

Objective Findings

Observation Thickened nodules may be observable in the palm of the hand in the early stages. This is followed by puckering of the skin and flexion contractures of the metacarpophalangeal and proximal interphalangeal joints of the affected fingers (5, 6, 9).

Active Movements Initially stiffness is encountered on extension of the fingers. In the later stages the patient will present with limitation of finger extension, which may be anywhere from a few degrees to 90% or more of the usual available range of motion (5, 7, 10, 17, 18).

Passive Movements Strong soft-tissue resistance is experienced at end range of available extension. It is possible to see increased puckering of the skin when end range of motion is achieved and sustained (5, 7, 17, 18).

Resisted Movements Strength is not affected until the later stages of the condition, and even then there is no major loss of muscle strength in the fingers or hand (7, 15, 18).

Palpation Thickened nodular tissue is palpable over the flexor tendons of the third, fourth, or fifth fingers in the palm of the hand. In the later stages of the condition it is possible to feel the thickened cords in the same area (4, 7, 23).

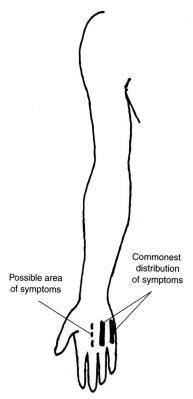

FIG. 3.24 Commonest distribution of symptoms for Dupytrens contracture in the right hand.

Treatment Ideas (1, 2, 4–7, 9, 15, 17, 18, 24)

In chronic cases where flexion contractures of the fingers exist the patient usually requires a surgical release. In the early stages of the condition or following surgery, the use of thermal modalities prior to passive stretching of the fingers into extension, combined with extension of the wrist, can be helpful in maintaining range of motion or reducing the speed at which contractures occur. Over the long term, gentle fascial type stretches prolonged over 2 to 5 minutes at a time may prove more useful than shorter-duration stronger stretches.

Muscle stimulation of the flexor muscles of the forearm while the patient holds the fingers extended as far as possible against the contraction applies effective stretch to the tendons in the palm of the hand. Massage of the skin with lanolin cream before stretches has been used to help soften the affected tissue. It is essential that the patient maintain a daily routine of stretching exercises for as many years as required to resist progression of the flexion contractures.

Restrictions The patient should be advised to avoid irritation of the palm of the hand, such as in the constant use of tools, and to this end the use of padded gloves or padded material on the handle of tools can be helpful. It is best if the patient also avoids any activity that requires the fingers to be flexed for extended periods of time. Whenever the fingers have been flexed for any period of time, the patient should be advised to passively extend them for an equal period of time whenever possible.

Wrist Sprain

This is a diagnosis that is made when all other causes of pain around the wrist, such as a fractured scaphoid, have already been ruled out by x ray. The findings therefore are of no bony injury, but the wrist remains sore and swollen. The likely pattern of pathophysiology is a tear or simply overstretching of fibers of the collateral ligaments or capsule of the wrist joint. Effective early treatment can prevent prolonged or recurrent symptoms, particularly in workers or athletes who are required to use their wrists strongly or continuously (3, 6, 9, 40).

Subjective Findings

Onset Onset is always sudden after trauma, usually following a fall onto the outstretched hand. The patient is usually under the age of 40 as after that age the patient is more likely to break a bone than injure soft tissue (6, 11, 12, 19).

Duration Patients are normally seen within a matter of days, but may present 2 to 3 weeks after onset.

Frequency Most commonly this only occurs once in any given patient, although on rare occasions it can be recurrent in nature, usually with a history of a previous wrist sprain that was untreated or poorly treated (3, 11–13).

Area of Symptoms Pain may be felt at the medial, lateral, or posterior wrist joint line, or in any combination of these areas (Fig. 3.25) (3, 9, 13, 16).

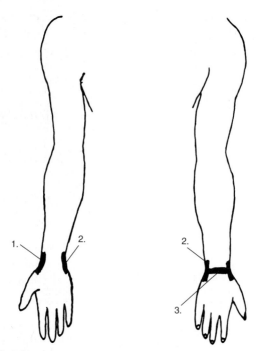

FIG. 3.25 Area of symptoms for sprain of right wrist at either:
1 - lateral aspect of wrist. 2 - medial aspect of wrist. 3 - posterior aspect
of wrist. Or symptoms can occur at two or three of these areas
simultaneously.

Type of Symptoms Sharp pain is usually produced on certain movements of the wrist or on putting pressure through the wrist, such as when
resting the hands flat on a tabletop (9, 13, 16).

Miscellaneous Recurrent wrist sprains are commonly associated with
arthritis of the wrist joint.

Objective Findings

Observation There may be a mild to moderate degree of swelling
around the wrist depending on how long after the injury the patient is first
seen (3, 9, 11).

Active Movement Movements of the wrist joint are normally near full range, although most movements will be stiff due to the presence of swelling. Pain will usually be produced on ulnar or radial deviation, or extension of the wrist, or any combination of these movements (9, 11, 12, 16).

Passive Movement Pain is most commonly experienced on extension of the wrist carried out passively and is felt at end range. In that case there is usually also pain on passive posterior/anterior glide of the forearm bones on the carpus. Pain may also be produced on either ulnar or radial deviation of the wrist (11, 12, 19).

Resisted Movement There will be no pain produced on lightly resisted isometric movements in any direction, but strong resistance will produce varying degrees of pain due to the tension applied to affected tissue, rather than due to any pathology of the muscles or tendons of the wrist (11, 12, 19).

Palpation Tenderness may be elicited over the proximal attachment of either the medial or lateral collateral ligaments of the wrist or over the posterior joint line (Fig. 3.7) (6, 12, 16, 23).

Specific Tests As noted, it is important that the possibility of bony injury has been ruled out through x-ray examination prior to making the assumption that the problem is purely soft tissue in nature.

Treatment Ideas (3, 6, 9, 11, 13, 16, 19, 40)

Initial treatment in the first 2 to 3 days following injury is rest in a splint or through the application of an ace bandage, with cessation of any pain-producing activities. Ice should be applied regularly five or six times per day during the first 2 to 3 days. If the patient is seen at a later date post injury, contrast bathing can be used, in which the patient uses ice-cold water in one basin and warm water in another, with the wrist immersed for 1 minute in the cold and 3 minutes in the hot, repeated three times. This may prove useful in reducing recalcitrant swelling around the joint, particularly if it is restricting movement. The patient should be instructed to maintain all active movements of the wrist, thumb, and fingers and of the inferior radial ulnar joint, pushing exercises to near the point of pain, but not into pain.

Progression is achieved by the application of thermal doses of ultrasound interferential and hot packs. Active wrist and hand exercises are supplemented by assisted exercises to make sure that full range of motion is gained as soon as possible. When active movements are near painless, resisted exercises can be started using small hand equipment for resistance of finger and thumb movements. Hand weights or an exercise band for isometric and then isotonic wrist movements can be used.

Winding a weighted rope around a pole using wrist and hand movements is a very effective way of both working and stressing the wrist joint. At this time the patient can also be instructed in passive distraction of the wrist joint to stretch the affected soft tissues and to help prevent the formation of adhesions and contractures.

The later stages of treatment consist of a work up into a generalized gym program for upper-extremity exercises, which should be designed to assimilate the patient's occupational, recreational, or sports activities. Weight work should be carried out with the patient's wrist in varying positions of flexion, extension, and ulnar or radial deviation.

Restrictions   In the initial stages following injury the patient should be advised to use a brace or bandage to protect the wrist, as well as to serve as a reminder of the problem, so that any activities that may unnecessarily exacerbate the symptoms will be avoided. Pushing, pulling, and carrying activities should be restricted to light weights (5–10 lb), depending on the build of the patient. Any twisting motions of the wrist and forearm, as in using a screw driver or torquing device, should be avoided.

Activities that produce heavy vibrations, such as using a jack hammer, will not be tolerated well in the first 1 to 2 weeks following injury. As the patient is able to cope with stronger resisted exercises in the clinic then similar activities at home or in the workplace can be attempted. Initially a wrist support should be worn while attempting these activities, but as the patient shows tolerance for the activity he should wean himself off the brace. The patient should only be released for normal activities after demonstrating that he is able to take his body weight on his hands when resting on a table and performing flexion, extension, ulnar deviation, and radial deviation movement while in that position. If the patient is able to tolerate this without any discomfort it is very unlikely that he will injure himself performing any other form of activity outside of the clinical setting.

REFERENCES

1. Salter R.B.: Textbook of Disorders and Injuries of the Muscular Skeletal System (3rd ed). Williams and Wilkins, Baltimore, Maryland, 1999
2. Braddom R.L. (ed): Physical Medicine and Rehabilitation. W.B. Saunders, Philadelphia, 1996
3. Payton O.D. (ed): Manual of Physical Therapy. Churchill Livingston, New York, 1989
4. Mercier, L.R.: Practical Orthopaedics (4th Ed). Mosby Yearbook, St Louis, 1991
5. Dandy D.J., Edwards D.J.: Essential Orthopaedics and Trauma (3rd ed). Churchill Livingston, New York, 1998
6. Crowther C.L.: Primary Orthopaedic Care. Mosby, St. Louis, 1999
7. Skinner H.B. (ed): Current Diagnosis and Treatment in Orthopaedics. Appleton and Lange, Norwalk, CT, 1995
8. Donatelli R.A., Wooden M.J. (eds): Orthopaedic Physical Therapy (2nd ed). Churchill Livingston, New York, 1994

9. Snider R.K. (ed): Essential of Musculoskeletal Care. American Academy of Orthopaedic Surgeons, Rosemont, IL, 1997

10. Goldie B.S.: Orthopaedic Diagnosis and Management: A Guide to the Care of Orthopaedic Patients (2nd ed). ISIS Medical Media, Oxford, U.K., 1998

11. Kasdan M.L. (ed): Occupational Hand and Upper Extremity Injuries and Disease (2nd ed). Hanley and Belfus, Philadelphia, 1998

12. Nicholas J.A., Hershman E.B.: Upper Extremity in Sports Medicine (2nd ed). Mosby, St. Louis, 1995

13. Kesson M, Atkins E.: Orthopaedic Medicine: A Practical Approach. Butterworth Heinemann, Oxford, U.K., 1998

14. Hadler N.M.: Occupational Musculoskeletal Disorders (2nd ed). Lippincott, Williams and Wilkins, Philadelphia, 1999

15. Apley A.G., Solomon L.: Apley's System of Orthopaedics and Fractures (6th ed). Butterworth, London, 1983

16. Prentice W.E.: Rehabilitation Techniques in Sports Medicine. WCB/McGraw Hill, New York, 1999

17. Anderson B.C.: Office Orthopaedics for Primary Care: Diagnosis and Treatment (2nd ed). W.B. Saunders, Philadelphia, 1999

18. Corrigan B., Maitland G.D.: Practical Orthopaedic Medicine. Butterworth London, 1983

19. Cyriax J.: Textbook of Orthopaedic Medicine: Vol.1, Diagnosis of Soft Tissue Lesions (8th ed). Bailliere Tindall Eastbourne, U.K., 1982

20. Gross J, Feeto J., Rosen E.: Musculoskeletal Examination. Blackwell Science, Cambridge, MA, 1996

21. Magee D.J.: Orthopaedic Physical Assessment (2nd ed). W.B. Saunders, Philadelphia, 1992

22. Konin J.G., Wilksten D.L., Isear J.A.: Special Tests for Orthopaedic Examination. New Jersey, Slack, 1997

23. Field D.: Anatomy: Palpation and Surface Markings (2nd ed). Butterworth Heinemann, Oxford, U.K., 1997

24. Malone T.R.., McPoil T.G., Nitz A.J. (eds): Orthopaedic and Sports Physical Therapy (3rd ed). St. Louis, 1997

25. Viikari-Juntura E.: Risk Factors for Upper Limb Disorders. Clin. Orthop., 351:39–43, 1998

26. Frostick S.P., Mohammad M., Richie D.A.: The Sports Injury of the Elbow. B. J. Sports Med. 33:301–311, 1999

27. Andrews J.R., et al.: Physical Examination of the Thrower's Elbow. J. Orthop. Sports Phys. Ther., 17 (6):279–288, 1993

28. Stroyan M., Wilk K.E.: The Functional Anatomy of the Elbow Complex. J. Orthop. Sports Phys. Ther., 17 (6):279–288, 1993

29. Wilk K.E., Arrigo C., Andrews J.R.: Rehabilitation of the Elbow in the Throwing Athlete. J. Orthop. Sports Phys. Ther., 17 (6):305–317, 1993

30. Galloway M., Demaio M., Mangine R.: Rehabilitative Techniques in the Treatment of Medial and Lateral Epicondylitis. Orthopaedics, 15:1089–1096 1992

31. Navak C.B., MacKinnon S.E.: Nerve Injuries in Repetitive Motion Disorders. Clin. Orthop., 351:10–20, 1998

32. Dellon A.L., Hammet W., Gittelshon A.: Non-Operative Management of Cubital Tunnel Syndrome: An 8-Year Prospective Study. Neurology 43:1673–1678, 1993

33. Boxenthka D.J.: Cubital Tunnel Syndrome Pathophysiology. Clin. Orthop. 351:90–94, 1998
34. Szabo R.M.: Carpal Tunnel Syndrome. Orthop. Clin. North AM., 23 (1):103, 1992
35. Kuhlman K.A., Hennessey W.J.: Sensitivity and Specificity of Carpal Tunnel Syndrome Signs. Phys. Med. Rehabil., 76 (6):451–457, 1997
36. Szabo R.M., Madison M.: Carpal Tunnel Syndrome. Orthop. Clin. North Am., 23 (1):103, 1992
37. Newland C.C.: Gamekeeper's Thumb. Orthop. Clin. North Am., 23:41–48, 1992
38. Wadsworth L.T.: How to Manage Skier's Thumb. Phys. Sports Med., 20: 69–78, 1992
39. Harvey F.J., Harvey P.M., Horsley M.W.: de Quervain's Disease: Surgical or Non-Surgical Treatment. J. Hand Surg., 15A:83–87, 1990
40. Mooney J.F., Siegel D.B., Koman C.A.: Ligamentous Injuries of the Wrist in Athletes. Clin. Sports Med., 11:129, 1992

The following tables contain test movements for examination of the cervical and thoracic spine. The starting positions and a description of each movement are given. These would be considered the optimal test positions in each case, which must be modified for individual patients who are unable to achieve or sustain a described position.

Active Movements of the Cervical Spine

Name of Movement	Starting Position	Movement
Flexion	Common position to test is in sitting, but the movement can be assessed in standing or half lying. The patient's head is in the neutral position (as in sitting and looking straight ahead).	The patient is instructed to take his chin to his chest, bending the head forwards. The patient should be able to touch their chin to chest. Average range of motion: 45°
Extension	Extension is usually tested in sitting, but can be tested in standing or side lying. The patient's head is in the neutral position.	The patient is instructed to take his head back so as to look at the ceiling, approximating the back of the skull to the upper back. Average range of motion: 40–45°
Side Flexion	This movement can be tested in sitting or standing, starting with the head in the neutral position.	The patient is instructed to take the right ear to his right shoulder. Correct any tendency the patient may have to either flex or rotate the cervical spine during this motion. The patient may also try to bring the shoulder to the ear, therefore the shoulder girdle may need to be stabilized. Average range of motion: 45°
Rotation	Rotation can be tested in sitting, standing, or supine lying, starting with the head in the neutral position.	The patient is instructed to look over one shoulder, looking behind himself as far as possible. The patient should not turn his shoulders (i.e., thoracic rotation), correct

(continued)

Active Movements of the Cervical Spine (*continued*)

Name of Movement	Starting Position	Movement
		any tendency towards side flexion or forward flexion during testing of this movement. Average range of motion: 50–60° (chin coming into line with the shoulder)
Protrusion	The movement is tested in sitting or standing starting with the head in the neutral position	The patient is instructed to push his face forwards in order to stick his neck out. No flexion or extension of the cervical spine should be allowed to occur (i.e., the plane of the face should remain in the same vertical alignment).
Retraction	The movement can be tested in sitting, standing, or if necessary in half lying, starting with the head in the neutral position.	The patient is instructed to draw the head backwards while tucking the chin in (so as to give himself a double chin). No flexion or extension of the cervical spine should be allowed to occur. Some patient's find it helpful to place the index finger on the chin to help guide it backwards.

Passive Movements of the Cervical Spine

Name of Movement	Starting Position	Movement
Flexion	The movement is tested in supine lying with the patient's head clear of the end of the treatment table. Support the patient's occiput with one hand and place the other hand on the anterior upper chest wall to stabilize the shoulder girdle.	The head is raised using the hand supporting the occiput to bring the patient's chin towards his chest.
Extension	The movement is tested in supine lying with the head clear of the end of the treatment table. Support the patient's occiput with one hand and grasp the patient's chin with the other hand.	Lower the head towards the floor while supporting the head with the hand at the occiput. Pressure is applied through the hand on the chin.
Side Flexion	The movement is tested in supine lying with the patient's head clear of the end of the treatment table. Support the occiput with both hands.	Carry the patient's head sideways to approximate the ear to the shoulder. Repeat on the other side.
Rotations	The movement is tested in supine lying with the patient's head clear of the end of the treatment table. Support the patient's occiput with one hand with the other hand grasping the patient's chin.	The head is turned to one side to bring the chin into alignment with the shoulder using combined pressure at occiput and chin. The movement is repeated to the other side.
Retraction	The patient is placed in supine lying with his head clear of the end of the treatment table. Support the patient's occiput with one hand, place the other hand over the anterior of the patient's chin.	Pressure is applied with the hand on the patient's chin to push the head backwards. The hand holding the occiput controls the movement to prevent any flexion or extension of the cervical spine.

Resisted Movement of The Cervical Spine

Name of Movement	Starting Position	Movement
Flexion	The movement is tested in sitting with the patient's head unsupported and in the neutral position Place one hand on the patient's forehead.	Apply pressure to the forehead so as to push the patient's occiput backwards and downwards. The patient resists the movement, maintaining the neutral position.
Extension	The movement is tested with the patient sitting with their head unsupported and in the neutral position Place one hand on the patient's occiput.	Apply pressure to the occiput, pushing the head forwards and downwards, while the patient resists the movement maintaining the neutral position.
Side Flexion	The movement is tested in sitting with the patient's head unsupported and in the neutral position. Place one hand above one of the patient's ears.	Apply pressure to the side of the head pushing the opposite ear towards the shoulder. The patient resists the movement maintaining the neutral position. The movement is repeated on the opposite side.
Rotation	The movement is tested in sitting with the patient's head unsupported and in the neutral position. For testing right rotation place your right hand on the right side of the patient's chin and the left hand on the left side of the occiput. Hand positions are reversed for left rotation	For right rotation apply pressure to the right side of the face and the left side of the occiput, attempting to turn the patient's head around to the left. The patient resists the movement maintaining the neutral position. Hand pressures are reversed to test left rotation.

Active Movements of the Shoulder Girdle

Name of Movement	Starting Position	Movement
Elevation	The movement is tested in sitting, but can be tested in standing, supine lying, or half lying. The patient's arms should be resting at his side.	The patient is instructed to shrug his shoulders in order to bring them up towards the ears.
Depression	The movement is tested in sitting, but can be tested in standing, supine lying, or half lying. The patient's arms should be resting at his side.	The patient is instructed to push his hands and arm down away from his shoulders as if attempting to make the arms longer, bringing the shoulders away from the ears.
Retraction	The movement can be tested in sitting or standing. The patient's arms should be resting at his side.	The patient is instructed to draw the shoulders backwards as if trying to bring the shoulder blades together.
Protraction	The movement can be tested in sitting or standing. The patient's arms should be resting at his side.	The patient is instructed to round the shoulders as if trying to make the points of the shoulders meet in front of the chest.

Active Movements of The Thoracic Spine

Name of Movement	Starting Position	Movement
Flexion	The movement is tested in sitting or standing. The patient sits upright with his back un-supported and his arms resting at his sides.	The patient is instructed to slump forwards, rounding the back as if trying to place his chest on his thighs. The cervical spine should remain as near as possible in the neutral position, although some forward flexion is inevitable.
Extension	The movement is tested in sitting or standing. The patient sits upright with his back unsupported and his arms resting at his sides.	The patient is instructed to arch his back, being careful to avoid extension of the cervical spine or retraction of the shoulder girdle.
Rotation	The movement is testing is sitting or half lying. The patient sits upright with his arms folded across their chest.	The patient is instructed to turn his upper body around to one side, making sure that his head turns with his body so as to avoid rotation in the cervical spine. The movement is repeated to the other side.
Side Flexion	The movement is tested in sitting or standing. The patient sits upright with his arms resting by his sides.	The patient is instructed to take one hand down towards the floor so that he tilts his body sideways. If tested in sitting both buttocks must remain in contact with the seat. The movement is then repeated to the other side.

	Onset			
Sudden Due to Trauma	Sudden Due to Overuse	Sudden Due to No Cause	Gradual Due to Overuse	Gradual Due to No Cause
Upper Trapezius Muscle Strain Latisimus Dorsi Muscle Strain Whiplash	Cervical Disc—No Radiculopathy Thoracic Facet Joint Locking	Cervical Disc—No Radiculopathy Cervical Disc—with Radiculopathy Cervical Facet Joint Irritation—with Radiculopathy Cervical Facet Joint Locking Thoracic Facet Joint Locking	Cervical Postural Strain	Cervical Facet Joint Irritation—No Radiculopathy Cervical Postural Strain Thoracic Outlet Syndrome Cervical Spondylosis

Typical Age Range					
20–50 Years	25–45 Years	35–55 Years	40–60 Years	50 + Years	All Ages
Cervical Facet Joint Locking	Upper Trapezius Muscle Strain Latisimus Dorsi Muscle Strain Thoracic Facet Joint Locking	Cervical Disc—No Radiculopathy Cervical Disc—with Radiculopathy Cervical Facet Joint Irritation—with or without Radiculopathy (Work—Related) Thoracic Outlet Syndrome	Cervical Spondylosis	Cervical Facet Joint Irritation—with or without Radiculopathy	Cervical Postural Strain Whiplash

(continued)

Examination Findings Related To Specific Conditions (continued)

Duration

1–7 Days	3 Days–3 Weeks	1 Week–3 Weeks	2 Weeks–4 Weeks	6 Weeks–3 Months	3 Months–6 Months+
Cervical Facet Joint Irritation	Cervical Facet Joint Irritation—with Radiculopathy	Upper Trapezius Muscle Strain	Cervical Disc—No Radiculopathy	Cervical Facet Joint Irritation—No Radiculopathy	Thoracic Outlet Syndrome
Thoracic Facet Joint Locking			Latisimus Dorsi Muscle Strain	Cervical Postural Strain	Whiplash
			Whiplash	Thoracic Outlet Syndrome	Cervical Spondylosis

Frequency

First Time with These Symptoms	Recurrent and Increasing Symptom for 1–2 Years	Previous Similar Problems but Never This Severe	Previous Symptoms in One Area Now Spread to Another Area	One Long Continuous Episode
Upper Trapezius Muscle Strain	Cervical Disc—with No Radiculopathy	Cervical Disc—with Radiculopathy	Cervical Disc—with Radiculopathy	Thoracic Outlet Syndrome
Latisimus Dorsi Muscle Strain	Cervical Facet Joint Irritation—with No Radiculopathy	Cervical Facet Joint Irritation—with Radiculopathy	Cervical Facet Joint Irritation—with Radiculopathy	
Cervical Facet Joint Locking	Cervical Spondylosis	Cervical Postural Strain	Cervical Postural Strain	
Thoracic Facet Joint Locking				
Whiplash				

Area of Symptoms

In Sides of Cervical Spine and Upper/Middle Shoulder Girdle	In Neck but Worse on One Side	Central Cervical Pain	One Side of Neck and Ipsilateral Shoulder Girdle	Pain Spreading from Shoulder Girdle into the Back	Mid to Low Back Pain on One Side	Mid Back Pain More Towards One Side	Neck and Radiating into Arm	In One or Both Arms Only
Cervical Disc—No Radiculopathy Cervical Facet Joint Irritation—No Radiculopathy Cervical Postural Strain Whiplash	Cervical Disc—No Radiculopathy Cervical Disc—with Radiculopathy	Facet Joint Irritation—with or without Radiculopathy Cervical Spondylosis	Upper Trapezius Muscle Strain Cervical Disc—No Radiculopathy	Cervical Postural Strain Whiplash Cervical Spondylosis	Latisimus Dorsi Muscle Strain	Thoracic Facet Joint Locking	Cervical Disc Radiculopathy Facet Joint—with Radiculopathy Whiplash	Thoracic Outlet Syndrome

(continued)

Examination Findings Related To Specific Conditions (*continued*)

Type of Symptoms

Stiff Aching Neck	Sharp Pain in Neck	Sharp Pain on Neck Movements	Ache in Neck and Shoulder Girdle At Rest	Sharp Pain in Mid Back	Ache in Mid Back At Rest
Cervical Disc—No Radiculopathy Whiplash	Cervical Disc—with or without Radiculopathy Whiplash	Facet Joint Irritation Trapezius Muscle Strain Whiplash	Upper Trapezius Muscle Strain Cervical Postural Strain	Thoracic Facet Joint Locking	Latisimus Dorsi Muscle Strain

Sharp Pain on Movements of Thoracic Spine	Tight Burning Sensation in the Upper Back and Shoulder Girdle	Pain In Arm	Tingling and Numbness In Arm and Hand	Painless Loss of Strength In Upper Extremity	Headache
Latisimus Dorsi Muscle Tear Thoracic Facet Joint Locking	Cervical Disc—No Radiculopathy Cervical Facet Joint Irritation Cervical Postural Strain Whiplash	Cervical Disc—with Radiculopathy Facet Joint Irritation—with Radiculopathy Thoracic Outlet Syndrome	Cervical Disc—with Radiculopathy Thoracic Outlet Syndrome Whiplash	Cervical Disc With Radiculopathy Thoracic Outlet Syndrome	Cervical Spondylosis Whiplash Cervical Postural Strain

Observation

Obvious Stiff Neck	Deviation of Neck to One Side	Neck and Head Held Slightly Flexed and Protruded	Spasm in Cervical Paravertebral Muscles	Spasm in Paravertebral Muscles and Upper/Middle Trapezius
Cervical Disc—with or without Radiculopathy Facet Joint Irritation—with Radiculopathy Upper Trapezius Muscle Strain Cervical Facet Joint Locking Whiplash	Cervical Disc—with Radiculopathy Cervical Facet Joint Irritation—with Radiculopathy	Facet Joint Irritation—with No Radiculopathy	Cervical Disc—with or without Radiculopathy	Cervical Disc—with or without Radiculopathy Cervical Facet Joint Locking—with or without Radiculopathy Whiplash

Spasm in Thoracic Paravertebral Muscles	Rounding of the Shoulders with a Forward Head Posture	Pronounced Soft Tissue Thickening at the Cervical Thoracic Junction	Nothing to be Observed
Thoracic Facet Joint Locking	Common in Most Patients but Specifically Found Related to: Thoracic Outlet Syndrome Cervical Spondylosis Cervical Postural Strain	Cervical Postural Strain Cervical Spondylosis	Latisimus Dorsi Muscle Tear

(continued)

Examination Findings Related To Specific Conditions (continued)

	Active Movements						
Cervical Flexion Most Limited and Painful Movement	Side Flexion of Cervical Spine Limited	Retraction of the Cervical Spine Stiff and Limited	Cervical Side Flexion to One Side Increases Symptoms	Cervical Flexion and Extension Both Limited—Flexion Produces More Symptoms	Cervical Extension Most Limited and Produces Symptoms	Side Flexion and Rotation to Same Side Limited and Increases Symptoms	Cervical Flexion Tight But Does Not Hurt
Cervical Disc—with or without Radiculopathy	Cervical Disc—with or without Radiculopathy Whiplash	Cervical Disc—with or without Radiculopathy Facet Joint Irritation—with or without Radiculopathy Whiplash	Cervical Disc—with or without Radiculopathy	Cervical Disc—with Radiculopathy	Facet Joint Irritation—with or without Radiculopathy	Facet Joint Irritation—with or without Radiculopathy Facet Joint Locking	Facet Joint Irritation

Pain on Side Flexion to One Side and Rotation to Opposite Side	Pain in Arm Decreases on Elevation of Arm	Movements of Neck Stiff Rather Than Painful	Pain in Back on Combined Arm and Back Movements	Rotation of Thoracic Spine Painful and Limited	No Pain on Testing Active Movements	Marked Limitation of all Movements	Mild Limitation of All Movements
Cervical Postural Strain Upper Trapezius Muscle Strain	Cervical Disc—with Radiculopathy	Cervical Postural Strain Cervical Spondylosis	Latisimus Dorsi Muscle Strain	Thoracic Facet Joint Locking	Thoracic Outlet Syndrome Cervical Postural Strain	Whiplash	Cervical Spondylosis

(continued)

Examination Findings Related To Specific Conditions (continued)

Passive Movements

Muscle Resistance on Overpressure Into Flexion and Rotation of Cervical Spine	Neck Pain on Overpressure into Retraction	Springy Block at End Range Cervical Flexion and Rotation	Solid Block to One Side Flexion	Muscle Resistance to Overpressure into Extension	Pain on Overpressure into Extension
Cervical Disc—with Radiculopathy	Cervical Disc—No Radiculopathy Whiplash Cervical Facet Joint—with and without Radiculopathy	Cervical Disc—with Radiculopathy	Cervical Disc—No Radiculopathy	Cervical Facet Joint—with or without Radiculopathy	Cervical Facet Joint Irritation—with Radiculopathy Cervical Facet Joint Locking

Pain In Neck and Arm on Overpressure into Flexion	Pain on One Side Flexion and Opposite Rotation of Cervical Spine	Pain in Back on Arm Abduction with Contralateral Trunk Side Flexion	Pain on Side Flexion and Rotation of Cervical Spine to Same Side	Pain at End Range of All Movements	Stiffness at End Range of All Movements
Cervical Disc—with Radiculopathy Cervical Facet Joint Irritation—with Radiculopathy	Upper Trapezius Muscle Strain Cervical Spondylosis	Latisimus Dorsi Muscle Strain	Cervical Facet Joint Locking Cervical Facet Joint Irritation—with and without Radiculopathy Cervical Spondylosis	Whiplash	Cervical Spondylosis.

Resisted Movements

No Pain and Good Strength	Discomfort on Cervical Flexion	Pain on Side Flexion	Painful Weakness on Shoulder Abduction	Pain in Back on Adduction and Medial Rotation Shoulder	Weakness of Hands and Fingers	Pain on All Movements
Cervical Disc—with or without Radiculopathy	Cervical Disc—with or without Radiculopathy	Upper Trapezius Muscle Strain	Upper Trapezius Muscle Strain	Latisimus Dorsi Muscle Strain	Thoracic Outlet Syndrome (Late Stage)	Whiplash
Cervical Facet Joint Irritation—with or without Radiculopathy	Whiplash	Whiplash				
Cervical Facet Joint Locking						
Thoracic Facet Joint Locking						
Thoracic Outlet Syndrome						
Cervical Spondylosis						

(continued)

Examination Findings Related To Specific Conditions (continued)

Palpation				
Tenderness at Both Sides of the Cervical Spine	Tenderness Cervical Paravertebral Muscles	Tenderness on One Side of Cervical Spine	Tenderness One Side of Shoulder Girdle	Tenderness over Upper and Middle Trapezius
Cervical Facet Joint Irritation—with or without Radiculopathy Whiplash Cervical Spondylosis	Cervical Disc—with or without Radiculopathy Cervical Facet Joint Irritation—with or without Radiculopathy Cervical Postural Strain	Upper Trapezius Muscle Strain Cervical Facet Joint Locking	Upper Trapezius Muscle Strain Cervical Facet Joint Locking	Cervical Disc—with or without Radiculopathy Cervical Postural Strain Whiplash Cervical Spondylosis

Tenderness at Medial Border of Scapula	Tenderness in Thoracic Spine	Soft Tissue Thickening at Cervical/Thoracic Junction	Loss of Skin Sensation in Arm	Pulsating Lump behind Clavicle
Cervical Disc—with or without Radiculopathy Cervical Postural Strain Whiplash	Thoracic Facet Joint Locking Cervical Postural Strain	Cervical Postural Strain Cervical Spondylosis	Cervical Disc—with or without Radiculopathy Thoracic Outlet Syndrome	Thoracic Outlet Syndrome (Not Common)

PALPATION OF THE THORACIC AND CERVICAL SPINE

In this section a description is given of the method of palpation each structure referred to in relation to the following conditions:

- Cervical Disc Signs
- Cervical Disc with Radiculopathy
- Cervical Facet Joint Irritation (with No Radiculopathy)
- Cervical Facet Joint Irritation (with Radiculopathy)
- Cervical Postural Strain
- Upper Trapezius Muscle Strain
- Latisimus Dorsi Muscle Strain
- Cervical Facet Joint Locking
- Thoracic Facet Joint Locking
- Thoracic Outlet Syndrome
- Cervical Spondylosis
- Whiplash

The structures described in the following sections must be identified:

Upper Fibers of Trapezius (Fig. 4.1): The hands are placed on each side of the neck, resting on the patient's upper shoulder girdle between the neck

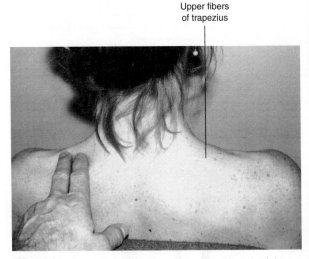

Upper fibers
of trapezius

FIG. 4.1 The bulk of the upper fibers of the trapezius at the right shoulder. The examiner's fingers are resting on the upper trapezius at the left shoulder.

and the point of the shoulder. If the patient shrugs his shoulders the upper trapezius will be felt to contract, making it possible to palpate the attachment of the muscle into the medial third of the nuchal line, the external occipital protruberance, and along the cervical spine laterally. The muscle belly needs to be initially palpated gently to elicit any tenderness, and then more deeply in order to identify the presence or absence of fibrous bands or nodules.

External Occipital Protruberance: With a finger placed on the cervical spine centrally move up towards the skull and the finger will enter a dip. Just above this point is a bony eminence, the external occipital protruberance (Fig. 4.2).

Nuchal Line: The nuchal line can be felt to spread out laterally from the occipital protruberance as a bony ridge. Following the nuchal line around the occiput, the finger will come to a rounded eminence lying behind the ear, which is the mastoid process (Fig. 4.3).

Spinous Processes: With the patient in supine lying and positioned so that the forehead is resting on the hands, palpate the cervical spine centrally starting at the occipital protruberance and working down. The first bony point that can be felt is the spinous process of C2. Each separate spinous processes is then quite easily identified down to the seventh cervical level (Fig. 4.4). The seventh cervical or first thoracic vertebrae will be the most prominent at the base of the neck. As a simple means of identifying a specific vertebrae at the base of the cervical spine it is worth remembering that the C6 spinous processes moves when the neck is flexed and extended, whereas the C7 spinous process does not.

Paravertebral Muscles: A ridge of muscle can be palpated immediately to each side of the cervical spine (Fig. 4.5). This is the mass of the paravertebral muscles and should be palpated for the presence of either tenderness or muscle spasm, either of which may well produce the other.

Facet Joints: The facet joints lie approximately one to two thumbs breadth (3/4–1 inch) lateral to the spinous processes. These should be palpated in order, starting at C2 and working downwards (Fig. 4.6).

Middle Fibers of the Trapezius (Fig. 4.7)*:* If the fingers are taken backwards from the lateral end of the clavicle over the shoulder they will encounter a bony ridge, the spine of the scapula, lying between the posterior lip of the acromion and the medial border of the scapula. Medial to the end of the spine of the scapula, lying between the scapula and the thoracic vertebrae, are the middle fibers of the trapezius.

Medial Border of the Scapula: This can be palpated approximately 2 inches lateral to the second to eighth thoracic spinous processes (Fig. 4.7).

Thoracic Spinous Processes: These are best palpated with the patient placed in the slumped sitting position. C7 and T1 are prominent at the base of the neck and it is possible to count down through the thoracic vertebrae from that point. As a rough guide T3 is approximately level with

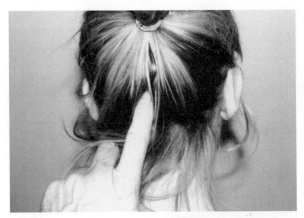

FIG. 4.2   The tip of the examiner's index finger is placed on the external occipital protruberance.

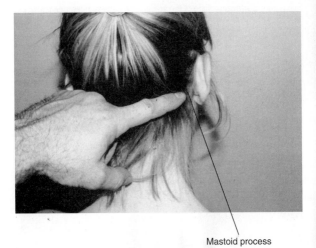

Mastoid process

FIG. 4.3   The examiner's finger is lying along the right nucal line and is pointing towards the right mastoid process.

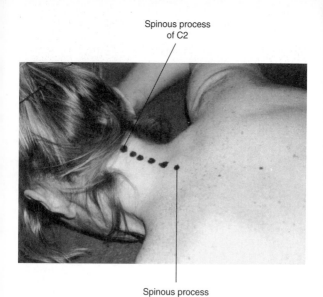

Spinous process
of C2

Spinous process
of C7

FIG. 4.4   Surface marking of the spinous processes in the cervical spine.

Cervical paravertebral
muscles

FIG. 4.5   The cervical paravertebral muscles shown on isometric
extension of the cervical spine.

Spinous process
of C3

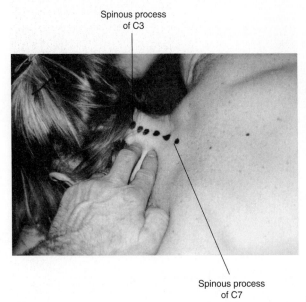

Spinous process
of C7

FIG. 4.6   The examiner has his finger tips on the area of palpation for the cervical facet joints.

the medial end of the spine of the scapula. T7 is level with the inferior angle of the scapula (Fig. 4.8).

Latisimus Dorsi Muscle: With the fifth finger resting on the iliac crest and the hand cupping the patient's side at the lumbar level, the patient is instructed to cough, making it possible to feel the latisimus dorsi muscle contract (Fig. 4.9). Once identified in this manner the muscle can then be palpated at leisure.

Iliac Crest: To identify the iliac crests the hands are placed on the patient's waist from behind and then drawn downwards, bringing them into contact with the bony ridges that are the iliac crests (Fig. 4.10). These can be difficult to find in the well-padded patient.

Lateral Processes: The levels of the cervical spine laterally are often hard to palpate because of the overlying tissues, but careful palpation in this area can provide useful information during the examination process. First, trace the jawline to the angle of the jaw and place another finger on the mastoid process—the transverse process of C1 lies half way between these two points (Fig. 4.11). Each transverse process can then be

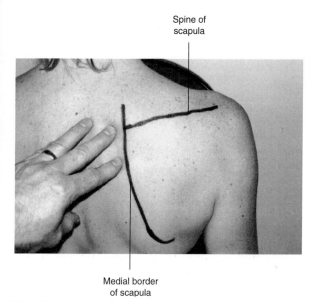

FIG. 4.7 Surface marking of the spine and medial border of the right scapula. The examiner's index and middle finger are placed on the middle fibers of the trapezius.

palpated in turn, working downwards and steadily more posteriorly (Fig. 4.12). These structures are often tender in the asymptomatic patient and it is important to compare the patient's reaction to palpation when compared to palpation of the other side, in order to confirm any difference in levels of discomfort experienced before any definitive conclusions are made.

Paravertebral muscles in the thoracic spine can usually be observed, and are easily palpated ridges, lying immediately lateral to the spine (Fig. 4.13).

Clavicles: Starting with the fingers placed on the patient's throat, take them downwards until they reach the notch in the superior part of the sternum (sternal notch). Lateral to the sternal notch is a bony protruberance that is the medial end of the clavicle. The curves of the clavicle can then be followed. These are initially convex medially and then concave laterally (Fig. 4.14).

Spinous process
of C7

Spinous process
of T1

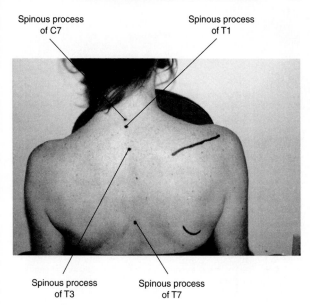

Spinous process
of T3

Spinous process
of T7

FIG. 4.8 The thoracic spinous processes and their relation to the spine and inferior angle of the scapula.

SPECIFIC TESTS OF THE CERVICAL AND THORACIC REGION (4, 7, 11, 15, 21, 25)

Reflexes

Biceps (C5-6)

With the patient in the sitting position, the elbow is supported in the examiner's hand with the forearm supported by the examiner's forearm. Identify the biceps tendon at the anterior aspect of the elbow in the cubital fossa and observe the biceps muscle bellies while striking the tendon with the reflex hammer.

Triceps (C7-8)

The patient sits with his arm by his side. One hand grips the patient's forearm and bends the elbow slightly. The triceps tendon lies proximal to the olecranon and the muscle bellies of the triceps can be observed in the upper arm posteriorly for signs of a twitch as the tendon is struck with the reflex hammer.

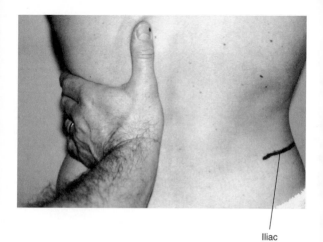

Iliac
crest

FIG. 4.9 The line marks the right iliac crest. The examiner's hand is placed over the patient's left latisimus dorsi to palpate it while the patient coughs.

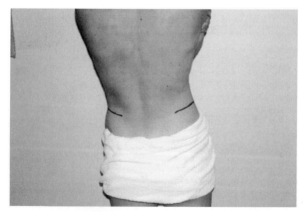

FIG. 4.10 Surface marking of the iliac crests.

Mastoid process

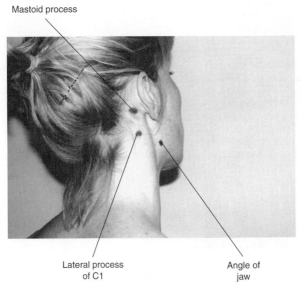

Lateral process
of C1

Angle of
jaw

FIG. 4.11 The relationship of the mastoid process and angle of the jaw to the lateral process of C1.

Vertebral Artery Test

Positive signs of vertebral artery problems are dizziness, lightheadedness, or visual disturbances on holding any of the following positions for a period of 30 seconds:

Full rotation of the head and neck to each side
Full extension of the head, neck and back
Combined rotation and extension of the cervical spine

Brachial Plexus Tension Test

With the patient in supine lying, the arm is passively abducted and slightly extended at the shoulder joint and then laterally rotated, the forearm is then supinated and the elbow extended. If symptoms are produced in the hand and arm (paraesthesia) then conformation of radial plexus tension is provided by side flexion of the cervical spine away from the test side,

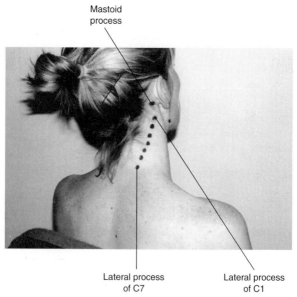

FIG. 4.12   Surface marking of the lateral processes of the cervical spine.

which will increase symptoms, whereas side flexion towards the test side will decrease symptoms in the hand and arm.

Dural Signs

1. The patient in supine lying is asked to actively flex his neck. If this produces the typical discomfort then a straight-leg–raise test is carried out, and the pain the patient is experiencing on neck flexion will increase sharply. Pain that only increases slightly or pain produced in an area other than that found on neck flexion are not conclusive dural signs.
2. The patient is placed in a slumped sitting position at the edge of the examination table. They are then asked to flex their neck followed by extension of one knee and then dorsiflexion of the ankle of the same leg. If these movements produce, and progressively increase, their typical symptoms then the findings are positive for dural impingement.

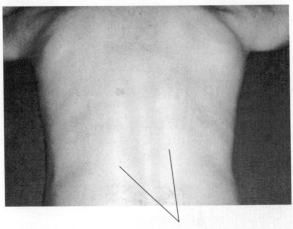

Thoracic paravertebral
muscles

FIG. 4.13 The thoracic paravertebral muscles on extension of the thoraco-lumbar spine.

Myotomes

Painless weakness on testing of the following muscles may suggest compression of the indicated nerve root. It is important to note the overlap between nerve roots supplying the same muscle groups.

C5: Muscles tested: deltoid and biceps, through shoulder abduction and elbow flexion with the forearm supinated.

C6: Muscles tested: biceps, brachialis, brachioradialis, and extensor carpi radialis longus, through flexion of the elbow in respectively supination, pronation, and the mid position, and wrist extension with radial deviation.

C7: Muscles tested: triceps, flexor carpi radialis, flexor digitorum radialis, and the wrist extensors, through the movements of extension of the elbow and flexion of the wrist.

C8: Muscles tested: abductors, pollicis longus and brevis, extensor pollicis longus and brevis, flexor carpi ulnaris, and the finger flexors, through extension and abduction of the thumb, flexion of the fingers, flexion and ulnar deviation of the wrist.

T1: Muscles tested: intrinsics of the hand, through attempting to grip the examiner's fingers between individual fingers of the hand (a scissorlike action).

Sternal notch

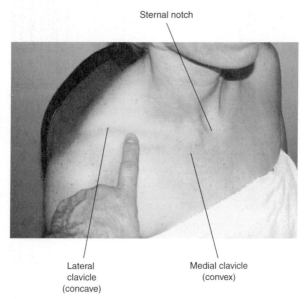

Lateral
clavicle
(concave)

Medial clavicle
(convex)

FIG. 4.14   The curves of the right clavicle and the sternal notch. The examiner's fingers is resting on the junction of the medial ⅔ of the upper clavicle with the lateral ⅓.

CERVICAL AND THORACIC CONDITIONS

Cervical Disc Signs (with No Radiculopathy)

It is often difficult to give a definitive diagnosis by attributing particular signs and symptoms to specific anatomical structure in the spine. Various texts often disagree on the relevance of individual findings, and we are hampered by a lack of clearcut evidence, as few of these conditions require the patient to undergo surgery or, for that matter, to be reviewed at autopsy. In the long run patients with spinal problems are often treated according to their presenting symptoms and how those symptoms change with treatment. However, it is still important to attempt to attribute symptoms to a particular structure, as it then becomes easier to investigate the correlation between symptoms, treatment, and the progression or regression of a condition. In this way we may eventually discover the specific causes of the many and varied symptoms arising in and from the structures of the spine. In this particular condition the signs and symptoms that

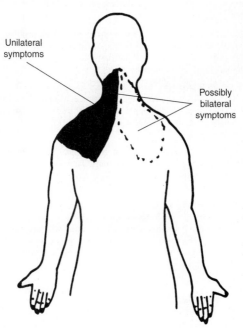

Unilateral symptoms

Possibly bilateral symptoms

FIG. 4.15 Area of symptoms for cervical disc problem (no radiculopathy).

arise could theoretically be expected to appear if the wall of an intervertebral disc were to bulge irregularly at an area of weakness, producing some degree of soft tissue damage and irritation in the spine itself, but with no direct pressure being placed on neural structures (3, 4, 11, 14, 18).

Subjective Findings

Onset The patient is most commonly between 35–55 years of age. Onset is sudden and usually due to no cause, although in some cases the patient may complain of an overuse type of syndrome such as working at a computer for a long period of time or sitting in a car for a long trip. Less commonly onset may be gradual with no cause (4, 6, 11).

Duration Patients may go weeks before seeking treatment, but most patients usually present within 2 to 4 weeks of onset, as initially they believe that they have a stiff or injured muscle, but then over time they begin to realize that this is not what they have and that it is showing no signs of going away.

Frequency   A common history is of recurrent neck problems of increasing severity and duration over many months or even 1 to 2 years. Patients will often complain that they have had similar symptoms before but that they have never been as bad as they are now (4, 5, 18, 24).

Area of Symptoms   These are poorly localized to the sides of the cervical spine, often more pronounced on one side compared to the other, with pain radiating into the upper and medial trapezius bilaterally, but again usually more severe on one side as compared to the other (Fig. 4.15) (1, 6, 11, 20).

Type of Symptoms   The patient normally describes a stiff and aching neck with sharp pain on some movements. They may also complain of a tight, burning sensation in the shoulder girdle and upper back either unilaterally or bilaterally (1, 5, 20, 24).

Miscellaneous   Headaches are quite commonly associated with this condition, usually starting in the occipital region and then spreading over the top of the head and into the eyes. The patient will also complain of having difficulty with any activity that requires him to have his neck flexed for any period of time, such as when reading a book or working at a bench (4, 5, 11).

Objective Findings

Observation   The patient's neck may be obviously stiff so that he first turns his shoulders instead of his head to look to the sides or the back. Muscle spasm may be observed in the cervical paravertebral muscles or in the upper shoulder girdle (6, 18, 24).

Active Movements   Flexion of the cervical spine is the most limited and most painful movement. Rotation to either side is stiff and usually produces pain, but will not be too limited in range. Side flexions will be stiff and limited bilaterally, but more so to the affected side, and they will not necessarily produce pain. Extension of the cervical spine may be stiff or painful, but will be less uncomfortable than flexion. Protraction of the cervical spine is usually of full range and pain free. Retraction produces discomfort centrally in the cervical spine and is stiff, but again not particularly painful (2, 3, 11, 13, 20).

Passive Movements   Muscle resistance is usually encountered towards the end range of flexion and on both rotations. There is a stiff end feel to extension and on side flexions, and retraction is usually stiff and produces neck pain on overpressure. Protraction will produce no symptoms, even on overpressure (1, 11, 17, 25).

Resisted Movements   No pain is experienced on light isometric resistance of any movement and good strength is normally encountered in the neck, shoulder girdle, and upper extremities. Any movement in the cervical spine that is strongly resisted may produce typical discomfort due to stress on inflamed tissue, rather than because of a specific muscular pathology (7, 24).

Palpation Tenderness is usually elicited over the upper trapezius bilaterally and over the mid trapezius or the medial border of the scapula on the affected side (Fig. 4.7). Marked muscle tension or possibly muscle spasm will be encountered in the cervical paravertebral muscles and the muscles of the shoulder girdle in most cases (Fig. 4.5) (22, 24, 25).

Specific Tests Reflexes in the upper extremity will be normal, and there will be no dural signs or vertebral artery signs (20, 21, 25).

Treatment Ideas

The patient usually gains comfort from the use of hot packs or heating pads applied to the neck and shoulder girdle. A cervical roll should be prescribed for use inside a pillow for sleeping, and the patient can be advised to use this during the night if pain either wakens him or keeps him awake. The most important treatment in the clinic in the initial stages is to find a position of the head and neck that alleviates the patient's symptoms, as this will indicate decreased pressure on the weakened area of the disc. Once this position has been found, and the initial assessment will have pinpointed the movements that are least uncomfortable, then active exercises can be instituted for the shoulder girdle, upper extremities, and lower extremities to promote and maintain muscle condition.

The application of laser to tender spots in the trapezius muscle can help alleviate tension in that area, thus decreasing the patient's overall level of discomfort. Transcutaneous electrical nerve stimulation or interferential are effective means of promoting muscle relaxation, particularly if the patient is positioned in a way that relieves the symptoms while these modalities are being applied. Postural re-education for the head, neck, and shoulder girdle should begin immediately, with exercises initially in supine lying, with the head and neck in a comfortable and well-supported position.

When the patient is able to control the symptoms by positioning of the head and neck, then active neck retraction and early-range extension, with the neck supported by a towel roll, can be started. Shoulder and shoulder girdle exercises can be progressed to the sitting position and the active neck exercises can be carried out in sitting with the use of a towel held around the neck for support while the exercises are being completed. The patient will find that this limits movement and affords a sense of comfort, as the patient is often unwilling to attempt full-range motions for fear of further injury.

Active exercises should be progressed to include retraction, extension, side flexions, and rotations, in lying initially and then in sitting. Resisted shoulder retraction using an exercise band to resist horizontal abduction is an effective way of promoting better posture, particularly when associated with retraction of the cervical spine. This particular exercise can be enhanced by the use of neuromuscular electrical stimulation for the middle and upper trapezius, as this will help to draw the patient's shoulders back into the preferred position.

Passive neck movements can also be started moving into pain-free ranges with light overpressure. Again, this is first attempted in lying and then progressed to sitting. Gentle manual traction can be attempted, and if successful in relieving symptoms, then mechanical traction using weights in the 10 to 20 pound range, depending on the build of the patient, is often more effective in the long term for relieving symptoms. Passive stretching of the shoulder girdle into depression and protraction is an effective means of stretching muscles that can become tight and painful as the patient endeavors to maintain a better head, neck, and shoulder girdle posture. Stretching of these muscles by the use of "bad movements" (flexion of the neck and protraction of the shoulders) is often forgotten. The patient may therefore begin to complain of increasing discomfort in the upper back associated with their exercise regime. It is important to maintain a balance between all movements in the area, while continuing to emphasize the movements of retraction and elevation of the shoulder girdle and retraction of the cervical spine.

The patient should be progressed onto a program of general resisted exercises for the trunk and upper extremities, again with an emphasis on postural muscle control. These exercises are often easily integrated into a home program using an exercise band or dead weights, and the patient needs to be instructed to continue these on a regular basis in order to prevent further recurrence of their neck problem. Active treatment must be backed up by a structured program of neck care education throughout the course of treatment.

Restrictions In the initial stages the patient should not work for any period of time with the head or neck flexed, such as when working with a computer or at a workbench. Repetitive flexion and rotation of the neck, which can occur when working with a computer while using a document that is lying on the desk, must also be avoided. The patient must be instructed not to maintain any one head and neck position for more than a few minutes at one time. The patient must be guided by his symptoms, and any increase in discomfort should immediately signal the necessity for a change in position. Patients will often find difficulty working with their arms at or above shoulder height, particularly when any degree of weight is involved, and again this activity should be restricted to an amount that does not produce or increase symptoms. As stated earlier, the patient should be instructed to use a rolled towel or a cervical roll in his pillow to support the neck while sleeping.

Driving should be done in short bursts wherever possible, if the patient is required to drive for any extended period of time then a soft collar is a consideration. The use of soft collars in general is a subject that can provoke quite a good deal of debate. Personally I tell patients that they must never wear the collar for more than 1 hour at a time and not more than 4 hours in a day, and that they should assume that they will no longer require the collar in 2 to 3 weeks. Anyone who has worn a cervical collar for any period of time will be able to tell you that it is very comforting, and that it makes the neck feel very vulnerable and weak when it is removed, particularly after it has been worn for an extended period of time. I forbid patients to come into the clinic wearing the collar, as that is often a sure sign that it is being worn virtually all the time at home. If the patient has been wearing a soft collar for an extended period of time before he is seen for assessment, the hardest job the therapist faces is to wean him from that support so that further active treatment can be instigated. This devise must be looked upon as a mixed blessing and used in a judicious manner.

Lifting, carrying, and handling weights with any degree of arm stretch will usually provoke symptoms in this type of patient. A weight restriction should be imposed, and must be one that the patient can cope with without producing any increase in symptoms. It should be remembered that even light weights can produce quite an intolerable degree of strain on the neck and shoulder girdle when the arms are extended, due to the leverage provided by the length of the arms. Pushing and pulling activities are not usually a problem, although if these need to be performed over any prolonged period of time the patient's head position will become a critical factor. Once more the therapist and patient must be guided by the patient's symptoms, and work or daily activities modified as required to prevent onset of discomfort. As symptoms subside the patient will be able to progress both the amount of time and the degree of weight or amount of resistance that is involved in any given activity.

Cervical Disc (with Radiculopathy)

Overview

In a case such as this, the symptoms suggest a definite protrusion of nuclear material from the disc, which is affecting a cervical nerve root or roots. The patient's symptoms are usually more severe in the arm than in the neck, although pain may be equally divided between both areas; in very rare cases the neck may be more painful than the arm. The patient's symptoms are often quite severe and muscle spasm may spread discomfort throughout a large area of the upper back, a factor that can often be misleading during assessment (4, 7, 14, 20).

Subjective Findings

Onset The patient is usually between 35 and 55 years of age. Onset is most often sudden with no known cause. In many cases the patient will state that he woke with the pain in the morning or that it started very soon after rising (9, 18, 20).

Duration The severity of the symptoms and the fact that they are functionally very limiting often means that the patient is seen within a matter of days following onset of the condition.

Frequency It is common for a patient to have a history of previous neck problems, often with no arm symptoms or with only minor symptoms compared to the present episode. In all likelihood this is the first time the patient will have experienced these particular symptoms (3, 6, 17, 24).

Area of Symptoms Symptoms are felt throughout the cervical region, but will be far worse on one side. Symptoms in the arm will be unilateral in distribution and can be felt anywhere from the shoulder to the fingers. Symptoms are also often felt around and over the scapula on the affected side. The distribution of the arm symptoms will often be specific to the area supplied by the affected nerve root and can then in themselves be diagnostic (Fig. 4.16) (3, 4, 21, 24, 25).

Type of Symptoms Sharp pain is usually felt in the neck and arm, and the neck and shoulder girdle will often be stiff, most particularly on

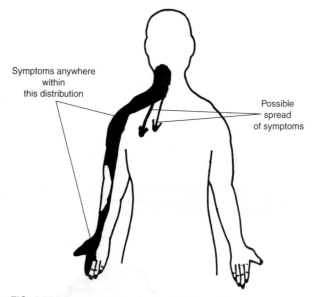

Symptoms anywhere within this distribution

Possible spread of symptoms

FIG. 4.16 Area of symptoms for cervical disc problem (with radiculopathy in the C6 distribution).

the affected side. An array of symptoms may be felt in the arm, with paraesthesia and numbness being the most common. Arm symptoms will often be localized to a specific dermatome, in severe cases loss of muscle strength may be found in specific muscles (myotomes) (2, 5, 6, 11, 20).

Miscellaneous   The patient may in some cases be found sitting in the waiting room with his forearm resting on his head, having found that this relieves the arm symptoms when they are due to pressure on a nerve root (usually C 5–6).

Objective Findings

Observation   The patient often presents with the neck held in either a degree of flexion or side flexion away from the affected side or a combination of the two. A lateral shift of the spine away from the affected side may be observed when viewing the patient from the rear (6, 7, 11).

Active Movements   In this condition there is usually one movement that is not only pain free, but that also tends to relieve either the arm symptoms, the neck symptoms, or both. Most commonly this is side flexion away from the affected side, and less commonly it can be rotation away from the affected side. Side flexion to the affected side is usually limited and produces immediate increase in both neck and arm symptoms. Flexion and extension will both be limited, with either one or both of these movements producing neck and arm symptoms. Rotation to the affected side may also exacerbate neck and arm symptoms, but is usually less of a problem than the other movements described (9, 11, 13, 17).

Passive Movements   The same pattern of restriction will be found on passive testing as found on active movements. A springy block may be noted at the end range of either flexion or rotation to the affected side. A solid block or muscle spasm may be elicited on side flexion to the affected side (2, 4, 11).

Resisted Movements   Isometric testing of the cervical spine and shoulder girdle does not usually produce any noticeable symptoms, although resisted flexion of the cervical spine may produce discomfort in the neck, particularly when resistance is strongly applied (5, 6, 24).

Palpation   There are often various tender points to be found in the sides of the cervical spine bilaterally and in the upper trapezius and around the medial border of the scapula on the affected side. Loss of sensation may be found in the arm, usually over the site of a specific dermatome (22, 24, 25).

Specific Tests   The patient may have decreased or absent reflexes at the elbow or wrist. Brachial plexus tension tests may be positive and dural signs may also be present (11, 21, 25, 26, 28).

Treatment Ideas
(2, 5, 6, 7, 9, 10, 14, 20, 29, 32–34)

The most important initial thrust of treatment is to find a position that the patient can assume that will alleviate his arm symptoms in particular, and both the arm and neck symptoms if you are lucky. This position is often given away by the patient's posture observed during assessment. If the patient is holding his head in right-side flexion, it is probable that if put in the supine lying position with his head and neck well supported, and the cervical spine side flexed to the right, then symptoms in the left arm will steadily resolve.

The patient should be encouraged to maintain this rest position at regular intervals throughout the day. No excuse regarding requirements of daily activities of work, sports, or leisure can be allowed to interfere with these regular rest periods—this cannot be stressed strongly enough to the patient. The patient will need to keep his head and neck well supported on a medium-sized pillow, with a cervical roll or a rolled-up towel placed in the cervical region and adjusted by the patient to the position of maximum comfort. It is equally important to instruct the patient not to remain in any position, even a position that relieves the symptoms, for too long a period, as this will eventually become painful and relief of symptoms will then become more difficult. This will also stop the patient's natural inclination to tighten up completely due to pain, stiffness, and muscle spasm.

The purpose of finding a relatively pain-free position is so that the patient can carry out exercises with the unaffected arm initially, then with the shoulder girdle, and finally with the affected arm, without producing symptoms brought on by the movements. Heat pads and ice packs are extremely useful ways of relieving the discomfort produced by muscle spasm, often enabling the patient to relax more effectively, particularly if in a comfortable position to begin with. The scenario of pain producing muscle spasm, producing stiffness, producing more pain, producing more muscle spasm, and so on, is one that familiar to any practitioner and is something that can be avoided by good patient education. This will be easier to achieve when you can prove to the patient that you can find a position or movement that alleviates the symptoms. A soft collar can be helpful in affording some comfort to the patient, but must be worn only sporadically, with a 1 hour maximum at any one time and a 4 hour maximum in a day, otherwise the patient comes to depend on the support and comfort provided, and loses range of motion and muscle strength as a result.

From the position of comfort, active movements of the cervical spine should be practiced, initially taking movements such as rotation and side flexion away from the affected side and back to the neutral position. Exercises can be continued with the arm and shoulder girdle, and a start should be made on postural correction. However, it is not uncommon to find that retraction of the cervical spine in sitting is uncomfortable for the patient and may provoke symptoms in the neck or arm. Again, the patient's rest position should be employed throughout treatment sessions to alleviate symptoms and to prevent provoking obstinate muscle spasm. Once the symptoms in the arm begin to decrease, gentle manual cervical traction can be attempted, but should be halted if any arm or neck symptoms are produced.

Active exercises that were initially carried out in lying can be progressed to sitting. The author has found that mechanical traction in sitting with the patient's head and neck in their most comfortable pain-free position is a simple and effective means of reducing symptoms. The position of the neck in this case is often one of a mild degree of flexion combined with protrusion. Traction that relieves symptoms should be followed immediately by postural correction, which in turn should be interspersed with gentle stretching of the muscles of the neck and shoulder girdle whenever possible. If the patient finds traction in the clinic an effective means of reducing symptoms, then a home traction unit should be prescribed, as short bursts of traction for 10 to 15 minutes at a time two to three times per day are usually more effective, and less likely to produce reaction, than one long dose of traction every other day.

Progression of exercises must always wait on symptom reduction, particularly in the arm. The temptation is to attempt all movements of the neck or arm simply because the patient is showing improvement. This all too often leads to an increase in symptoms lasting hours or even days, and the patient may start to show a lack of faith in the therapist. The patient must be advised to maintain a program of regular rest periods for relief of symptoms, accompanied by active exercise into the pain-free ranges of movement. Further progression of exercise can be made by carrying out resisted movements into pain-free ranges for the arm and shoulder girdle; this can be done even before all active movements are of full range.

Once the patient is able to complete all the active movements of the cervical spine and arm through full range, then he can progress into a gym exercise program for general trunk and extremity strengthening. Emphasis is on postural correction and maintenance of the correct posture throughout an exercise session. Education of the patient regarding the common causes of the condition and how to prevent reoccurrence is an important part of the treatment plan, and should be a ongoing component of any treatment program. Patients are usually more amenable to education when the symptoms are starting to improve, rather than in the early stages when progress may be slower.

Restrictions Activities that may exacerbate symptoms usually involve sustained positioning of the neck, most commonly either flexion, side flexion to the affected side, rotation to the affected side, or any repetitive motions into these ranges. The patient must avoid these types of activities in the early stages of treatment, otherwise progress will become painfully slow. Driving should be carried out for the minimal amount of time possible; while driving the patient may benefit from the use of a soft collar, as the vibration inherent in any vehicle can quickly exacerbate symptoms. The patient's work and leisure activities need to be reviewed, with particular attention to sustained positions and repetitive movements of the head and neck. Computer or assembly work are two areas where symptoms are often exacerbated by poor ergonomic design. Work site or home visits are often impractical, so the patient must be shown relevant educational material to enable him to effectively assess the situation himself. All daily activities must be paced so that rest positions and stretches can be employed *before* symptoms are aggravated.

Cervical Facet Joint Irritation (No Radiculopathy)

Overview

Again, this is a condition that is possibly more described than real, as there is no way of actually proving that the facet joints are irritated. However, the history and objective examination tend to show that the patient's symptoms increase with movements or activities that put pressure on the facet joints. When this occurs in combination with the absence of other soft tissue signs, it seems reasonable to assume that these small but important joints are the probable cause of the patient's symptoms. Similarly treatment aims to relieve pressure on these joints (3, 4, 36).

Subjective Findings

Onset   Onset is gradual, with no known cause or occasionally due to overuse, such as working with the arms above the head while having to look up for a period of time. The patient is usually over 50, but may be younger if the work that he does involves prolonged periods of neck extension (e.g., welders and electricians) (3, 11, 17).

Duration   The patient often suffers symptoms for a prolonged period of time before seeking therapy. A period of several weeks to several months is common.

Frequency   There is usually a history of recurrent neck problems over a 1- to 2 year period, with steadily increasing intensity and duration of symptoms with each subsequent episode (4, 13).

Area of Symptoms   Symptoms are felt centrally in the cervical spine and to one or both sides. If both sides are affected one side will usually be more painful than the other. Pain may also radiate into the area of the upper trapezius or over the scapula, unilaterally or bilaterally (Fig. 4.17) (1, 11, 17).

Type of Symptoms   Pain is sharp on movements and felt in the cervical spine. A general ache, stiffness, and occasionally a burning sensation may be felt in the upper and middle shoulder girdle to one or both sides (1, 11).

Miscellaneous   Male patients will often complain of difficulty shaving, as they experience discomfort when they look up into the mirror to shave under their chin. Women may have a similar problem while trying to apply eye makeup. Patients may also complain of cracking or grating in the neck on movements of the cervical spine, particularly rotation. These may sound very loud to them, but are more felt than heard on examination.

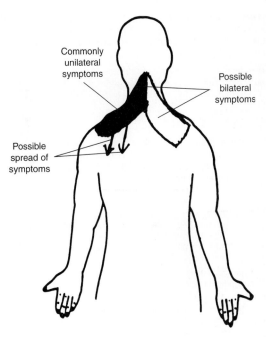

FIG. 4.17 Area of symptoms for facet joint irritation (no radiculopathy).

Objective Finding

Observation In either very acute cases or where an episode has lasted for a prolonged period of time patients tend to hold their neck slightly flexed and noticeably protracted (forward head posture) (3, 4, 8).

Active Movements There is marked restriction of extension and the movement will produce the patient's typical symptoms. Flexion is usually mildly limited, with stiffness and a pulling sensation felt in the sides of the cervical spine. Both side flexions are usually limited, with sharp pain felt in the neck on the side of the affected joint on flexion to that side and a pulling sensation felt on the side of the affected joint with flexion away from the affected side. Active rotation of the cervical spine is usually stiff, but not particularly limited or painful (4, 11, 12, 17).

Passive Movements Muscle resistance is usually encountered on overpressure into extension, with a stiff soft tissue end feel to all other movements.

Resisted Movements   There is no pain on isometric testing of any movements in the cervical spine or shoulder girdle. Strength in the muscles of the neck, shoulder girdle, and upper extremities will be within normal limits (7, 9, 11).

Palpation   Tenderness is normally elicited over the affected joints, usually most noticeably over the C4–5, C5–6, and C6–7 segments (Fig. 4.6) (4, 9, 22, 25).

Treatment Ideas
(1, 3, 4, 8, 9, 14, 32, 35)

Heat application usually has a soothing effect on the patient's symptoms and promotes muscle relaxation. Pulsed ultrasound over the affected joints can also help to relief discomfort. The author has found that laser over a tender joint can produce some temporary relief of symptoms. The patient's sleeping habits should be examined carefully and he should be instructed to use a rolled-up towel or cervical roll inserted into the pillowcase to support the curvature of the cervical spine in the lying position. With this condition, a slightly larger pillow, which produces mild flexion of the cervical spine, often proves most effective in producing a position of comfort. Once the patient is made comfortable in the lying position, active shoulder and shoulder girdle exercises can be started with the patient's head well-supported and in the pain-free position.

Gentle manual traction of the cervical spine with the head maintained in the position of maximum comfort can produce surprisingly quick relief of symptoms. This form of traction can be used as an irritation test, if the patient tolerates it well over two or three sessions of treatment and reports relief of symptoms, then progression to mechanical traction is indicated. This should be started with weights in the 7–10 pound range, depending on the build of the patient, and increasing to 15–20 pounds as the symptoms decrease. At this time gentle pain-free active neck flexion, rotation, and side flexion exercises can be employed with the patient initially in the supine lying position, and then in sitting. A smooth surface such as a plastic sheet will enable the patient to carry out side flexion in lying more effectively than on a pillow or sheet. A pillow should be used under the plastic sheet so that extension of the neck is avoided. At this stage light resisted upper-extremity exercises can be introduced, with the patient performing them in a position of comfort.

Neck retraction should be introduced slowly in supine lying, if tolerated, progression can be made to retraction and extension, still in lying. If the patient's symptoms continue to decrease then the same exercises can be attempted in sitting. At that time postural re-education can commence, with the aim of strengthening the muscles of the shoulder girdle and the cervical paravertebral muscles. The use of a strap fixed around the head with a velcro fastener and a loop for the application of exercise band is a very effective way of providing resisted work for the cervical musculature. Traction should be continued throughout the recovery period and the patient can also be progressed onto a general strengthening and conditioning regime. Again, the emphasis is on postural re-education and is combined with ongoing education so that the patient has an enhanced understanding of the causes of the problem (which is often related to postural strain), and therefore the most effective ways of preventing reoccurrence. The solving of one episode of symptoms is only a victory in a minor battle in the war against what is essentially a recurrent problem.

Restrictions   The patient must be instructed to avoid all neck extension in their daily activities, and also any sustained or repetitive flexion or rotation as these movements often cause exacerbation of symptoms, even if they are not actual causative factors. The patient should be instructed to change position often so as to prevent onset of symptoms, rather than having to use change of position to alleviate symptoms after they have occurred. The time spent in any one position can be slowly progressed as long as symptoms are not provoked. If they are provoked, the patient must rest in a position that relieves them until they have cleared completely. Once the patient's condition is improving, neck extension activities can recommence. Initially this has to be counterbalanced by frequent gentle flexion of the cervical spine, which should become a routine daily activity in what is essentially a change of lifestyle for the patient. Once these joints have shown themselves susceptible to irritation they are going to prove to be equally susceptible in the future unless the patient changes the activities and postures that produced the problem.

Cervical Facet Joint Irritation (with Radiculopathy)

Overview

In this condition the signs and symptoms suggest irritation of a nerve root by posterior structures in the neck, or simple referral of pain into the arm because of common innervation with an affected joint in the cervical spine. This is a diagnosis that can be made in the absence of specific x-ray findings, such as foraminal encroachment due to osteophyte formation. The overall picture is one of symptoms produced in the arm mainly by extension of the neck (8, 9, 13).

Subjective Findings

Onset   This is usually sudden with no known cause and is found most commonly in patients over the age of 50 (4, 9).

Duration   As the symptoms are very limiting as regards daily activities the patient is often seen in the early stages, often within a few days of onset or at the most 2 to 3 weeks.

Frequency   This is usually the first time the patient has had symptoms affecting the arm. There may be a history of previous episodes, but with symptoms localized to the neck and shoulder girdle.

Area of Symptoms Symptoms are found either centrally, or to one or both sides of the cervical spine and radiating into one arm. Pain may be referred any distance down the arm up to and including the hand and fingers (Fig. 4.18). The neck symptoms usually precede the arm symptoms, but the arm symptoms are often of greater concern to the patient as they are often more intense than the neck symptoms (1, 11, 17, 36).

Type of Symptoms Pain and stiffness are experienced in the cervical spine with pain, numbness, paraesthesia, dysaesthesia in the arm and hand (1, 3, 8, 9, 11).

Miscellaneous The patient's x-rays may show degenerative changes in the facet joints, as well as "degeneration" of the cervical discs. Unfortunately these findings can also be normal in older patients, and therefore may or may not have any clinical significance. The patient very commonly claims that his neck makes noises, particularly creaking and

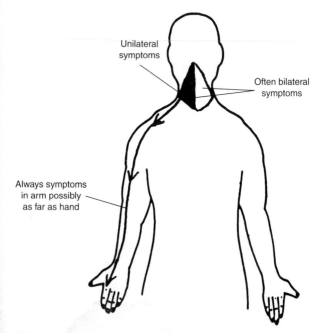

FIG. 4.18   Area of symptoms for cervical facet joint problem (with radiculopathy).

cracking, during all movements, but most noticeably when turning the head to look over the shoulder.

Objective Findings

Observation The patient's neck is usually held in mild flexion, often with some degree of side flexion away from the affected side. Muscle spasm is often observable in the upper shoulder girdle and in the cervical paravertebral muscles (1, 8, 9).

Active Movements Extension of the cervical spine and side flexion to the affected side will both be very limited and will produce radiation of symptoms into the arm. Flexion is usually moderately restricted and may also produce radiation of pain into the arm. Side flexion away from the affected side may be painful in the neck, but will tend to reduce the arm symptoms. Rotations may be symptom free bilaterally, or may produce symptoms on rotation to the affected side, again with the symptoms usually being provoked in the arm rather than in the neck. Even when of full range the movements of rotation will still tend to be reported as stiff by the patient on active testing (3, 9, 12).

Passive Movements Overpressure at end range of extension will produce marked arm pain, and muscular resistance to the movement (spasm) will be noted. Overpressure on flexion will tend to produce neck pain followed by arm pain. All movements will feel stiff at end range and any movement producing arm symptoms will also provoke muscle spasm (3, 9).

Resisted Movements Good strength will be found in the neck, shoulder girdle, and arms, with no particular discomfort on isometric testing. However, strongly resisted movements of either flexion or extension of the cervical spine will tend to produce neck pain because of the stress applied to the irritated joint.

Palpation Muscle spasm will be palpable in the cervical spine and upper shoulder girdle, and is often more noticeable on the opposite side to the symptoms. Tenderness is also usually elicited over the affected joints lateral to the spinous processes in the cervical spine, most commonly over C4–5, C5–6 or C6–7 (Fig. 4.6). It is not unusual to find tenderness over two or even all three segments. It is important not to confuse this tenderness with the tenderness of a paravertebral muscle in spasm or the natural tenderness experienced on any deep palpation in this area (1, 13, 15, 22).

Treatment Ideas
(3, 4, 9, 11, 13, 14, 17, 32, 35)

It is usually necessary to find an effective rest position for the patient so that he can sleep comfortably at night. This is often achieved by having the patient lie on the unaffected side with a fairly small pillow containing a rolled towel or cervical roll so that the neck is slightly side flexed away from the painful side, but at the same time supported by the roll.

Position of the affected arm is often important in relief of symptoms; the position of maximum relief can only be found by trial and error. This is difficult to achieve following initial assessment as the patient's condition is often irritated by the tests applied during assessment. In that case application of heat or ice to the neck and shoulder girdle will often produce a more relaxed and cooperative patient.

Once a position of rest is established active movements of the neck, shoulder girdle, and arms can be started through pain-free ranges. Often the only neck movements available are those into pain-free ranges, such as side flexion away from the affected side and either or both rotations. The author has found the use of pulsed ultrasound over the affected segments of the cervical spine to be helpful in many cases, again mainly through promotion of relaxation and subsequent relief of muscle spasm.

If is often worth trying light manual cervical traction early in the treatment regime. If the patient is placed in a lying position that already relieves the neck and arm symptoms, then traction will usually increase the period of time for which pain relief is experienced. If traction produces any typical discomfort it should be discontinued at once. Active exercises for the cervical spine can be progressed into the sitting position, again moving into pain-free ranges for rotation, side flexion, and flexion. Interferential therapy or transcutaneous electrical nerve stimulation applied at the end of the treatment session helps to alleviate any discomfort in the shoulder girdle muscles produced by the exercises. If the patient does gain pain relief with these modalities, then they will also prove very useful prior to the application of traction. If the patient responded well to manual traction, then mechanical traction can be attempted, again carried out in the position of symptom relief, initially with light weights, gradually progressing the weight as tolerated.

Active arm exercises in sitting can be commenced once the patient is able to control his arm symptoms by movement or positioning of the neck. If arm symptoms are produced by the exercises and cannot be relieved by movement or positioning of the neck, then they must be stopped. Assisted stretches of the cervical spine into rotation and side flexion away from the painful side can be taught to the patient, and are followed by assisted flexion carried out initially in lying and then in sitting. This will help to stretch tight muscles and may help to alleviate pressure on the affected joint or joints.

By this time the patient should be able to tolerate a certain degree of movement into extension, retraction, and side flexion to the affected side. These should be tackled individually, in whichever order proves to be least uncomfortable. As soon as a degree of retraction is possible then postural re-education can begin with strengthening of the postural muscles of the neck and shoulder girdle with the aid of neuromuscular electrical stimulation. The patient is instructed to assume pain-relieving positions as and when required to alleviate any onset of symptoms. Exercises should not be restarted until the symptoms are once again under control.

A program of active exercises for all movements of the cervical spine, shoulder girdle, and upper extremities should be instigated, with a bias in repetitions towards those movements that have been shown to relieve the patient's symptoms. However, the overall aim of treatment is to restore full normal active range of motion in the cervical spine, which must include those movements that previously produced symptoms. A regime of upper extremity and upper body strengthening related to the patient's normal level of daily activities should be started at this time. Cervical traction should be maintained throughout the course of treatment, and the author has found it to be most effective at the end of each treatment session, with the weights progressed to the maximum the patient can tolerate for a 15-minute period. It may be necessary to continue to traction the patient in their position of comfort, even in the final stages of the course of treatment. Patient education regarding the causes of neck problems and the means of preventing them is essential and is usually better received once the patient is showing progress with treatment. However, it can also be very useful where a patient shows a tendency towards continuing with those activities in daily life that initially provoked the symptoms, as the folly of their ways is often brought home to them more vividly via videotape or slide presentations than through the badgering of the therapist.

Restrictions The patient should be instructed to avoid all overhead work in the early stages, with no sustained static positioning of the head, as even a "good" position will become uncomfortable with time. The patient should be instructed to continue with activities as normally as possible, but in short bursts and avoiding neck extension. The patient should rest with the head or arm in whatever position is most effective in relieving symptoms, as required. Once the symptoms ease they may go back to the activity again, but not if it produced a rapid onset of their symptoms. The patient's work habits and activities of daily living must be examined, as the best prevention of recurrence of symptoms is a change in lifestyle. This condition is seldom if ever due to a single injury, but rather to repeated stresses and strains. Areas of particular concern are use of computers, particularly the positioning of the screen or any documents that are being reviewed. People in high-risk occupations, such as welders or electricians, have a daunting task attempting to modify their work habits, but nevertheless the attempt must be made, otherwise recurrence is almost inevitable.

Cervical Postural Strain

Overview

When the correct lordotic curve is maintained in the cervical spine, the weight of the head passes through the discs and vertebral bodies as intended. If this curvature is flattened out, as in the mild to moderate forward head posture that can be found in the majority of patients, then the weight of the head hangs on the ligaments and muscles of the postero-lateral cervical region and the middle and upper shoulder girdle. Over time the tension on these tissues produces pain and muscle spasm, which can spread as far as the lower margins of the ribcage posteriorly. The patient who is experiencing the degree of discomfort that this condition can produce will not for one minute believe that it is due simply to a faulty posture (5, 9, 37).

Subjective Findings

Onset   Onset is gradual and usually the patient cannot attribute it to a particular cause, but a clearly taken history will indicate overuse in the form of a static posture or specific positioning of the neck and arms sustained for periods of time. The condition seems to affect patients of all ages, from high school students hunched over a desk to 70-year-old retirees hooked on the internet (5, 8, 9, 11).

Duration   The condition usually persists for several weeks before the patient seeks medical attention. It is not uncommon for them to have a history of an episode lasting many months.

Frequency   The condition is by nature recurrent and symptoms usually increase in intensity with time, as does the size of the area over which the symptoms are experienced (7, 9, 11).

Area of Symptoms   These usually start in the sides of the cervical spine and the upper or middle trapezius. It is commonly bilateral in nature, although one side is often more uncomfortable than the other. Spread of symptoms will occur into the interscapular area, over the scapulae, and down as far as the lower ribs posteriorly (Fig. 4.19) (5, 9, 20, 22).

Type of Symptoms   The patient typically complains of aching and tenderness, with lumps or knots felt or experienced in the affected musculature. The patient will also complain of a feeling of pressure, particularly in the cervical spine. Headaches are a quite common sequel to the other symptoms (5, 11, 20).

Miscellaneous   Pain generally worsens as the day goes on, particularly a workday, and particularly with sedentary occupations (9–5 syndrome). The symptoms are most commonly associated with sitting or standing with the head slightly flexed, and the pain is worse if the arms are raised and unsupported, as in standing working at a workbench or sitting using a computer keyboard with no support for the arms (8, 9, 11, 20).

Objective Findings

Observation   The patient usually has a poor posture with rounding of the shoulders and protrusion of the cervical spine (forward head posture) (9, 37).

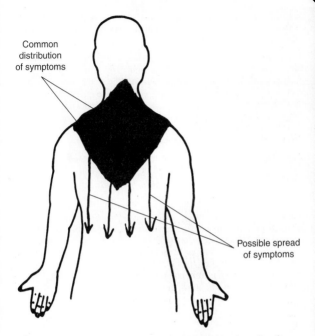

Common distribution of symptoms

Possible spread of symptoms

FIG. 4.19 Area of symptoms for cervical postural strain, notice the distance symptoms can spread down the thoracic spine.

Active Movements Movements of the cervical and thoracic spine should be within normal limits, although stiffness may be reported at end range of any or all movements. This stiffness is normally felt in the neck, but can be felt anywhere within the normal distribution of the symptoms. If the symptoms are noticeably one sided then pain may be produced in the affected musculature of the shoulder girdle by side flexion of the cervical spine away from the affected side and on rotation towards the affected side (1, 7, 14).

Passive Movements Overpressure applied at the end range of any of the movements will usually produce a tightness or pulling pain in the neck, shoulder girdle, or mid back. This is usually most pronounced at the end range of flexion of the cervical spine (5, 8).

Resisted Movements The patient may complain of some mild discomfort, usually on either isometric resisted flexion or extension of the cervical spine; however, this pain is not usually in the typical distribution of their symptoms. Muscle strength is always normal in the neck, shoulder girdle, and upper extremities.

Palpation There is usually diffuse tenderness present throughout the muscles of the neck, shoulder girdle, and upper back. Some specific points may be particularly tender, such as the middle of the upper trapezius, bilaterally in the neck at the C6–7 level, along the medial border of the scapula, and at the junction between the middle and upper trapezius. Small fibrous nodules may be found in and around the same regions, which are quite tender to the touch and may have been discovered by the patient and pointed out prior to the objective examination.

Specific Tests If the patient is instructed to sit with their head hanging forward (chin to chest) for a period of 1 to 2 minutes, the symptoms should start to be clearly reproduced (9, 20, 25).

Treatment Ideas
(5, 7–11, 14, 20, 33)

The initial thrust of treatment is always postural correction. This should start in supine lying with the use of a towel roll in the cervical spine to re-inforce the natural lordotic curve and active exercises for neck retraction, shoulder girdle retraction, and elevation with extension. The thoracic spine should be extended if rounding of the shoulders is a marked feature of the patient's posture, in which case the use of a towel roll along the length of the thoracic spine may initially prove more effective than the use of a cervical roll.

Active neck and arm exercises are used to promote retraction and elevation of the shoulders and retraction of the cervical spine with a mild degree of thoracic extension. Patients will often benefit from reversal of these movements from time to time, so that the neck is flexed and the shoulders fully protracted in order to stretch tense and painful muscles in the neck and upper back. Application of heat produces decrease in immediate discomfort in the majority of patients. Interferential therapy to relax the muscles of the shoulder girdle is also helpful. Some patients experience more marked relief from the use of ice, but I advise them never to use this particular physical agent prior to either work or exercise.

The patient is progressed onto active and light resisted exercises in sitting, again concentrating on cervical protraction and shoulder girdle retraction and elevation. A general light-intensity workout using free weights or an exercise band for the shoulder girdles and upper extremities will also help to improve the patient's overall muscular tone. They should be advised to exercise for short periods frequently throughout the day, rather than attempting 20 or 30 minutes of exercises once or twice per day. One exercise the author favors for counteracting slumping of the shoulders in the 9–5 syndrome is short bursts of resisted horizontal abduction of the shoulder using a light resistance band for 15–20 repetitions, repeated once every hour during the work day.

This 9–5 syndrome is the natural deterioration of a person's posture through the workday, as fatigue in the postural muscles allows the head to poke forward more and the shoulders to slump, producing increased flexion of the thoracic spine. This diurnal variation becomes more noticeable as the work week progresses (Monday to Friday syndrome). Where a patient's muscle tone seems to remain obstinately poor, the use of neuromuscular electrical stimulation on the middle and upper trapezius is an effective way of improving function when combined with a resisted exercise program.

The patient has to be educated thoroughly as regards the causes of their symptoms and the prevention of recurrence by postural awareness, postural correction, and changes in work or life habits. A general exercise program, which also includes cardiovascular training, should be prescribed, with the patient continuing exercising in a gym setting. This program need only be repeated for some 30–40 minutes two to three times per week, but the enhanced physical activity will then reinforce the postural re-education if the patient is willing to undertake the effort involved.

Restrictions

Any activity that requires the neck to be flexed to any extent for any period of time, particularly when the arms are used away from the body, can still be continued from the outset but only if sufficient time is allowed for regular rest and stretch periods so that symptoms are not produced. Many patients state that they do stretch when they feel tired and sore and their education should stress that they stretch *before* the symptoms occur and not just as a result of them. Studying at a desk, using a computer, working on an assembly line, etc. are all common causes of exacerbation of this condition but they need not be if the ergonomic set up is correct. Even when ergonomic changes have been made the patient must continue to break up static positions for short rest breaks and stretching routines. Usually lifting and carrying weights is not a problem for patients suffering from this condition and in fact it is usually found that active work, such as light to moderate lifting and carrying, is beneficial to their condition and in many cases should be encouraged, particularly if it breaks up static positioning.

Upper Trapezius Muscle Strain

Overview

The upper part of the trapezius muscle can be injured by sudden or forceful movements of the head, neck, or shoulder girdle. Because of the extent of the muscle and poor pain localization, symptoms can be spread over a wide area, which may cause confusion when trying to determine the diagnosis (8, 13).

Subjective Findings

Onset   Onset is sudden due to trauma. A clear description of the injury will usually show that force was applied to the head or shoulder girdle, forcing separation of the two. Patients are typically 25–45 years of age.

Duration   This is a moderately limiting condition functionally, so patients normally seek treatment within a matter of 1 to 3 weeks.

Frequency   It is unusual to find this occurring more than once in a given patient, although the patient may reinjure a healing muscle quite easily and may not refer themselves for treatment until the second injury because at that time they become more concerned about long-term effects.

Area of Symptoms   Only one side of the neck is affected. Pain can be felt from the occipital ridge, along the lateral aspect of the cervical spine, into the upper shoulder girdle, across the shoulder, over the deltoid region, and into the scapular area (Fig. 4.20). The patient often displays the area of discomfort by placing the hand so that it covers the side of the neck and the upper part of the trapezius muscle. On odd occasions the pain may also pass up behind the ear to the area of the mastoid process.

Type of Symptoms   Pain is usually sharp on movements of the neck and head with a poorly defined ache at rest, which is particularly noticeable in sitting when the head is unsupported.

Miscellaneous   The injury will often have involved forceful side flexion away from the side of pain or rotation toward the side of pain. The shoulder may also have been forcefully depressed (as in making a tackle in football or rugby).

Observation   The patient often presents with a stiff neck, turning the thoracic spine and shoulders instead of the head when looking over the shoulder. The cervical spine may be shifted laterally towards the painful side.

Active Movements   There will be limitation of side flexion of the cervical spine away from the painful side and on rotation towards the painful side. Discomfort on movement should be well localized to the point of injury and occurs at the end of available range of motion. Flexion and extension tend to be uncomfortable and limited to some degree or other, but on testing these movements the symptoms are not as marked as on the other movements described. Side flexion to the painful side may be uncomfortable at end range, as the muscle contracts more powerfully to produce further movement. However, rotation away from the affected side is always pain free, although the patient may describe the movement as being stiff.

Passive Movements   Muscle resistance is experienced at the end range of all painful movements, with the same pattern of restriction as that described for active movements.

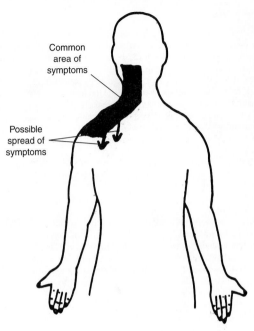

FIG. 4.20 Area of symptoms for left upper trapezius muscle strain.

Resisted Movements Pain is experienced on resisted side flexion of the cervical spine towards the painful side and on rotation away from the painful side. Strongly resisted shoulder girdle elevation may also produce discomfort on the affected side, but is only diagnostically significant if this pain is not reproduced by the same degree of resistance on the unaffected side. Isometric abduction of the shoulder at 90 degrees will produce discomfort in the upper shoulder girdle region.

Palpation Tenderness can be elicited in the muscle mass of the upper trapezius (Fig. 4.1) often with a focal tender point near the neck. Muscle tension or outright muscle spasm will be produced on palpation of the upper trapezius muscle mass. Tenderness can often also be elicited in the lateral aspect of the cervical spine over the insertion of the muscle, and in very severe cases along the occipital ridge on the affected side.

Treatment Ideas
(8, 13)

If the patient is seen within 1 to 2 days of injury then ice and rest should be advised, with gentle shoulder girdle circumduction (rolling the shoulders) carried out within pain-free range. A soft cervical collar may help during the first few days in some cases, although many patients find that the pressure of the collar on the shoulder girdle is too uncomfortable. This drawback often outweighs any benefits that are derived from use of the collar. The collar should never be worn for more than 4 days after the injury as muscle stiffness develops very easily.

By the third or fourth day following injury the patient should be capable of active exercises for all movements of the cervical spine, shoulder girdle, and upper extremities. The patient should be instructed to carry out the movement only to the point at which discomfort begins, and no further. At this time pulsed ultrasound applied to the site of injury may help to stimulate repair; interferential therapy will decrease discomfort in many cases.

As active movements become relatively pain free auto-assisted stretching can be commenced. This should begin with flexion of the neck, with the patient's hands placed on the back of the head and the elbows brought forward and together to apply a traction force to the cervical region. Once this is well tolerated, the patient can progress to auto-assisted side flexions and rotations. This can be done to both sides for both movements, starting with the painless movements. Pressure should be applied lightly at the end range of motion and held for 10–15 seconds. For right side flexion the patient places the right hand on the left side of the head to apply overpressure at the end of available range of motion. The left hand is then used on the right side of the head to assist in left-side flexion. For right rotation the heel of the left hand pushes on the left side of the jaw, and visa versa for left rotation.

A stronger stretch can be applied to the affected muscle by having the patient sit in a chair and grip the seat with the hand of the affected side, while side flexing the cervical spine away from the painful side. Further stretch can be applied by the patient placing his other hand over the top of his head and applying light pressure at the end range of available range of motion. At this time resisted exercises can be started for the arms and shoulder girdle, progressing to resisted work for the cervical spine using a head halter and exercise band. Postural re-education forms an important part of the treatment protocol as few people have a truly satisfactory head, neck, and shoulder girdle posture, and any opportunity to improve this will help in the prevention of other neck problems not necessarily related to this specific muscle injury.

The patient should be progressed onto a general resisted gym exercise program for the upper extremities and trunk, which should relate to the level of daily activities enjoyed prior to the injury. Muscle work should be a blend of endurance and power training, with progression to explosive movements of the head, neck, shoulder girdle, and arms, as and when tolerated.

Restrictions Initially the patient should be instructed to avoid working with his arms at or above shoulder height, particularly where any weight is involved or if it is for a prolonged period of time. Repeated rotation, side flexion, or flexion of the neck will often exacerbate symptoms; this type of activity should be broken up into short periods with rests and stretches as required to prevent onset of symptoms.

Where the injury is caused by specific sports activities the type of circumstances that lead to the injury should be avoided for at least 3 to 4 weeks post injury and until the patient is capable of sustaining strong explosive types of exercise without experiencing discomfort. Lifting heavy weights, and more particularly the carrying of weights over distance, should be modified by reducing the weight or distance until the patient has demonstrated comfort with this type of action in the protected environment of the clinic. Exercises should simulate and exceed the physical demands that the patient faces in his daily activities before those activities can resume. The author has found that patients can usually tolerate the majority of their normal daily activities if they simply break up tasks, allowing adequate rest in order to prevent onset of discomfort.

Latisimus Dorsi Muscle Strain

Overview

This condition can produce confusion in diagnosis because of the site of pain, normally in the patient's side in the thoracolumbar region and therefore distant from the causative action, which normally occurs at the shoulder. Pain can be very acute, particularly in the first few days following injury, and can often be confused with a fractured or bruised rib. However, the condition does tend to resolve quickly, although reinjury is commonplace, particularly in the first 1 to 2 weeks following onset.

Subjective Findings

Onset The patient is most commonly a male between 25 and 45 years of age and onset is always sudden due to trauma. The classic history given is one of pulling on something heavy, such as when taking timber out of the back of a truck, and experiencing immediate pain in the side, or of two people carrying a heavy load and one of them allows their end to drop, with the other taking the full strain as the load falls (24).

Duration Patients normally spend the first 2 to 3 weeks waiting for the pain to disappear because they quite correctly diagnose it themselves as being "muscular," and are therefore sure that it will resolve in its own time. When this does not happen, or more commonly when they hurt themselves again by straining on an incompletely healed muscle, they turn up for treatment, usually believing that they have a back problem.

Frequency This is commonly one isolated incident and recurrence is uncommon once the condition has cleared fully, although, as already stated, reinjury of a healing muscle is not unusual.

Area of Symptoms Pain is experienced in the area between the inferior angle of the scapula and the lower ribs as far distally as the iliac crest (Fig. 4.21).

Type of Symptoms Pain is very sharp on movement with a steady and often quite severe aching pain at rest, particularly following any marked degree of activity.

Miscellaneous Patients may complain of pain on taking a deep breath. There may also be discomfort when coughing, sneezing, and straining on the toilet.

Observation There is usually nil of note to be observed in the affected area, although if the patient is in severe discomfort he may present with a

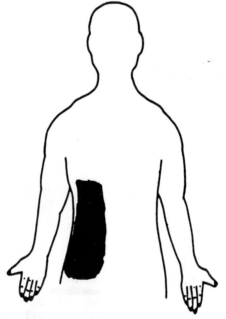

FIG. 4.21   Area of symptoms for left latisimus dorsi muscle strain.

slight degree of side flexion of the spine towards the affected side in an attempt to relieve the pain.

Active Movements No pain or limitation of movement will be experienced on testing of movements of the thoracic spine, cervical spine, or arm, independently of each other, except in rare cases when pain may be felt on full abduction of the arm or on side flexion of the thoracic spine away from the painful side. The patient's typical pain is usually reproduced by a combination of side flexion of the thoracic spine away from the side of pain, with full abduction and lateral rotation of the arm on the affected side.

Passive Movements The pattern of restriction of motion will be the same passively as actively, with the patient's typical pain produced by overpressure into abduction of the shoulder on the affected side when the thorax is side flexed away from the painful side.

Resisted Movements Pain is produced in the patient's side on combined isometric adduction and medial rotation of the shoulder. This is particularly marked if the movement is tested with the shoulder in the abducted and laterally rotated position so that the latisimus dorsi muscle is slightly stretched.

Palpation Specific tenderness is often difficult to detect and this in part differentiates this condition from an injury to a rib, as the site of injury in that case is always exceptionally tender and usually very easy to find. Tenderness in the muscle belly of the latisimus dorsi is often easier to find when the patient is lying on the unaffected side with the arm abducted, so that the arm rests against the side of their head. The tenderness still tends to remain diffuse and is spread over a large area between the scapula and the pelvis on the affected side. However, diligent search will often find a focal point of tenderness in the injured muscle belly (Fig. 4.9).

Treatment Ideas

The patient should first be advised to ice the painful area and rest the affected muscle. Three or four days postinjury the patient can progress to the use of heat. At that time the patient can also start individual active movements of side flexion and rotation of the thoracic spine and abduction and lateral rotation of the arm. This can be followed by slow gentle stretches combining side flexion of the thoracic spine away from the side of injury with full abduction of the arm. It is usually best to side flex the spine first, and then use the arm movement to apply further pressure, as this allows better control of the degree of weight being applied to the injured tissue at the end of movement as full stretch is applied to the muscle.

The patient can progress to resisted exercises for the injured muscle followed by stretch. Resisted exercises should emphasis combination movements of adduction with medial rotation of the arm; proprioceptive neuromuscular facilitation techniques are often extremely useful at this stage of treatment. Resisted exercises should be both proceeded and followed by a thorough stretching of the muscle. The continued use of heat often enables patients to exercise more effectively and with less discomfort. If residual discomfort is felt after exercise then ice can be a useful adjunct to treatment.

The patient is progressed onto a general upper extremity exercise program, with emphasis placed on pushing and pulling activities for both endurance and power training. Any residual discomfort experienced on full stretch of the muscle can be addressed by the use of sustained distraction of the abducted and laterally rotated shoulder, with the patient in side lying over pillows, so that the thoracic spine is side flexed away from the injured side.

Restrictions In the initial stages patients should be advised against any forceful pushing and pulling activities, or raising themselves by use of their arms. Any weight training activities will also have to be modified. Testing the patient with light weights for each piece of equipment that is being used, gradual progression of the weights used, and instructions to immediately stop any exercise that produces discomfort in the affected area will all help to negate the likelihood of recurrent injury. A clear explanation of the time scale involved for repair and healing of the muscle is the best means of maintaining a patient's compliance with the treatment protocol.

Cervical Facet Joint Locking

Overview

The name for this condition is, unfortunately, a complete misnomer, as the facet joints are mechanically incapable of locking. The patient's problem is, in fact, muscular, with spasm preventing movement. However, the examination findings suggest a facet joint problem, the muscle spasm appears to be a reaction to the joint problem, rather than an intrinsic muscular problem. Since the facet joints therefore do give the appearance of having "locked up," I do not feel it is necessary to be too pedantic in attempting to find a more anatomically correct title for the condition (6, 8–10, 19).

Subjective Findings

Onset This is sudden with no known cause of onset. In the majority of cases the patient will have experienced onset of symptoms on waking, having had no problem with the neck prior to going to sleep. Patients are typically between 20 and 50 years of age (1, 5, 8).

Duration The patient is usually seen within a matter of days to a week following onset, as the pain can be quite excruciating and both functionally and socially limiting.

Frequency Usually this will be the first time that the patient has experienced these symptoms, although he may have had a few bouts of neck discomfort that previously cleared quite quickly.

Area of Symptoms The patient is able to localize the symptoms to the side of the neck and the ipsilateral upper shoulder girdle region, although some pain may also be felt centrally in the cervical spine (Fig. 4.22) (4, 8, 9).

Type of Symptoms Pain is sharp in nature and occurs on movements of the neck, particularly when turning the head to look over the shoulder. The patient will also complain of a constant stiffness and aching in the neck, particularly when sitting with the head unsupported (8, 9, 24).

Miscellaneous The author has often found that patients will state that they slept particularly well during the night prior to waking with the symptoms. A very typical picture is that of a patient having been to a late-night barbeque, where he enjoyed one or two beers and then slept very soundly, but woke with a stiff neck, which became painful on attempted movement.

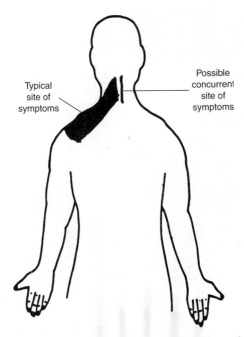

Typical site of symptoms

Possible concurrent site of symptoms

FIG. 4.22   Area of symptoms for cervical facet joint locking on the left side.

Objective Findings

Observation   It will be observed that the patient has a stiff neck as he will move the thoracic spine and shoulder girdle to turn to look over the shoulder; however, there is usually no lateral deviation of the spine on examination (9, 11).

Active Movements   There is marked limitation of side flexion and rotation to the affected side. Both of these movements will produce sharp pain felt both laterally in the neck and in the upper shoulder girdle on the same side. Extension of the cervical spine will be less limited, but equally painful. All other movements are stiff, but do not produce any sharp discomfort. The closer to onset of the condition that the patient is seen the more obvious this pattern of restriction, but after a period of several days the patient will begin to demonstrate more discomfort and stiffness on attempting what were previously pain-free movements. However, even later the same basic pattern should still be discernible (1, 9, 11, 24).

Passive Movements   The pattern of limitation of movement is the same as that found on active testing. Muscle spasm and guarding will be felt on side flexion and rotation of the cervical spine to the affected side, and also commonly on extension. The patient tends to resist overpressure on any movement, but palpation of the upper and middle trapezius on the affected side during passive testing will quickly indicate that the above movements are the ones that are producing the greatest distress (9, 11, 24).

Resisted Movements   All movements of the cervical spine, shoulder girdle, and shoulders will be strong and pain free on isometric testing.

Palpation   Marked tenderness is usually elicited lateral to the spinous processes of the cervical spine on the affected side, most commonly at the C4–5, C5–6, or C6–7 levels (Fig. 4.6). Muscle spasm can usually be palpated in the upper, and occasionally the middle, portions of the trapezius muscle, as well as in the cervical paravertebral muscles, often bilaterally (11, 12, 22, 25) (Figs. 4.1, 4.5, 4.7).

Treatment Ideas
(1, 5, 8–11, 19, 24)

Application of heat will provide some relief from the pain and muscle spasm that the patient is experiencing, although in rare cases better results are obtained with the use of ice. Where rotation to one side is noticeably free from pain and restriction compared to the other side, the one exercise that the patient needs to carry out is active rotation to the pain-free side. This should be carried out 30–40 times once or twice per hour throughout the day. The patient must avoid rotation to the painful side in particular, and all other painful movements in general. Some patients have quite a hysterical reaction to this condition because of the level of discomfort. In these patients the prescription of a soft collar for 48 hours is helpful, although they should remove the collar every hour to carry out the active exercises described above. Within 2 to 3 days the patient's discomfort should have eased considerably. It is wise to continue with heat and local applications of modalities such as ultrasound and laser over the tender areas in the cervical spine. The active exercises can be extended to include flexion and side flexion away from the painful side. Shoulder girdle circumduction is a useful loosening up exercise both before and after the neck exercises.

Within a week to 10 days the patient should be experiencing minimal discomfort on movements to the affected side and no discomfort at rest. At this time auto-assisted stretches should be attempted for side flexion and rotation away from the painful side. These stretches are progressed further by auto-assisted side flexion and rotation to the affected side, but only when these movements are pain-free on active testing, although they may still be stiff.

Sustaining static positioning of the neck and head should be avoided in any position during the first few days following onset. Rotation and side flexion into pain must also be avoided, as these reinforce the pain and muscle spasm that is already present. A soft collar can be an effective restraint on movement if the patient finds he is unable to stop the movements without some form of external assistance. As symptoms subside the patient will naturally attempt more movement and will be able to tolerate static positions for longer periods of time.

Thoracic Facet Joint Locking

Overview

As in the cervical spine, the thoracic facet joints cannot mechanically lock. The probable cause of symptoms in this condition is strain or acute irritation of a facet joint with subsequent muscle spasm, which effectively prevents the joint or joints in one or more segments of the spine from moving. However, since as a result of the muscle spasm there is effectively a block on motion of the affected joints, there is no reason why the term facet joint locking should not be used to describe the signs and symptoms.

Subjective Findings

Onset Onset is often sudden with no known cause of origin. Occasionally the patient will describe a degree of overuse, particularly sustaining one position, usually slumped sitting or standing or an unaccustomed level of activity involving use of the trunk. The condition occurs most commonly in patients 25 to 45 years of age (1, 11).

Duration The patient normally presents for treatment within a few days of onset or within 1 to 2 weeks, as the pain produced by this condition is always acute and therefore of immediate concern to the patient.

Frequency Normally patients only suffer this particular problem on one occasion. Very rarely these symptoms will occur two or three times in one individual, but in these cases the symptoms can often be traced to another source, usually in the cervical region.

Area of Symptoms Symptoms are felt over the central thoracic spine and the thoracic paravertebral muscles, usually more marked on one side compared to the other. In some cases pain may pass around the ribcage, but no further than the midaxillary line (Fig. 4.23) (11, 22, 39).

Type of Symptoms Discomfort is sharp in nature and usually occurs only on certain movements, most commonly rotation and extension.

Miscellaneous The pain can be very severe at onset and patients often state at that time that they are unable to take a deep breath. Coughing and sneezing will often produce pain directly at the site of the lesion.

Observation Muscle spasm is usually observable in the thoracic paravertebral muscles around the affected area and often for several

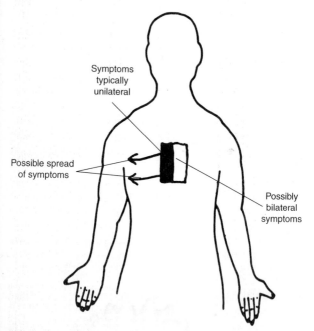

FIG. 4.23 Area of symptoms for thoracic facet joint locking on left side.

segments above and below that point. There should be no observable deviation of the spine.

Active Movements Rotation and side flexion to the affected side will be noticeably limited and will produce the patient's typical discomfort. Rotation away from the affected side will often produce pain, but will be less obviously limited. Side flexion away from the affected side may be stiff, but should not produce the patient's typical discomfort and will be only mildly limited. Flexion of the thoracic spine might be slightly limited, but may well be full and pain free. In fact, the patient may state that he feels better when carrying out this movement. Extension is usually moderately limited, but does not produce any particular pain (1, 11).

Passive Movements Testing of passive movements is not applicable in this condition, although overpressure applied to any painful movement should produce specific localized discomfort at the site of the lesion.

Resisted Movements There is no pain or loss of strength found on isometric testing of movements of the thoracic spine, cervical spine, shoulder girdle, or arms.

Palpation Tenderness will be elicited over one, two, or three segments of the thoracic spine on posterior/anterior pressure applied to the spinous processes (Fig. 4.8). There will also be diffuse tenderness over the thoracic paravertebral muscles around the affected area. There is often poor local intervertebral movement found on posterior/anterior pressure at several segments both above and below the affected area (11, 22, 25).

Treatment Ideas
(1, 11, 17, 39)

If the therapist has sufficient knowledge and suitable training, then a forceful posterior/anterior mobilization of the affected joints and the segments immediately above and below can, on many occasions, produce immediate relief of symptoms. This is particularly true if the movement is accompanied by a satisfactory click. The author normally applies a heat pack to the affected area before attempting this maneuver, as it gives the patient the time and incentive to relax after the discomfort of the assessment.

A more conservative approach to treatment in this condition is the use of heat combined with thoracic extension exercises, using a rolled towel placed along the spine with the patient in supine lying. Movements of the arms into elevation with shoulder girdle retraction will then produce a slow mobilization of the joints in the desired direction. This can be progressed by using straight arm raises with the patient in prone lying with the arms stretched out in front of them and further progressed by head and chest raises also done in prone lying.

Once the immediate discomfort decreases, resisted shoulder retraction initially done in supine lying and then in sitting helps to reduce pain by improving upper back posture. The resistance should be mild to moderate, as this relatively gentle form of exercise also helps to restore normal function to the muscles in the region. The use of electrical modalities over the affected joints and muscles is indicated if the patient's level of discomfort precludes the use of either exercises or passive mobilization. The relaxation and pain relief afforded by these modalities will then allow the introduction of mobilization in one form or another.

Restrictions This condition is often self limiting as regards the avoidance of activities that provoke symptoms, as the degree of discomfort experienced by the patient usually prevents him from sustaining, or often even attempting, any symptom-provoking activities or movements. The patient should be advised to change positions or activities as and when necessary to avoid exacerbation of symptoms. The condition is fairly short lived by nature and the patient will not have to tolerate restriction of activity for any extended period of time.

Thoracic Outlet Syndrome

Overview

The thoracic outlet is bordered by the scalenus anterior muscle anteriorly, the scalenus medius muscle posteriorly, and the first rib inferiorly. The brachial plexus and its accompanying subclavian artery may be compressed in this area by a cervical rib, a fibrous band in place of a cervical rib, or tendinous bands extending between the scalenus anterior and scalenus medius. On rare occasions callus from a healing clavicular fracture can compress this neurovascular bundle. It appears that the most common causes of this condition are congenital, but onset often occurs in patients in their 30s, as their shoulder girdle posture starts to deteriorate (1, 5, 14, 16, 18, 40).

Subjective Findings

Onset Onset is gradual with no known cause, although on rare occasions it can occur gradually after trauma (specifically a fractured clavicle). Patients are usually between 35 and 55 years of age; it is very uncommon to find this condition in a patient under the age of 30 (5, 7, 13, 18).

Duration The patient will often suffer the symptoms for many weeks or even months before seeking medical attention.

Frequency The history is of one long continuous episode, although the patient may report periods of decreased symptoms lasting approximately a week to a month. However, the patient will state that the symptoms are always present to some extent, and simply vary in intensity from week to week (4, 5, 16, 24).

Area of Symptoms Symptoms are felt diffusely in the arm, often in the distribution of the C8/T1 dermatome (Fig. 4.24) (13, 16, 18).

Type of Symptoms Pain and paraesthesia are felt in the arm and may progress to weakness in the intrinsic muscles of the hand. In some cases

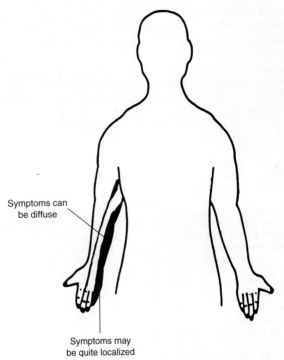

Symptoms can
be diffuse

Symptoms may
be quite localized

FIG. 4.24 Area of symptoms for thoracic outlet syndrome (these may be unilateral as depicted or can be bilateral, in a similar distribution).

vascular signs may be present in the upper extremity, such as excessive sweating or coldness and cyanosis of the fingers (4, 13, 18, 24).

Miscellaneous The patient often complains that he is unable to carry weight in the hand with the arm hanging at his side (such as in carrying groceries in a bag). Women who carry heavy purses slung over their shoulders may find that this produces their typical symptoms.

Objective Finding

Observation The patient commonly has a poor posture, with rounding of the shoulders and protrusion of the head (forward-head posture). Wasting of the intrinsic muscles of the hand may be observed in chronic or severe cases (18, 24, 40).

Active Movements Movements of the neck, shoulder girdle, and affected arm are all full range and pain free (1, 4, 16, 18, 24).

Passive Movements Again, full range of motion will be present on passive testing and there will be a normal end feel to all movements.

Resisted Movements In severe or chronic cases a painless weakness may be found in the hand and fingers. All other movements of the neck, shoulder girdle, and arm are pain free and of normal strength (8, 16, 18, 24).

Palpation Usually there is nil of note to be found on palpation, although a pulsating lump may be found in the hollow behind the clavicle on the affected side if the subclavian artery is elevated over a cervical rib or fibrous band (1, 13, 18).

Specific Tests Symptoms may be produced by sustained depression of the shoulder with traction of the arm. Conversely, in some cases, symptoms are produced by elevation of the shoulder girdle. In either case the opposite movement to the one that produces symptoms should abolish the symptoms rapidly. Adson's test is carried out with the patient in sitting. First find the patient's radial pulse and then have the patient turn his head towards the side of the arm being tested while extending the neck. Then, passively extend and laterally rotate their shoulder. Finally, ask the patient to take a deep breath and hold it. The test is considered positive if the radial pulse disappears during these maneuvers. X-rays are required to exclude the presence of a cervical rib, however, the presence of a fibrous band, which can act like a cervical rib, will not be observable on x-ray (8, 13, 21, 24, 25).

Treatment Ideas
(1, 5, 7, 8, 13, 14, 19, 23, 26, 40, 41)

The aim of treatment is to restore and sustain the correct postural alignment of the head, neck, shoulder girdle, and upper back. Active exercises are done in lying, with small towel rolls in the cervical and thoracic spine to help passively position the spine while the patient uses his postural muscles in a relaxed and pain-free manner. Active stretching exercises should be taught for the cervical spine, shoulder girdle, shoulders, and upper back because even though there is normally no particular restriction of active movement, increased flexibility in the area will enable the patient to achieve and sustain a correct posture with less difficulty.

The patient progresses to resisted exercises for elevation of the arms through abduction and flexion, shoulder girdle elevation and retraction, cervical retraction, and thoracic extension. These movements are performed in supine lying initially and progressed to sitting or standing. The exercises are aimed at endurance training using relatively light resistance and high repetitions. Any exercise that produces the patient's typical arm symptoms should be stopped immediately and modified so that this no longer occurs. Neuromuscular electrical stimulation of the shoulder girdle muscles will assist the patient in achieving and sustaining the correct position for postural correction, which can then be reinforced by the resisted exercises.

Observable improvement in the patient's posture is normally accompanied by decreased symptoms in the arm. Once this occurs the patient is progressed into a gym exercise program for further strengthening of the postural muscles. At this time the program should include both endurance and power work to facilitate normal muscle function. The patient must be instructed to continue with some form of resisted exercise and to maintain postural awareness as long as there are any indications of symptoms in the arm.

Restrictions The only restriction the patient needs to follow is change of position or activity when the symptoms are produced in the arms. The patient can continue with any activity that does not produce symptoms. The patient should find that modification of his posture will allow him to attempt activities that would otherwise produce the arm symptoms, and should be encouraged to do this in a pro-active manner. He must be repeatedly advised that persisting in activities that produce the typical arm symptoms will either prolong or prevent the eradication of the symptoms.

Whiplash

Overview

This term was initially used to describe the mechanism of a particular injury to the cervical spine. It has now become a diagnosis in its own right, and one with an unfortunately bad reputation caused by the occasional abuse of insurance coverage following motor vehicle accidents, etc. The cervical spine can sustain injury by sudden acceleration or deceleration forces producing hyperextension or hyperflexion injuries. This commonly occurs when a patient is the occupant of a car that is either rear-ended or involved in a head-on collision, but can occur in any circumstance where the head continues to move rapidly forward and backwards when the body's motion is stopped. In severe cases fractures or dislocations can occur, but in the cases that are commonly seen in orthopaedic clinics the injury occurs in the soft tissues of the cervical spine and shoulder girdle. This can involve the ligaments, intervertebral discs, and muscles of the neck, shoulder girdle, upper thoracic region, and chest wall. Symptoms can either be local in nature or very widespread; unfortunately, there is no way of determining how genuine these symptoms might be. The therapist therefore has to accept at face value the problem as described by the patient and treat accordingly (1, 5, 11, 24, 42, 43).

Subjective Findings

Onset Onset is usually sudden due to trauma, although often symptoms will not reveal themselves until 1 to 2 hours, or occasionally 1 to 2 days, following injury. This injury can occur at any age (5, 7, 8, 24).

Duration Hopefully the patient is seen within 2 to 3 weeks of the injury; however, this depends on the patient and attending health practitioner. In some cases it could be as long as 3 to 6 months after injury before the patient is referred for treatment. Patients who are still suffering severe symptoms 3 months after the injury usually have a very poor prognosis for recovery (4, 8, 11, 24).

Frequency This is something that usually happens on only one occasion to any given patient. However, the author has encountered a few patients over the years who have been sufficiently unlucky to sustain this injury on two, and in one memorable case, three occasions.

Area of Symptoms Symptoms are felt in the cervical spine, the shoulder girdle, the anterior chest wall, the side of the head or face, down one or both arms, and down the back as far as the base of the ribcage (Fig. 4.25). Headaches are also a common symptom in the majority of cases (4, 5, 7, 10).

Type of Symptoms Pain is the main presenting symptom, but there may also be complaints of paraesthesia and anesthesia in any or all of the areas described above (7, 8, 10, 13).

Miscellaneous The patient may complain of a variety of symptoms, such as visual disturbances, vertigo, nausea, dysphasia, hoarseness, and temporomandibular joint problems (1, 5, 7, 24).

Objective Findings

Observation The patient often presents with an observable degree of stiffness in the neck, which may be marked on occasions. (The author had one patient who was discovered sitting in the waiting room supporting her head with both hands, her thumbs under her jaw and her fingers supporting her occiput. She was unwilling to relinquish this degree of support even during testing of her movements and palpation of the spine.) Muscle spasm is often observable in the cervical paravertebral muscle and in the upper and middle trapezius bilaterally. There may be a lateral shift of the cervical spine away from the site of pain, if the pain is more unilateral in nature (1, 2, 11, 43).

Active Movements Usually all movements of the cervical spine are limited, some to an extreme degree. Depending on the mechanism of injury, either flexion or extension will be most limited, although on occasions both movements are equally limited. Side flexions are always, at least moderately, and often severely, limited. The degree of limitation of rotation to either side can vary considerably from case to case, some being near full, although painful, others being extremely limited. Retraction is always painful and limited to at least a moderate degree. Protraction may be the only movement that is not limited; however, it is still likely to be uncomfortable (7, 12, 18, 24).

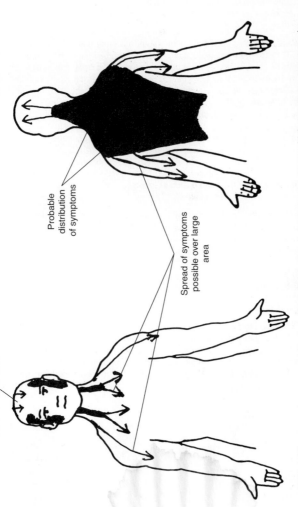

FIG. 4.25 Area of symptoms following whiplash injury, note the large area over which symptoms can spread.

Probable distribution of symptoms

Spread of symptoms possible over large area

Passive Movements Overpressure at end range of any of the movements will produce muscle spasm and voluntary guarding. The pattern of movement restriction should be the same as that encountered on active testing.

Resisted Movements Pain should be most marked on isometric side flexion of the cervical spine with the pain being experienced on the side that the patient is attempting to move towards. Again, all movements are likely to produce some degree of discomfort. Rotation, flexion, and extension are all likely to produce pain in the sides of the neck, the upper shoulder girdle, the anterior chest, or anterior neck (in the region of the sternomastoid muscle unilaterally or bilaterally). The degree of pain will vary from patient to patient, but should not be as great as that produced by either active or passive testing. Resisted elevation and retraction of the shoulder girdle may be uncomfortable, but should not be markedly so. All other movements of the shoulder girdle should be pain free. Isometric abduction of the shoulder at 90 degrees will tend to produce discomfort in the region of the upper trapezius muscle and at the base of the cervical spine on the affected side (4, 7, 13).

Palpation Tenderness is usually pronounced and may be both general and specific. Diffuse tenderness is felt in the paravertebral muscles of the cervical, and occasionally thoracic, spine, also in the region of the upper and middle trapezius, particularly around the medial border of the scapula. Tender points are usually found laterally in the cervical spine, in the muscle mass of the upper trapezius, and along the medial border of the scapula. Diffuse tenderness is usually experienced on palpation of all the muscles in the affected region, possibly because of the effects of prolonged muscle spasm (11, 13, 22).

Specific Tests X-rays are usually taken to preclude other more serious pathology before it is assumed that the patient is suffering from entirely soft-tissue injuries. There should be no neurological signs; if there are, whiplash should be considered as a separate issue that is combined with radiculopathy, as described in other conditions in this chapter, and treatment would therefore need to be reviewed and revised accordingly (13, 25, 38).

Treatment Ideas
(1, 4, 5, 7, 8, 10, 24, 34)

Where the patient demonstrates extreme discomfort, one option is to prescribe a soft cervical collar, which can be particularly useful in the very early stages. However, this option should not be considered lightly, as it may eventually prove impossible to wean the patient off this device. It is necessary to explain in detail (and write down for the patient) when the patient can wear the collar. This should be restricted to a maximum of 16 hours out of 24 for the first few days, then 50% of the time for a further week or two. The patient must be educated as regards the time required for healing of a soft-tissue injury, and it must be made clear that there will be no need to use a collar after that time period. The patient will usually get maximum pain relief from use of the collar if his neck is in a slightly flexed position when the collar is on. The patient can also be advised as regards the use of heat or ice at home to relieve both pain and muscle spasm.

Active exercises should be encouraged from an early stage, particularly movements of unaffected areas of the arms, trunk, and legs. Movements should first be attempted through pain-free ranges wherever and whenever possible. The patient should be advised to rest between sets of exercises with his head and shoulder girdle in a position that affords the least discomfort. This will usually be in lying with the head well supported by a soft pillow and the cervical spine in either a neutral or slightly flexed position. It is important not to be overly gentle or considerate at this time, otherwise progress will never occur. A plan of progression of active exercise should be written out for the patient and explained in terms of soft-tissue healing and restoration of function. The patient should also be advised to always sustain a moderate degree of exercise, as patients usually experience exacerbation and remission of their symptoms from time to time. The tendency is for them to increase and decrease their exercise levels as their symptoms increase and decrease, which simply accentuates the "good day/bad day" syndrome. It is better for the patient to continue with a steady rate of exercises, neither decreasing the amount of exercise when in pain nor increasing it when the pain decreases. In that way the change in level of symptoms will become less pronounced with time.

The use of any modality may be attempted to determine if it enables the patient to exercise more effectively or with less discomfort. There is often a tendency for the patient to become dependent on these passive modalities; this should be avoided by educating the patient as regards their use and constant reenforcement of an understanding of the beneficial effects of early active exercises. Exercises can be progressed by applying resistance to unaffected areas such as the legs, and then light resistance to the affected joints, particularly the upper extremities and shoulder girdle, with the use of light weights or a light exercise band initially used in lying, followed by progression into sitting or standing. The use of resisted exercises in non-affected areas is also a good test of patient compliance (if this happens to be an issue).

As pain levels decrease or localize, then manual stretching techniques for traction of the cervical spine and stretching of the shoulder girdle muscles into protraction and depression can be attempted to help loosen tense muscles. The main thrust of the active exercises is towards restoration of a good posture with retraction of the cervical spine and retraction and elevation of the shoulder girdle. These exercises should initially be carried out in lying and then in sitting and standing. Active exercises should progress to include all movements of the cervical spine, shoulder girdle, and upper extremities, with further progression to resisted exercises, initially for the shoulders, then the shoulder girdle, and finally the cervical spine. The patient will usually require constant encouragement and motivation to maintain these exercise levels. It is important to maintain progress in exercise no matter how slowly, and the patient should not be allowed to slide back into a reliance on passive modalities.

When the patient is able to cope with active stretches and resisted exercises using resistance bands or free weights, he should be progressed to functional exercises for lifting, carrying, pushing, and pulling-type activities with steadily increasing weights. This can be combined with a general gym exercise program with a mixture of cardiovascular exercise, endurance work, and strength training. As the patient progresses onto a resisted exercise program any persistent stiffness in the neck or shoulder girdle can be treated by passive movements with steady overpressure into the restricted ranges. The pressure applied should be light, but sustained for 30 to 60 seconds for each movement. The gym exercise program and functional resisted exercises should be progressed to a point that is suitable for the patient's normal lifestyle.

Restrictions The patient will usually restrict themselves adequately enough during the initial stages of this condition and the use of a soft collar helps in that respect. The patient should avoid prolonged static positioning of the neck and shoulder girdle or repeated movements of the neck. Use of the arms at or above shoulder height for any length of time, or with any more than light weights, will usually prove difficult and should be discontinued at the point when discomfort begins. It is very useful with this type of injury to put time limits on restrictions so that the patient realizes that these are not permanent. As the patient progresses through the treatment regime the restrictions should be modified to reflect the patient's objective improvement rather than his subjective complaints.

Cervical Spondylosis

Overview

There does not seem to be any general agreement on the description of either the pathophysiology or signs and symptoms relating to this condition. Various causes for the condition are postulated, including degenerative disc disease, facet joint arthropathy, and synovitis of the facet joints. The literal translation from the Latin would be "a problem with the joints of the neck." In the absence of other definitive evidence to indicate any other condition this is as good a description as any to cover the presenting signs and symptoms. In this case then we will adhere to the most benign description of the condition, which could best be stated as neck and shoulder girdle symptoms probably related to the normal process of wear and tear.

Over 90% of people at 50 years of age show signs of degenerative disc disease on x-ray examination of the cervical spine, but not all these people have symptoms in their neck and shoulder girdle. Radiological evidence of hypertrophic changes in the facet joints, such as the presence of osteophytes, is also not uncommon, and again are often present in the symptom-free individual. However, it is also hypothesized that irritation due to pressure from bony exotosis, or inflammatory reaction at the discs or ligaments and in the joints of the spine, could produce these sort of symptoms in the neck and shoulder girdle. Therefore, if a patient presents with signs and symptoms not typical of any other condition and in the absence of any other specific investigative results, there can really be no better description of the condition than "a problem with the joints of the neck" or cervical spondylosis. Conservative treatment is very effective in the majority of these cases (1, 2, 6, 11, 18).

Subjective Findings

Onset Onset is gradual with no known cause and occurs in patients usually between 40 and 60 years of age (11, 13, 18).

Duration The patient will have suffered their symptoms for at least a few weeks, and more often months or even years before seeking the advise of a health professional.

Frequency The patient typically gives a history of recurrent, gradually worsening symptoms occurring over a prolonged period of time, and of steadily increasing frequency and severity (2, 6, 13, 24).

Area of Symptoms The patient usually reports spread of symptoms starting in the cervical spine, where they are felt centrally or to either one or both sides. Pain will then radiate over the upper trapezius to the point of the shoulder and occasionally across the area of the scapula, unilaterally or bilaterally, and into the upper thoracic spine. Pain radiating over the head from the occiput to the frontal region is common and is often described as a form of headache (Fig. 4.26) (1, 2, 13).

Type of Symptoms The patient will describe an aching pain with increasing stiffness that is usually worse in the mornings. Headaches are a common complaint, although their frequency and duration can vary considerably from patient to patient.

Miscellaneous The patient often complains of crepitation (usually described as cracking and creaking) on movements of the neck, particularly rotation.

Objective Findings

Observation The patient's posture is usually poor, with protrusion of the head and rounding of the shoulders. A typical finding, particularly in the older patient, is a noticeable protrusion at the cervical/thoracic junction, commonly known as a "dowager's hump" (1, 2, 4, 18, 25).

Active Movements Normally all movements will be somewhat limited and the patient will complain of stiffness, but not necessarily any

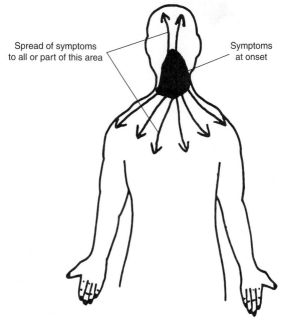

Spread of symptoms
to all or part of this area

Symptoms
at onset

FIG. 4.26   Area of symptoms in cervical spondylosis.

great deal of pain, at end range of motion. Protrusion of the neck is the exception to the rule, as it is seldom limited to any great extent and is usually pain free (18, 24).

Passive Movements   There is a stiff end feel to all limited movements and the patient will complain of pain at end range of one or two movements, most commonly rotation or side flexion to either or both sides (4, 11, 24).

Resisted Movements   There will be good strength on isometric testing of the musculature of the cervical spine and shoulder girdle. There should be no pain reported even when quite heavy resistance is applied to the movements.

Palpation   Diffuse tenderness can be elicited throughout the cervical spine and in the upper trapezius bilaterally. The muscles of the upper shoulder girdle and neck may feel tight and tense. Soft-tissue thickening may be palpable centrally at the lower cervical and upper thoracic region (dowager's hump) (2, 11, 22, 25).

Special Tests All neurological tests of the upper extremities should be unremarkable. X-ray studies may show degenerative changes (as they will in 90% of the population in the typical age range for patients suffering from this condition). A CAT scan or MRI studies may show foraminal impingement or other significant disc or joint problems, but in that case the patient's signs and symptoms should indicate one of the other conditions described previously in this chapter.

Treatment Ideas
(4, 6, 10, 11, 13, 14, 24, 35)

If the patient is suffering from a marked degree of discomfort then prescription of a soft cervical collar may help in the early stages of the condition. The patient should be advised to wear the collar for 1 hour on and 1 hour off, during the day for the first 2 to 3 weeks. The use of heat may be helpful, particularly before exercise or to promote relaxation at the start of treatment. Laser or ultrasound can be applied where point tenderness is elicited. Initially active exercises should be carried out through 50–75% of available range to loosen up the muscles, as the patient is often stiff due to pain and muscle tension or spasm. The patient should be instructed in the use of a towel roll or cervical roll, placed inside their pillowcase for sleeping, in order to support the natural curvature of the cervical spine.

By the second or third session of treatment it should be possible to try manual cervical traction; if the patient responds positively then mechanical traction, with light weights over 10 to 15 minute periods, will often produce quite prolonged periods of symptom relief. Active exercises can be progressed to full available range, with emphasis placed on those movements that prove to be least painful. A simple rule of thumb is to have the patient do twice as many movements into the pain-free ranges as they do into the ones more likely to produce discomfort. No movement should be carried beyond the point of onset of pain.

Further progression can be made by the use of passive movements or auto-assisted movements to apply stretch at the end range of pain-free movements. These passive movements should be carried out in short bursts, with long rests between each set of exercises. In many cases at this point in the treatment program the gains in mobility will be quite significant.

When the patient is comfortable with the active exercises then postural re-education should be started, with the use of neuromuscular stimulation to provide elevation and retraction of the shoulder girdle while the patient works on resisted exercises to strengthen the muscles of the neck and shoulder girdle. A program of neck education is essential and should contain information on the common causes of neck problems and how to avoid them. This is then related to the patient's exercise program in the clinic and at home. Initially isometric neck exercises should be employed with the patient sitting or lying in their most pain-free position; this is then progressed to isotonic strengthening with a headband attached to resistance band.

Further progress can be achieved by a general upper extremity and upper body workout with appropriate cervical, thoracic, and upper extremity stretches interspersed throughout the resisted exercise program. This sort of resisted exercise program should only be used when the patient's symptoms are decreasing and there are signs of better posture, as strengthening exercises used while the patient still demonstrates a poor head, neck, and shoulder girdle posture will only help to strengthen that poor postural position. Because of the nature of this condition, and its probable relationship to degeneration through wear and tear in the cervical spine, it will be necessary for the patient to continue with a home exercise program of stretching and strengthening exercises for an indefinite period. For that reason the program should be made as simple and as short as possible to encourage ongoing compliance with the treatment program once the patient has finished attending the clinic.

Restrictions   If a soft collar is used in the early stages of treatment it will usually be an effective form of restriction as regards any activities that are likely to reproduce the patient's symptoms. Repetitive movements of the cervical spine, awkward postures, or sustained positioning of the neck and shoulder girdle are usually self limited by discomfort; nevertheless, the patient should still be advised to avoid or revise these activities. In most cases the patient simply needs to be reminded of the fact that as the symptoms decrease he will find that he is able to carry out more activities without producing any discomfort. The patient should then use pain as a guide and stop activities that produce discomfort at that time. Continuing with an activity or sustaining a position that produces the symptoms will inevitably lead back down the road to further treatment, and if a patient wishing to avoid this must then remain constantly aware of the condition and revise his daily activities accordingly. He should keep the soft collar handy, particularly for long car journeys, and as a temporary measure for pain relief when the condition is exacerbated, as may happen from time to time, particularly if the patient exercises less consistently.

REFERENCES

1. Payton O.D. (ed): Manual of Physical Therapy. Churchill Livingston, New York, 1989
2. Braddom R.L. (ed): Physical Medicine and Rehabilitation. W.B. Saunders, Philadelphia, 1996
3. Salter R.B.: Textbook of Disorders and Injuries of the Muscular Skeletal System (3rd ed). Williams and Wilkins, Baltimore, 1999
4. Skinner H.B. (ed): Current Diagnosis and Treatment in Orthopaedics. Appleton and Lange, Norwalk, CT, 1995
5. Crowther C.L.: Primary Orthopaedic Care. Mosby, St. Louis, 1999

6. Dandy D.J., Edwards D.J.: Essential Orthopaedics and Trauma (3rd ed). Churchill Livingston, New York, 1998

7. Mercier, L.R.: Practical Orthopaedics (4th ed). Mosby Yearbook, St Louis, 1991

8. Bland, J.H.: Disorders of the Cervical Spine: Diagnosis and Medical Management (2nd ed). W.B. Saunders, Philadelphia, 1994

9. McKenzie R.A.: The Cervical and Thoracic Spine: Mechanical Diagnosis and Therapy. Spinal Publications (N.Z.), Waikanae, New Zealand, 1990

10. Grant R.. (ed): Physical Therapy of the Cervical and Thoracic Spine (2nd ed). Churchill Livingston, New York, 1994

11. Corrigan B., Maitland G.D.: Practical Orthopaedic Medicine. Butterworth, London, U.K., 1983

12. Gross J., Feeto J., Rosen E.: Musculoskeletal Examination. Blackwell Science, Cambridge, MA, 1996

13. Snider R.K. (ed): Essential of Musculoskeletal Care. American Academy of Orthopaedic Surgeons, Rosemont, IL, 1997

14. Donatelli R.A., Wooden M.J. (eds): Orthopaedic Physical Therapy (2nd ed). Churchill Livingston, New York, 1994

15. Mertagh J., Kenna C.J.: Back Pain and Spinal Manipulation (2nd ed). Butterworth Heinemann, Oxford, U.K., 1997

16. Hadler N.M.: Occupational Musculoskeletal Disorders (2nd ed). Lippincott, Williams and Wilkins, Philadelphia, 1999

17. Kesson M., Atkins E.: Orthopaedic Medicine: A Practical Approach. Butterworth Heinemann, Oxford, U.K., 1998

18. Apley A.G., Solomon L.: Apley's System of Orthopaedics and Fractures (6th ed). Butterworth, London, 1983

19. Prentice W.E.: Rehabilitation Techniques in Sports Medicine. WCB/McGraw Hill, New York, 1999

20. Anderson B.C.: Office Orthopaedics for Primary Care: Diagnosis and Treatment (2nd ed). W.B. Saunders, Philadelphia, 1999

21. Konin J.G., Wilksten D.L., Isear J.A.: Special Tests for Orthopaedic Examination. Slack, New Jersey, 1997

22. Field D.: Anatomy: Palpation and Surface Markings (2nd ed). Butterworth Heinemann, Oxford, U.K., 1997

23. Malone T.R., McPoil T.G., Nitz A.J. (eds): Orthopaedic and Sports Physical Therapy (3rd ed). St. Louis, 1997

24. Corrigan B., Maitland G.D.: Practical Orthopaedic Medicine. Butterworth, London, 1983

25. Magee D.J.: Orthopaedic Physical Assessment (2nd ed). W.B. Saunders, Philadelphia, 1992

26. Moses A., Carman J.: Anatomy of the Cervical Spine: Implications for the Upper Limb Tension Test. Aus. J. Physiother., 42 (1):31–35, 1996

27. Hall T., Quinter J.: Response to Mechanical Stimulation of the Upper Limb in Painful Cervical Radiculopathy. Aus. J. Physiother., 42 (4):277–285, 1996

28. Lewis J., Ramot R., Green A.: Changes in Mechanical Tension In the Median Nerve: Possible Implications for the Upper Limb Tension Test. Physiotherapy, 84:254–261, 1998

29. Saal J.S., Saal J.A., Yurth E.F.: Non-Operative Management of Herniated Cervical Intervertebral Disc with Radiculopathy: An Outcome. Spine, 21: 1877–1883, 1996

30. Lu J., et al. Cervical Intervertebral Disc Space Narrowing and Size of Intervertible Foramina. Clin. Orthop., 370:259–264, 2000

31. Debois V., et al. Soft Cervical Disc Herniation: Influence of Cervical Spine Canal Measurements on Development of Neurological Symptoms. Spine, 24:1996–2002, 1996.

32. Zylbergold R.S., Piper M.C.: Cervical Spine Disorder: A Comparison of Three Types of Traction. Spine 10:867–871, 1985

33. Grant R., Jull G., Spencer T.: Active Stabilization Training for Screen-Based Keyboard Operators: A Single Case Study. Aus. J. Physiother., 43 (4):235–242, 1997

34. Carter V.M. et al. The Effect of a Soft Collar Used as Normally Recommended or Reversed on Three Planes of Cervical Range of Motion. J. Orthop. Sports Phys. Ther., 23:209–215, 1996

35. Sweezey R.L., Sweezey A.M., Warner K.: Efficacy of Home Cervical Traction Therapy. Am. J. Phys. Med. Rehabil. 78 (1):30–32, 1999

36. Meyer J.R.: Diffuse Idiopathic Skeletal Hyperostosis in the Cervical Spine. Clin. Orthop., 359:49–57, 1999

37. Grimmer K.: An Investigation of Poor Cervical Resting Posture. Aus. J. Physiother., 43 (1):7–16, 1997

38. Yeung E., Jones M., Hall B.: The Response to The Slump Test in a Group of Female Whiplash Patients. Aus. J. Physiother., 43 (4):245–252, 1997

39. P: The T4 Syndrome: Some Basic Science Aspects. Physiotherapy, 83: 186–189, 1997

40. Karas S.E.: Thoracic Outlet Syndrome. Clin. Sports Med., 9:296–310, 1990

41. Leffert R.D., Perlmutter G.S.: Thoracic Outlet Syndrome: Results of 282 Transaxillary First Rib Resections. Clin. Orthop. 368:66–79, 1999

42. Laporte C. et al. Severe Hyperflexion Sprains of the Cervical Spine in Adults. Clin. Orthop., 363:126–134, 1999

43. Livingston M.: Common Whiplash Injury: A Modern Epidemic. Charles C. Thomas, Spring Field, 1999

The following tables contain test movements for examination of the low back and pelvis. The starting positions and a description of each movement are given. These would be considered the optimal test positions in each case, but should be modified for individual patients who are unable to achieve or sustain a described position.

Active Movements of The Low Back

Name of Movement	Starting Position	Movement
Flexion	The movement is best tested in standing and then repeated in supine lying. Standing: The patient stands erect with his hands resting at his sides. Supine Lying: The patient lies flat on his back with knees bent and feet flat on the treatment table.	Standing: The patient is instructed to bend forwards, sliding his hands down the anterior aspect of his thighs and lower legs to try and touch his feet. Supine Lying: The patient is instructed to bring both knees up towards his chest with his hands remaining at his sides throughout the movement.
Extension	The movement is best tested in standing and then in prone lying. Standing: The patient stands erect with his hands placed on his buttocks. Prone Lying: The patient lies flat on his stomach with his hands placed palm down and level with his shoulders.	Standing: The patient is instructed to arch his back, leaning backwards as far as possible while keeping his hands on his buttocks. Prone Lying: The patient is instructed to raise his head and shoulders by pushing up on his arms while keeping his pelvis on the treatment table, so as to arch the lower back (a "sloppy push-up").

(continued)

Active Movements of The Low Back (*continued*)

Name of Movement	Starting Position	Movement
Side Flexion	The movement is best tested in standing, but can also be tested in sitting or supine lying.	The patient is instructed to take one hand down the outside of the leg on the same side, moving as far down towards the floor as possible.
	The patient stands with his feet slightly apart and his hands resting at his side.	The movement is repeated on the opposite side.

Rotation is normally tested during examination of the low back and is carried out as described in the thoracic spine. No rotation occurs in the lumbar spine because of the alignment of the surfaces of the facet joints laterally and medially. However, rotation in the thoracic spine can torsion soft-tissue structures in the low back and pelvis and therefore should be testing during examination.

Resisted Movements in the Low Back

Name of Movement	Starting Position	Movement
Flexion	The movement is tested in supine lying with the patient's knees flexed so that his feet are flat on the treatment table. Hands are placed at the side.	The patient is instructed to place his hands on his thighs, then raise his head and slide his hands up the thighs towards the knees. Pressure can be applied to the anterior of the patient's chest to further resist movement.
		The patient may instead be instructed to raise his feet off the treatment table while keeping the knees bent. Pressure is applied to the knees to increase resistance.
Extension	The movement is tested with the patient in prone lying with a hand placed over each scapula. The patient's hands are placed at his side.	The patient is instructed to try and raise his chest off the treatment table while downward pressure is applied to prevent the movement from occurring.

Resisted Movements in the Low Back (*continued*)

Name of Movement	Starting Position	Movement
Rotation	The movement is tested in sitting. The patient sits upright with his arms folded across his chest. Place your right hand at the posterior of the right shoulder and your left hand at the anterior of the left shoulder to test right rotation. The hand positions are reversed when testing left rotation.	To test right rotation push the patient's right shoulder forward while pulling the left shoulder backwards. The patient resists the movement to maintain the neutral position. Hand pressures are reversed to test left rotation.
Side Flexion	The movement is tested in sitting with the patient sitting upright with his arms resting at his sides. The right hand is placed on the lateral aspect of the patient's right upper arm over the deltoid muscle to test right-side flexion. The left hand is placed on the left deltoid to test left-side flexion.	To test right-side flexion, push the patient toward the left side while the patient resists the movement maintaining the neutral position. Pressure is applied to the left side to push the patient towards the right in order to check left-side flexion.

Examination Findings Related to Specific Conditions of the Low Back and Pelvis

	Onset			
Sudden Due to Trauma	Sudden Due to Overuse	Sudden with No Cause	Gradual Due to Overuse	Gradual with No Cause
Sacroiliac Joint Strain Lumbar Muscle Strain Lumbar Facet Joint Strain Combined Lumbar Disc/Facet Joint Problem	Lumbar Disc (with Radiculopathy) Sacroiliac Joint Strain Lumbar Muscle Strain Combined Lumbar Disc and Facet Joint Irritation	Lumbar Disc (with Radiculopathy) Lumbar Disc (no Radiculopathy) Combined Lumbar Disc/Facet Joint Irritation	Facet Joint Irritation (no Radiculopathy) Low Back Postural Strain	Facet Joint Irritation (no Radiculopathy) Low Back Postural Strain Facet Joint Irritation (with Radiculopathy) Spinal Stenosis Chronic Spinal Instability

	Typical Age Ranges			
15–35 Years	20–40 Years	20–50 Years	35–55 Years	50 Years +
Chronic Spinal Instability	Sacroiliac Joint Strain	Lumbar Muscle Strain Low Back Postural Sprain Lumbar Facet Joint Strain	Lumbar Disc (no Radiculopathy) Lumbar Disc (with Radiculopathy)	Facet Joint Irritation (no Radiculopathy) Facet Joint Irritation (with Radiculopathy) Spinal Stenosis

Duration

1–3 Weeks	1–6 Weeks	3–6 Weeks	6 Weeks–3 Months	3 Months–6 Months +
Lumbar Disc Lesion (with Radiculopathy)	Lumbar Disc Lesion (no Radiculopathy)	Sacroiliac Joint Strain	Facet Joint Irritation (no Radiculopathy)	Spinal Stenosis
Lumbar Muscle Strain	Combined Lumbar Disc/Facet Joint Irritation	Low Back Postural Strain	Facet Joint Irritation (with Radiculopathy)	Chronic Spinal Instability
Lumbar Facet Joint Strain				

Frequency

Steadily Increasing Episodes over 1 or More Years	Recurrent Back Problems, but First Time with Leg Symptoms	First Time Suffering These Symptoms	Previous Back Problems, but These Symptoms are Different
Lumbar Disc (no Radiculopathy)	Lumbar Disc (with Radiculopathy)	Sacroiliac Joint Strain	Combined Lumbar Disc/Facet Joint Problem
Facet Joint Irritation (no Radiculopathy)	Facet Joint Irritation (with Radiculopathy)	Lumbar Muscle Strain	Spinal Stenosis
Sacroiliac Joint Strain		Lumbar Facet Joint Strain	
Low Back Postural Strain			
Spinal Stenosis			
Chronic Spinal Instability			

(continued)

Examination Findings of Specific Conditions of the Low Back and Pelvis (*continued*)

Area of Symptoms

Across Low Back	In Low Back—More To One Side	Low Back—One Side Only	Pain in Back and Buttock	Lateral Hip Region	Pain Spreading to Thoracic Region
Low Back Postural Strain	Lumbar Disc (no Radiculopathy)	Lumbar Disc (no Radiculopathy)	Lumbar Disc (no Radiculopathy)	Lumbar Disc (no Radiculopathy)	Low Back Postural Strain
Spinal Instability	Lumbar Disc (with Radiculopathy)	Sacroiliac Joint Strain	Lumbar Disc (with Radiculopathy)	Lumbar Disc (with Radiculopathy)	
	Facet Joint Strain	Lumbar Muscle Strain	Sacroiliac Joint Strain	Spinal Instability	
	Spinal Stenosis		Facet Joint Irritation (with Radiculopathy)	Combined Lumbar Disc/Facet Joint Problem	
	Lumbar Muscle Strain		Spinal Instability		
	Combined Lumbar Disc/Facet Joint Problem				

In Leg to Knee	In Leg to Foot	Both Sides of Back Equally	Central Lumbar Pain
Lumbar Disc (with Radiculopathy)	Lumbar Disc (with Radiculopathy)	Low Back Postural Strain	Facet Joint Irritation (with Radiculopathy)
Sacroiliac Joint Strain	Combined Lumbar Disc/Facet Joint Problem	Facet Joint Irritation (no Radiculopathy)	Facet Joint Irritation (no Radiculopathy)
Facet Joint Irritation (with Radiculopathy)		Facet Joint Strain	Facet Joint Strain
Combined Lumbar Disc/Facet Joint Problem			Spinal Stenosis

Type of Symptoms

Constant Ache in the Low Back	Occasional Sharp Pain in Back	Sharp Pain on Back Movements	Constant Sharp Pain in Back	Occasional Ache in Low Back	Ache in Back And Buttocks	Aching Back Just Sitting
Sacroiliac Joint Strain	Facet Joint Irritation (no Radiculopathy)	Lumbar Disc (no Radiculopathy)	Lumbar Disc Lesion (with Radiculopathy)	Facet Joint Strain	Sacroiliac Joint Strain	Low Back Postural Strain
Lumbar Disc (no Radiculopathy)	Facet Joint Irritation (with Radiculopathy)	Facet Joint Irritation (with Radiculopathy)		Low Back Postural Strain	Facet Joint Irritation (with Radiculopathy)	Lumbar Disc Lesion (with Radiculopathy)
Facet Joint Irritation (no Radiculopathy)	Facet Joint Strain	Facet Joint Irritation (no Radiculopathy)		Sacroiliac Joint Strain		Lumbar Disc Lesion (no Radiculopathy)
Low Back Postural Strain		Lumbar Muscle Strain		Spinal Stenosis		
		Facet Joint Strain				

Ache in Back after Activity	Tingling/Numbness in Leg	Pain in Leg	Sense of Heaviness in Both Legs	Bilateral Symptoms in Legs	Sensation of a Lump in the Back	Spasm in Back Muscles
Lumbar Muscle Strain	Lumbar Disc Lesions (with Radiculopathy)	Lumbar Disc (with Radiculopathy)	Sacroiliac Joint Strain	Spinal Stenosis	Low Back Postural Strain	Any of the Back Conditions
	Spinal Stenosis	Facet Joint Irritation (with Radiculopathy)	Spinal Stenosis			
		Spinal Stenosis				

(continued)

Examination Findings of Specific Conditions of the Low Back and Pelvis (continued)

	Observation					
Flattening of Lumbar Lordosis	Increased Lumbar Lordosis	Shift of Spine to One Side	Sitting with Weight Taken Off One Buttock	Spasm in Paravertebral Muscles	Spasm More Pronounced on One Side	Limp Favoring One Leg
Lumbar Disc Lesion (with Radiculopathy)	Facet Joint Irritation (with Radiculopathy)	Lumbar Disc (with Radiculopathy)	Lumbar Disc (with Radiculopathy)	Can Occur in Any of the Back Conditions	Lumbar Disc (with Radiculopathy)	Lumbar Disc (with Radiculopathy)
Lumbar Disc Lesion (no Radiculopathy)	Facet Joint Irritation (no Radiculopathy)	Facet Joint Strain			Lumbar Muscle Strain	Sacroiliac Joint Strain
Sacroiliac Joint Strain	Sacroiliac Strain					
Lumbar Muscle Strain	Spinal Stenosis					
Low Back Postural Strain	Spinal Instability					
Facet Joint Strain						
Combined Lumbar Disc/Facet Joint Problem						

Active Movements

Lumbar Flexion Limited and Produces Typical Symptoms	Lumbar Extension—No Symptoms or Less Symptoms	Lumbar Flexion and Extension are Limited and Produce Typical Symptoms	Extension Limited and Produces Typical Symptoms	Flexion Stiff but No Typical Symptoms	Pain Mainly on Rising From Flexion
Lumbar Disc Lesion (with Radiculopathy)	Lumbar Disc (with Radiculopathy)	Combined Lumbar Disc/Facet Joint Problem	Facet Joint Irritation (no Radiculopathy)	Facet Joint Irritation (with Radiculopathy)	Sacroiliac Joint Strain
Lumbar Disc Lesion (no Radiculopathy)	Lumbar Disc (no Radiculopathy)	Lumbar Disc (with Radiculopathy) (Large Protrusion)	Facet Joint Irritation (with Radiculopathy)	Facet Joint Problems (no Radiculopathy)	
Combined Lumbar Disc/Facet Joint Problem		Facet Joint Strain	Sacroiliac Joint Strain	Spinal Stenosis	
			Combined Lumbar Disc/Facet Joint Problem		
			Spinal Stenosis		

(continued)

Examination Findings of Specific Conditions of the Low Back and Pelvis (continued)

Side Flexion to One Side Produces Typical Symptoms	Rotation Stiff with Pulling Sensation	Straight Leg Raising Limited and Painful	All Movements Full and Pain Free
Lumbar Disc (with Radiculopathy)	Facet Joint Strain	Lumbar Disc (with Radiculopathy)	Low Back Postural Strain
Facet Joint Irritation (with Radiculopathy)		Combined Lumbar Disc/Facet Joint Problem	Spinal Instability
Facet Joint Irritation (no Radiculopathy)			
Sacroiliac Joint Strain			

Passive Movements

Back Pain on Flexion Overpressure	Only Leg Pain on Flexion Overpressure	Back and Leg Pain on Flexion Overpressure	Back and Leg Symptoms on Extension Overpressure	Pain on Both Flexion and Extension Overpressure	Pain in Low Back on Rotation Overpressure
Lumbar Muscle Strain	Lumbar Disc Lesion (with Radiculopathy)	Lumbar Disc Lesion (with Radiculopathy)	Facet Joint Irritation (with Radiculopathy)	Combined Lumbar Disc/Facet Joint Problem	Sacroiliac Joint Strain
Lumbar Disc Lesion (with Radiculopathy)		Combined Lumbar Disc/Facet Joint Problem	Spinal Stenosis	Sacroiliac Joint Strain	Lumbar Muscle Strain
Lumbar Disc Lesion (no Radiculopathy)				Facet Joint Strain	

Solid Block to Extension	Poor Intervertebral Mobility on P/A Pressure	Pain on P/A Pressure Lumbar Spine	Excessive Degree of Flexibility	No Pain and Full Range of Movement
Facet Joint Irritation (with Radiculopathy)	Lumbar Disc Lesion (with Radiculopathy)	Lumbar Disc Lesion (no Radiculopathy)	Spinal Instability	Low Back Postural Strain
Facet Joint Irritation (with no Radiculopathy)	Lumbar Disc Lesion (no Radiculopathy)	Lumbar Disc Lesion (with Radiculopathy)		Spinal Instability
Combined Lumbar Disc/Facet Joint Problem	Facet Joint Irritation (no Radiculopathy)	Facet Joint Irritation (with Radiculopathy)		
Spinal Stenosis	Facet Joint Problem (with Radiculopathy)	Facet Joint Problem (no Radiculopathy)		
	Combined Lumbar Disc/Facet Joint Problem	Combined Lumbar Disc/Facet Joint Problem		

Resisted Movements

No Pain and Good Strength	Strongly Resisted Movements Produce Back Pain	Pain on Extension of Back or Hips	Painless Weakness in Legs
Lumbar Disc (with Radiculopathy)	Facet Joint Irritation (with Radiculopathy)	Lumbar Muscle Strain	Lumbar Disc (with Radiculopathy)
Lumbar Disc (no Radiculopathy)	Facet Joint Problems (no Radiculopathy)		
Facet Joint Irritation (with Radiculopathy)	Sacroiliac Joint Strain		
Facet Joint Irritation (no Radiculopathy)	Lumbar Facet Joint Strain		
Low Back Postural Strain	Combined Lumbar Disc/Facet Joint Problem		
Combined Lumbar Disc/Facet Joint Problem			
Spinal Stenosis			
Spinal Instability			

(continued)

Examination Findings of Specific Conditions of the Low Back and Pelvis (continued)

	Palpation					
Poor Lumbar Intervertebral Mobility	General Tenderness over Paravertebral Muscles	Tenderness Central Lumbar Spine	Specific Tender Points in the Paravertebral Muscle	Tenderness around Posterior Superior Iliac Spine	Excessive Intervertebral Mobility	Muscle Spasm/Tension in Low Back
Lumbar Disc Lesion (with Radiculopathy)	Lumbar Disc Lesion (with Radiculopathy)	Facet Joint Irritation (with Radiculopathy)	Lumbar Muscle Strain	Sacroiliac Joint Strain (or Associated with Chronicity in any of the Other Conditions)	Spinal Instability	Any of the Back Conditions
Lumbar Disc Lesion (no Radiculopathy)	Lumbar Disc Lesion (no Radiculopathy)	Facet Joint Irritation (no Radiculopathy)				
Facet Joint Irritation (with Radiculopathy)	Facet Joint Irritation (no Radiculopathy)	Combined Lumbar Disc/Facet Joint Problem				
Facet Joint Irritation (no Radiculopathy)	Combined Lumbar Disc/Facet Joint Problem	Lumbar Muscle Strain				
Combined Lumbar Disc/Facet Joint Problem	Sacroiliac Joint Strain					
Low Back Postural Strain	Low Back Postural Strain					
Lumbar Facet Joint Strain						
Spinal Stenosis						

PALPATION OF THE LOW BACK AND PELVIS

In this section a description is given of the method of palpating each structure referred to in relation to the following conditions:

- Lumbar disc lesion (no radiculopathy)
- Lumbar disc lesion (with radiculopathy)
- Lumbar facet joint irritation (no radiculopathy)
- Sacroiliac joint strain
- Lumbar muscle strain
- Low back postural strain
- Lumbar facet joint irritation (with radiculopathy)
- Lumbar facet joint strain
- Combined lumbar disc/facet joint problem
- Spinal stenosis
- Chronic spinal instability

Iliac Crests

With the patient standing, the hands are placed on the patient's waist from the rear. The hands are then taken down caudally until they reach the bony ridges that are the iliac crests (Fig. 5.1). These may be quite difficult to identify in the obese patient.

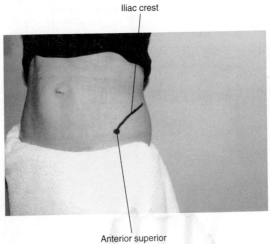

FIG. 5.1 Surface marking of the right iliac crest and the anterior superior iliac spine.

Anterior Superior Iliac Spine (ASIS)

Having identified the iliac crests, bring the hands forward so they move onto a protrusion at the anterior of the iliac crest, which is the anterior superior iliac spine (Fig. 5.1).

Posterior/Superior Iliac Spine (PSIS)

These are most easily identified with the patient lying prone, but can also be found with the patient in the standing position. The hand is taken around the iliac crest posteriorly to the point where a dimple can be seen and palpated at the posterior extent of the crest (Fig. 5.2). This marks the position of the posterior superior iliac spine where the subcutaneous tissues attaches directly to the bone. These are harder to identify in men and are far closer to the spine in men than in women.

Sacroiliac Joint

This is not truly palpation of the sacroiliac joint as such, but a finger placed a thumb's-breadth medial and distal to the posterior superior iliac spine is over the posterior extent of the sacroiliac joint (Fig. 5.2).

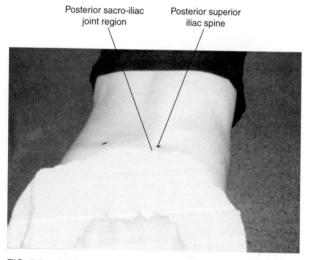

FIG. 5.2 Dimples marking the position of the posterior superior iliac spines and point for palpation at the posterior of the sacroiliac joint.

Thoracolumbar Paravertebral Muscles

These are easily palpated muscular ridges on either side of the spine that can be observed with the patient in the standing, sitting, or prone lying position (Fig. 5.3). After observing many normal spines it is possible to differentiate between well-developed muscle, good muscle tone, poor muscle tone, muscle spasm, and muscle tension in this area.

Spinous Processes (Fig. 5.4 and 5.7)

These processes will stand out better with the patient lying prone with one or two pillows placed under the abdomen and pelvis to provide some flexion of the spine. Starting with the fingers on the posterior superior iliac spines, move to the mid line of the sacrum, at which point a finger will be at the level of the second sacral vertebrae (S2). Palpating up two spinous processes the finger will lie on the fifth lumbar spinous process. This is often described as being like a steeple in a valley, as the body of L5 lies slightly anterior to the others and it's process is shorter. Careful palpation is required when moving up the spine from one spinous process to another. Constant referral to a model of the spine while doing this will improve proficiency.

Thoraco-lumbar
paravertebral muscles

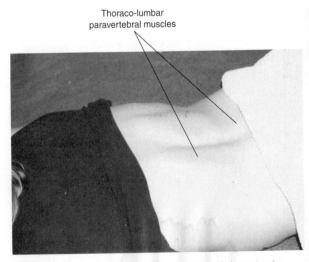

FIG. 5.3 Thoraco-lumbar paravertebral muscles during extension of the back.

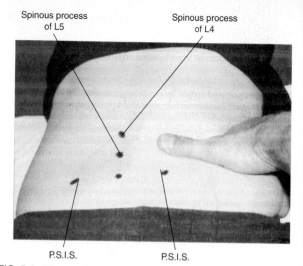

FIG. 5.4 The posterior superior iliac spines and spinous processes of L4 and L5. The examiner's hand is resting on the right iliac crest and thumb points towards the L4-5 interspace.

Spinous process of L5

Spinous process of L4

P.S.I.S.

P.S.I.S.

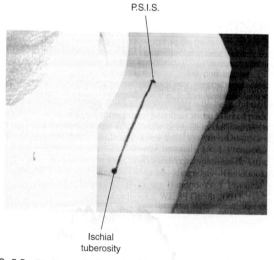

P.S.I.S.

Ischial tuberosity

FIG. 5.5 The line marks the area of the sacro-tuberous ligament, between the posterior superior iliac spine and the ischial tuberosity.

L4–L5 Interspace

The space between the fourth and fifth lumbar vertebrae is at the center of a line drawn horizontally across the back at the level of the highest point on the iliac crests. With the hands resting palms downward on the top of the iliac crests, the thumbs will point towards this interspace (Fig. 5.4).

Sacrotuberus Ligament (Fig. 5.5)

This ligament lies along a straight line passing distally down from the posterior superior iliac spine to the ischial turberosity.

Ischial Tuberosity

The easiest way to find the ischial tuberosity is to have the patient sit on your hands so that you can feel these rounded bony processes that bear the patient's weight during sitting. They can also be felt with the patient lying prone, although this requires moderately deep palpation at the medial side of the lower half of the buttock (Fig. 5.5 and 5.6).

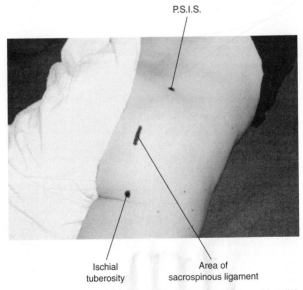

P.S.I.S.

Ischial tuberosity

Area of sacrospinous ligament

FIG. 5.6   The line marks the area of the sacrospinus ligament (medial to a line between the posterior superior iliac spine and the ischial tuberosity).

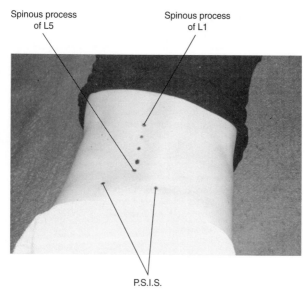

Spinous process of L5

Spinous process of L1

P.S.I.S.

FIG. 5.7 Spinous processes of the lumbar spine.

Sacrospinous Ligament (Fig. 5.6)

This ligament lies just medial to a line drawn between the posterior superior iliac spine and the ischial tuberosity, at about the halfway point.

Skin Sensation

It is important when assessing the back to assess the patient's skin sensation over the area of the dermatomes in the lower extremities. Tools required are a sharp pin for pinprick and a fine brush for light touch. Instruct the patient to close his eyes and respond whenever he feels contact, either with a pinprick or a brush. The patient should not be asked each time if he feels the touch. Rather, he should be told to respond each time he feels it, so that there is no misleading hint. It is best to instruct the patient to say "yes" every time something is felt Any area of apparent loss of sensation should be retested. Sometimes there may be outright numbness, but sometimes the patient may feel that there is simply a difference between one side as compared to the other, which is a sign of paraesthesia rather than anesthesia.

SPECIFIC TESTS FOR THE LOW BACK AND PELVIS

Knee Reflexes

Reflexes are best tested in the sitting position with the patient's lower leg hanging over the edge of a bed or treatment table and the feet clear of the floor. The patella tendon is struck sharply with a reflex hammer, which should produce a twitch in the quadriceps muscle. If there is difficulty eliciting a response in both knees the patient should be instructed to clasp his hands together and grip tightly, while at the same time try to pull the hands apart while clenching the teeth. This will produce a more marked reflex response. Decreased or absent knee reflexes unilaterally suggest an L3/L4 nerve root conduction deficit.

Ankle Reflexes

The patient can either be tested lying prone or kneeling with the feet off the end of a treatment table or chair. Strike the Achilles tendon with a reflex hammer and a twitch should occur in the calf muscle. This is most easily observed by watching the forefoot for the movement of plantar flexion. Again, if difficulty is encountered in eliciting the response bilaterally, then the patient is told to grip the bed, treatment table, or chair while clenching the teeth. Decreased or absent ankle reflexes suggest a problem with the L5/S1 nerve root.

Myotomes

The muscle groups listed in Table 5.1 are tested isometrically for the presence of painless weakness, which would indicate involvement of the specified nerve root:

TABLE 5.1 Myotomes in the Lower Extremity

Nerve Root	Specific Muscle Weakness
L3	Hip Flexion
	Knee Extension
L4	Ankle Dorsiflexion
	Great Toe Extension
L5	Great Toe Extension
	Foot Eversion
	Hip Abduction
	Knee Flexion
S1	Ankle Plantar Flexion (this is tested by having the patient attempt a heel raise in single-stance weight-bearing)
	Knee Flexion
	Foot Eversion
S2	Toe Flexion
	Ankle Plantar Flexion
	Knee Flexion

Straight Leg Raising

This test is performed with the patient lying supine. Support the patient's leg at the ankle and posterior of the knee. Raise the leg (hip flexion), keeping the knee straight. When the point is reached at which the patient feels discomfort, lower the leg slightly to the point where the discomfort eases. Then passively dorsiflex the foot. The discomfort should recur. During the first 70 degrees of movement stretch is applied to the L4–L5 and S1–S2 nerve roots, therefore pain that occurs on testing after 70 degrees of range is likely to be arising from the lumbar/pelvic joints. Pain arising before 70 degrees of hip flexion suggestion impingement or irritation of the above-mentioned nerve roots.

Cross Over Sign

If the patient complains of pain in the affected leg during straight leg raise testing of the unaffected leg, a central posterior bulging of the disc is suggested.

Dural Signs

Pinching of the dura can be tested for by holding the straight leg raise at the point of discomfort and then having the patient flex his neck. This will produce a sharp increase in pain if the dura is impinged. Another form of this test is to carry the straight leg raise to the point of pain, then lower the leg fractionally so that the discomfort disappears. If it reappears on flexion of the neck while the leg is held at that point, dural impingement is indicated.

Femoral Stretch (Prone Knee Bending)

With the patient lying prone, flex the knee as far as possible. With the knee held in the fully flexed position passively extend the patient's hip. If pain is produced in the patient's back or thigh on this maneuver, a lesion of the third lumbar, or more rarely second lumbar, nerve root is suggested.

Stressing the SI Joints

There are a great many tests described for the sacroiliac joint, unfortunately, false positives and false negatives are very common. Three of the passive tests and two of the resisted tests are listed. Pain on testing, felt at the sides of the low back at the level of the lumbar/sacral junction, would suggest a sacroiliac problem:

1. With the patient lying prone apply pressure to the apex of the sacrum (the palm of the hand is placed on the sacrum at the level of the posterior superior iliac spines). The pressure is applied to produce a posterior/anterior gliding effect of the sacrum.
2. With the patient lying supine place the palm of the hands on the anterior/superior iliac spines. To apply the most effective pressure

cross the arms over so that the right hand is on the left ASIS and visa versa. With the hands in this position attempt to push the pelvis, which will apply a compression force to the sacroiliac joints.

3. With the patient lying supine the hands are placed on the lateral aspect of the anterior superior iliac spines bilaterally, then inward pressure is applied, which will produce a distraction force at the sacroiliac joints.

4. The patient lying supine with the knees flexed is told to squeeze the knees together while you try to push the knees apart by applying pressure to the medial aspect of each knee (resisted hip adduction).

5. With the patient in the same position as for test number 4, press on the outsides of the knees, pushing them together, as the patient tries to push the knees apart (resisted hip abduction and lateral rotation).

LOW BACK AND PELVIS CONDITIONS

Lumbar Disc Lesion (No Radiculopathy)

Overview

This condition can be considered as some form of disruption of the posterior or posterolateral portion of a lumbar disc, or of the tissue that supports this area of the disc. No disc material has protruded and the nerve tissue in the area has not suffered any direct pressure. This condition is often self limiting in nature and will clear spontaneously in about 6 weeks, unless the patient is continuing with activities or undergoing treatment that exacerbates the condition. However, despite the fact that this episode will clear on its own, the condition itself is both recurrent and progressive in nature. The final goal of treatment therefore is to prevent recurrence, rather than to simply relieve the symptoms from the present episode (1–3, 13, 20, 31).

Subjective Findings

Onset The patient is commonly between 35 and 55 years of age. Onset is usually sudden with no cause, but can often be attributed to either overuse or trauma. However, on further questioning, it may be found that the activity that produced onset of symptoms was normally not out of the ordinary considering the patient's lifestyle (3, 4, 7, 8, 13).

Duration Patients normally present within 1 to 6 weeks of onset of symptoms; however, if the symptoms are mild, this time period can be extended to 2 or 3 months. Notice the discrepancy with the time limit of 6 weeks required for spontaneous recovery. The reason for this variance is often the patient's stubborn refusal to alter his daily routine enough to avoid activities that exacerbate the condition.

Frequency The patient will usually complain of recurrent episodes over a 1- to 2-year period with the history suggesting steadily increasing severity of symptoms, which also spread over a greater area as time progresses (1, 5, 6, 19, 20).

Area of Symptoms   The patient's major symptoms will be confined to the low back, usually more on one side than the other, and often with referral into the buttock and lateral aspect of the hip, either unilaterally or bilaterally (Fig. 5.8) (2, 4–6).

Type of Symptoms   Patients usually describe an aching type of pain in the back, buttocks, and hips. Pain is occasionally sharp on movements and is then felt mostly in the back, but also possibly in the buttocks (4, 6, 12).

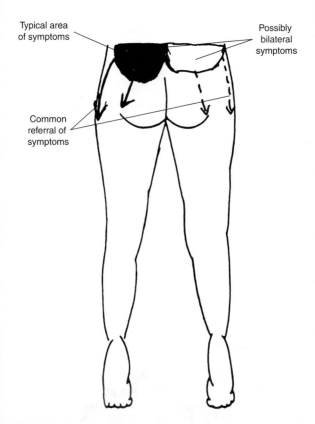

FIG. 5.8   Area of symptoms for a lumbar disc lesion (no radiculopathy).

Miscellaneous In general the history will suggest that the patient's symptoms are worse on repetitive or sustained flexion activities such as sitting, bending, and lifting.

Objective Findings

Observation Increased muscle tension or outright muscle spasm is often observed in the paravertebral muscles of the lumbar region and possibly also in the lower thoracic spine. Flattening of the normal lumbar lordosis is also common and may be related to the muscle spasm (12, 13, 33).

Active Movements Flexion of the lumbar spine will be limited to some degree and will produce the patient's typical pain. Extension of the lumbar spine may or may not be limited, but will either be pain free or will decrease the typical symptoms, particularly when carried out in the prone lying position. Side flexions and rotations should be of full range and pain free bilaterally (1, 11, 13, 14, 43).

Passive Movements Results of passive testing of movements of the lumbar spine in this type of condition are often either misleading or uninformative. It will usually be found that increase in typical symptoms is produced by overpressure at end range of flexion of the lumbar spine. On passive posterior/anterior gliding movements of the individual segments of the lumbar spine there should be some diffuse discomfort produced on movements. Occasionally there may be sharp pain felt directly at the offending segment. One or two segments of the lumbar spine will normally have decreased range of motion on posterior/anterior pressure compared to the other segments; this loss of range of motion should correspond to the segmental level suggested by the rest of the physical examination (12, 19, 20, 23).

Resisted Movements There should be no pain and good strength demonstrated on isometric testing of all back and leg movements, as long as the position in which the patient is tested is initially pain free (3, 13, 20).

Palpation Tenderness may be elicited over muscles that are in spasm in the thoracic and lumbar region and some discomfort may also be associated with pressure applied to stiff spinal segments. Otherwise there is nil of note to be found on palpation of the affected spinal region (12, 23, 24).

Specific Tests Straight leg testing should be full and pain free, although on occasions it may produce some discomfort in the low back only. However, even in this case sciatic stretch will be negative (6, 20, 22, 23).

Treatment Ideas
(6–8, 11–14, 19, 20, 27–30, 49–52)

Immediately following assessment the treatment should be aimed at establishing exactly what position the patient needs to assume in order to decrease the discomfort in the back. This position will most commonly be lying prone with some degree of extension of the lumbar spine. However, in some cases extension of the spine may also produce discomfort, in which case the patient is usually most comfortable in a neutral position, such as lying prone with one or two pillows under the pelvis. Some patients may find relief resting on their forearms and elbows, as if they are reading a newspaper or magazine while lying in the prone position. Most patients will have already found that they can get reasonably comfortable in a side lying position with the knees and hips flexed to one degree or another, usually with a pillow for the head and a pillow between the knees.

When the correct positioning for pain relief has been established, the patient should be encouraged to maintain this position for 10–15 minutes every hour while at home. The exact amount of time that is required will depend on the severity of the symptoms. The use of ice, hot packs, or a judicious mix of both, often helps to relieve discomfort. Transcutaneous electrical nerve stimulation or interferential therapy may be used for relief of pain and muscle spasm.

Once a position of comfort has been established, the patient can be started on simple active exercises. Commonly, leg extension in either the prone or side lying position, abduction combined with lateral rotation of the leg with the hip and knee flexed and the patient lying supine, and gentle swinging of the legs from side to side with the knees bent and the feet on the bed with the patient lying supine, are all exercises that the patient should be able to carry out without any undue discomfort. These exercises should initially be attempted in short bursts, but repeated several times per day. The patient will often then be able to progress to extension of the back, either using a head and chest raise in the prone lying position or continuing with single-leg raises in the prone lying position, but adding back extension in the standing position.

Once the patient's pain starts to decrease he can commence a general active non-weight bearing exercise program for all movements of the lumbar spine with the use of rest positions, or pain-easing movements, before, during, and after the other exercises. The patient must be instructed to stop any exercise immediately if it produces the typical symptoms. When this happens the exercise program must be reviewed in the light of further assessment and revised to eliminate those movements that produce typical pain.

Once the patient can successfully complete the active exercise program he can progress to general upper and lower extremity resisted exercises using a resistance band or wrist and ankle weights. These exercises are best done initially in the lying position, then in the standing and sitting positions. The patient will still require rest in a pain-free position, or use of a pain-relieving movement, in the initial stages of resisted exercise training. The application of heat prior to exercise can be used to relax the patient. Interferential therapy, transcutaneous electrical nerve stimulation, or ice following exercise may help to relieve any muscle stiffness.

Further progress consists of a gym exercise program aimed at strengthening the muscles of the trunk and all four extremities. The patient should continue with ongoing back-care education, with the exercise program relating specifically to maintenance of correct posture during functional activities. The relief of symptoms associated with this present episode should not be considered any major victory. The main task should always be considered to be the prevention of recurrence of symptoms, in which case successful treatment can only be measured by not having to see that patient again for the same type of symptoms.

Restrictions   Initially the patient should use pain as a guide: any position that produces the typical symptoms should be changed at once, as should any symptom-producing activity. For example, if the patient is sitting and the pain starts, he should stand or lie down, if he is washing the dishes and the pain starts he should stop and then position himself, or use an exercise to relieve the discomfort before continuing the activity. The patient must also be advised to avoid repetitive or sustained flexion of the spine, and initially should lift only light weights such as 1 to 2 pounds or less. The patient should never hold a weight away from the body, as it has been shown that a weight held in front of the body at chest height with the elbows 50% extended produces five times its weight in pressure on the lumbar discs. For example, a 20-pound baby, held at arms length because of a dirty diaper, can produce 100 lb. of pressure or more on the lumbar discs.

Sitting should be limited to an amount of time that does not produce symptoms. This needs to be strictly stressed where driving is concerned, as the patient's natural desire is not to break up a journey into 20- or 30-minute segments. Sustained flexion, even if only to a small degree, can produce quite severe symptoms. Activities such as brushing teeth, applying makeup, and so on, may need to be modified considerably to allow for adequate rest breaks. Any degree of forward flexion in either sitting or standing, such as working on a production line, at a workbench, vacuuming the floors, or washing dishes should only be attempted with caution. The patient needs to be advised to counteract all flexion activities by a sufficient degree of extension stretches in order to prevent, rather than relieve, symptoms. The need for these restrictions has to be explained clearly and positively to the patient, as he will have to continue to maintain back-care discipline for an indefinite period of time, even after the symptoms have completely cleared.

Lumbar Disc (with Radiculopathy)

Overview

The symptoms that the patient suffers in this condition appear to relate to the bulging of the intervertebral disc or an actual protrusion of nuclear material through cracks in the annulus. In this condition, leg symptoms will predominate and will be directly related to an affected nerve root or, in rare cases, two nerve roots. This may be a result of direct pressure on the nerve root or indirect irritation of it due to the inflammatory process. Symptoms will often spontaneously subside gradually over a period of a few weeks, but recurrence is common, particularly when the patient continues with the habits and activities that contributed to the original onset of the condition (1, 4, 7, 40–42).

Subjective Findings

Onset The patient is typically between 35 and 55 years of age. Onset is sudden, usually for no cause or through overuse (normally bending and lifting). Pain in the back or leg will typically increase over a period of hours. One of the classic presentations is of a patient gardening in the afternoon, having a stiff back that evening, then being unable to move the following morning (1, 5, 11, 13).

Duration The patient typically presents as an acute case within 1 to 3 weeks of onset of symptoms, as the pain is often severe and the condition is very functionally limiting. In some cases the patient may, in fact, be stuck in one position and almost unable to function, even in a limited manner.

Frequency Most commonly this is the first time that the patient has suffered this particular degree of discomfort, but will often have a history of recurrent, although less severe, back symptoms occurring over a period of months or even years (11, 16, 18).

Area of Symptoms Pain must be felt in the leg, but can also be felt in the back and buttock. Leg symptoms are normally confined to the distribution of a particular nerve root, most commonly in the posterior or lateral aspects of the leg (Fig. 5.9) (11–13, 20, 23, 36).

Type of Symptoms Pain will be the predominant symptom, but the patient may also complain of paraesthesia, anesthesia, or dysaesthesia in the affected limb (2, 3, 5, 13).

Miscellaneous It is not uncommon in these cases for the patient to be unable to sit long enough to give a history. The patient's sleep is also disturbed by symptoms and the pain is generally worse in the early hours of the morning or, in less severe cases, on rising (5, 11, 18, 20).

Objective Findings

Observation In the majority of cases flattening of the normal lumbar lordosis will be observed. Classically there is a lateral shift of the spine, normally away from the site of the pain, but occasionally towards it. The patient may hold the affected leg somewhat flexed at the knee and will sit with the weight transferred onto the buttock of the unaffected side. Muscle spasm may be observable in the lumbar and thoracic paravertebral musculature (10, 13, 15, 18, 20).

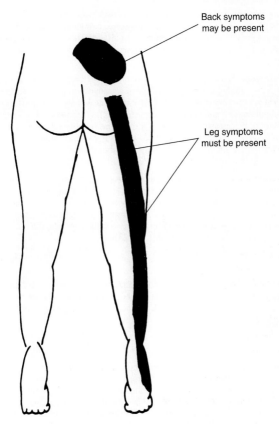

FIG. 5.9 Area of symptoms for a lumbar disc lesion (with radiculopathy in S1 distribution).

Active Movements Flexion is the most limited movement and should produce typical leg, and possibly back, symptoms. Extension is less limited and will either have no effect on, or may ease, the symptoms. With a large herniation, movement into greater range of extension may reproduce the typical leg and back symptoms. Where a lateral shift of the spine is observable side flexion towards the side of the shift is either pain free or pain relieving, whereas side flexion towards the other side will usually produce some leg or back symptoms. However, in the majority of cases side flexion is only mildly affected and usually does not produce pain. Rotation of the spine, carried out in sitting, should be of full range and pain free (3, 10–13, 26).

Passive Movements Posterior/anterior pressure over the spinous processes of the lumbar spine will produce pain over one or two segments locally. Often one or more segments of the spine will also be found to have poor intervertebral mobility compared to other segments of the spine. Passive overpressure on flexion of the spine should exacerbate the leg symptoms, but in the majority of cases this is an unnecessary maneuver, as the active movements will have already established a clear pattern of symptom distribution (3, 20, 23).

Resisted Movements Isometric resisted movements of the back and lower extremities should be pain free as long as they are carried out in a reasonably pain-free position. There may be specific weakness in the legs related to pressure on a particular nerve root. This weakness is painless in nature, and will often come as a surprise to the patient who did not, until that point, realize that it existed (3, 20, 23).

Palpation The findings on palpation will be the same as those described for a disc problem with radiculopathy.

Specific Tests Straight leg raising may be positive for sciatic stretch, but if the lesion is high in the lumbar spine, femoral stretch may be positive. There is usually absence of a reflex at the knee or ankle and positive dural signs may be present (12, 13, 22, 23).

Treatment Ideas
(1, 3, 4, 6, 8, 11–13, 15, 17, 19, 20, 30, 34, 37–39, 49–52)

Initial treatment consists of finding a position or movement that reduces the patient's leg symptoms, most commonly either in the prone lying position or the side lying position on the unaffected side. This may simply accentuate a position that the patient has already adopted, having found the quickest way to relieve pressure on the affected structures. The use of modalities or physical agents applied in this position often helps to relieve spasm and helps the patient to relax, particularly if the patient had been previously stiff and frightened for a period of time. None of these modalities will directly affect the discs in the lumbar region as they lie too deep under the surface.

Once the patient has been established in a comfortable position, active movements of the legs can be commenced. These should be attempted only within the range that does not produce symptoms. Following the work of Robin McKenzie, a protocol of mainly extension exercises is now the generally accepted approach, with extension usually accomplished in the prone lying position if this has been shown to reduce symptoms. If a particular position or movement does reduce the patient's symptoms, it must be stressed firmly to the patient that he must carry out this activity continuously throughout the day, no matter how annoying or time consuming this may be. (11)

Once pain control has been established, general active exercises can be commenced for both the arms and the legs, as this helps to promote movement of the joints throughout the trunk. Arm exercises are particularly useful, as they allow for a fair degree of activity without producing any discomfort and will help to reassure those patients who are very stiff and fearful of movement. Pain-relieving modalities can be continued for symptoms of muscle spasm or those resulting from stiffness and lack of movement. The usual progression of leg exercises is to go from leg extension in the prone lying position to hip abduction, in the supine lying position initially and then in the side lying position, followed by rolling of the flexed knees from side to side in the supine lying position with the patient's feet kept on the bed. Each exercise should be proceeded by an extension exercise for the lumbar spine.

At all times the patient should be encouraged to move around on the treatment table, up and down the table and from lying to sitting to standing and back. Just because the patient appears to be very stiff and in a great deal of pain does not mean that he should be treated as if made of glass. It is very easy to reinforce patient's fears of the seriousness of the underlying condition, and much more difficult to assure them that they are not going to be crippled for life. The last progression of active exercises is to hip and knee flexion in the supine lying position, once this is achieved without producing any increased symptoms, the patient can be progressed to weight-bearing exercises such as step ups on a small step (6 inches), 50% squats, and transference of weight from leg to leg, with and without support.

At this stage, the patient's symptoms, particularly in the leg, should be decreasing steadily and under control through the use of positioning or exercise. It becomes very important to then stress to the patient the dangers of unrelieved back flexion, as it is at this point in the recovery process that the patient is most likely to reinjure himself, not through heavy lifting because they are aware of that danger, simply through maintaining a flexed position for too long. Education using audiovisual aides can never really be overdone and is best given to the patient in short bursts throughout the treatment program.

At this time the patient should be moving into a full flexibility program for the spine and the lower extremities, resisted exercises using dead weights or a resistance band at home, and exercises on weight-training equipment in the clinic. Emphasis throughout these exercises should be on maintenance of the correct spinal posture. It is worth noting and stressing to the patient that there is no such thing as a bad movement of the spine. Flexion of the spine is not a problem unless it is repeated and sustained without relief over a period of time. A healthy spine should move comfortably in all directions and must be supported by a solid framework of muscles, particularly the back extensors and the abdominals.

The final stages of treatment will involve functional exercises to simulate the patient's lifestyle in work, daily activities, and recreational activities. Back education should be continued, with postural correction and the use of regular rest and stretch breaks throughout the day to relieve strain on the spine. Again, it must be made clear to the patient that this is not something that is just going to be continued while the symptoms last, but rather a lifestyle change that is necessary to prevent recurrence of the same symptoms within the next year or two. Before discharge the patient should also be instructed in what might be called "first aid," because return of symptoms of one degree or another is likely in the majority of cases, usually within a year of completion of treatment.

The patient needs to be taught how to find a pain-free position and to start again with the simple exercises that were found to be helpful in the initial stages of treatment during this episode. It is common for patients to stop all the exercises once they feel better and then to restart all the exercises when the pain restarts. Since this will include some movements that are likely to increase their symptoms in the early stages of an episode, they naturally will get worse. They therefore stop exercising and eventually end up returning for treatment in the clinic. Patients need to be taught to progress slowly through the program, as they did in the clinic, in order to effectively cope with any recurrent symptoms. They should start with pain relief, then work into flexibility exercises for movements that don't produce symptoms, so that any exacerbation of symptoms will usually only last for a few days and will be brought under control easily. They can then attempt the whole home program of exercises that they were taught at the clinic and continuing these exercises will help to reduce the frequency and duration of any further episodes.

Restrictions   In the early stages this condition is effectively self limiting because of the degree of discomfort that the patient experiences on attempting any activity that is likely to worsen the condition. However, the patient must be warned against any repetitive or sustained back flexion, particularly sitting. I usually tell a patient that for the first 2 to 3 weeks he can either lie down or stand, and forget about sitting altogether. This is, of course, unreasonable, but it does carry home the message of the dangers of sitting and that this particular stress should be minimized whenever possible.

Bending of the back should be avoided until back flexion is shown to be painless in treatment in the clinic, and then it should only be attempted with no weights. Again, it is unreasonable to expect the patient not to bend his back at all in the course of his daily activities. One classic example is of a young mother who must lift her baby out of the crib, as well as carry out all the other activities that the baby demands, which is impossible without flexing the lumbar spine. Taking it for granted that some degree of back flexion must occur throughout the day, the patient needs to be instructed to carry out extension stretches following any flexion activity, which should become routine.

Awkward postures and positions such as those involving torsion of the lumbar spine through rotation have to be avoided for several weeks, particularly if there is also any flexion component associated with the position. When the patient does return to these sorts of postures, it must be done on a graduated basis, with only 1 to 2 minutes spent in a position initially at any one time, with several minutes rest in between. This presents a particular problem in some occupations, such as a mechanic, but needs to be adhered to in order to prevent recurrence of the previous symptoms.

Patients often inquire about the efficacy of walking, but although walking is good for general health, it is wise to point out to them that the lumbar spine is a series of weight-bearing joints, and that walking any great distance is therefore likely to exacerbate their symptoms. From a health point of view regular short walks are much better for the back than one or two long walks during a day. Swimming is often more comfortable, as weight is relieved from the spine. Some patients with this condition find that swimming relieves their discomfort, while others will find that it increases it, so it is best to advise them to use the activity as tolerated and in short bursts, as for walking.

Lumbar Facet Joint Irritation (No Radiculopathy)

Overview

This diagnosis is more descriptive than real. It is made on the findings that movements that would presumably place pressure on the posterior spinal structures tend to produce the patient's typical symptoms, whereas those movements that would be expected to stress the intervertebral discs, ligaments, or muscles of the low back do not produce symptoms. This is possibly a more truly degenerative condition than so-called degenerative disc disease, considering the typical age and history of the patient. Treatment is aimed at relieving the stress placed on those posterior structures and restoring normal posture, which usually means reducing an increased lumbar lordosis (3, 7, 12).

Subjective Findings

Onset This is gradual with no cause or following overuse, particularly maintaining an extended position of the back for a period of time. Patients are normally aged over 50, but it is also a condition that can be found in younger women, when it is then usually related to pregnancy (3, 12, 15, 21).

Duration The patient has typically been suffering symptoms for 2 to 3 months or more before arriving for treatment, as the pain is usually not acute in nature and is often easily relieved in the early stages of the condition by the patient simply changing position.

Frequency   There is usually a history of a series of episodes of steadily increasing intensity and duration of symptoms over a period of one to two years. In an expectant mother it would be directly related to the pregnancy and there may be no previous history of other similar episodes (4, 15, 19).

Area of Symptoms   Symptoms are generally well localized to the central lumbar region, with some pain radiating across the back as the

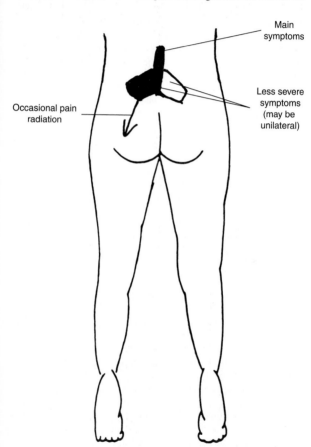

Main symptoms

Less severe symptoms (may be unilateral)

Occasional pain radiation

FIG. 5.10   Area of symptoms for lumbar facet joint irritation (no radiculopathy).

condition progresses. Usually this will be more noticeable on one side than the other, and referral of pain into the buttock on the more affected side is not uncommon (Fig. 5.10)(4, 7, 12, 19).

Type of Symptoms The patient often complains of a nagging ache in the low back, with occasional sharp pain either centrally or radiating into one buttock. These sharp pains are usually associated with extension activities or rotations taken to full range or repeated over a period of time (15, 19).

Miscellaneous Typically the patient's symptoms will be brought on by walking and are relieved by sitting or standing in a slumped position, as in leaning on a fence or other support. The patient will also usually have found that he can decrease the symptoms by lying flat on his back with the knees bent, or on his back with his feet up on a sofa or some similar support (4, 7, 13).

Objective Findings

Observation Patients will typically demonstrate a mild to moderately increased lumbar lordosis and some degree of lumbar paravertebral muscle spasm, or at least increased muscle tension in that area.

Active Movements There will be moderate to severe limitation of extension, which will also produce the patient's typical symptoms. Flexion is normally near full range, although there may be some back discomfort, usually a pulling sensation at end range of motion that is felt centrally in the lumbar spine. This will also be true of a sustained flexed standing position that although it helps to decrease symptoms for a period of time, will produce a pulling pain if held for too long. If a patient is experiencing unilateral back pain, then side flexion to that side is usually limited and produces the typical discomfort. Rotation should be of full range and pain free; however, the patient may complain of stiffness at the very end of movement to either side (7, 12, 13).

Passive Movements Overpressure on extension may produce a sensation of a bony-type block to movement and will reproduce and increase the patient's typical symptoms. Stiffness could be experienced at end range of motion of all other movements of the lumbar spine, but in general results gained from testing the passive movements in patients with this condition are not of any great significance (19, 23, 25).

Resisted Movements All isometric resisted movements of the lower extremities and trunk should be pain free and full strength. If the patient is in a position that produces discomfort to start, then any isometric testing is likely to increase that discomfort due to increased pressure through muscle work being applied to already irritated tissues.

Palpation There is usually very poor intervertebral mobility found on posterior/anterior pressure over the spinous processes throughout the lumbar spine, but particularly in the lower two or three segments. A moderate degree of pressure applied just laterally to the spinous processes in the lumbar spine can produce discomfort at each segment tested. Care needs to be taken during this type of examination, as any deep palpation in this area will always produce pain, even in the asymptomatic patient. The lumbar paravertebral muscle will be tender if they are in spasm (12, 13, 24).

Specific Tests The main findings in this condition are that all specific tests, such as straight leg raising and femoral nerve stretch are negative.

Treatment Ideas
(1, 3, 4, 7, 12, 13, 15, 19, 21, 49, 50–52)

A position needs to be found that will relieve the patient's symptoms when they occur. It was noted earlier that the patient has often already discovered this for himself, the position being one that produces slight flexion of the lumbar spine or at least reduced lordosis of the lumbar spine. This can be achieved lying supine with pillows placed under the knees for support, or lying supine with the legs raised onto a coffee table, for example. The patient should also be shown fully supported slumped sitting, where he can lean forward with his elbows resting on his thighs or on one or two pillows placed on the thighs.

Initial exercises that are most comfortable for the patient are usually single hip and knee flexion in the supine lying position, hip abduction in the supine lying position, initially with a flexed hip and knee and progressing to a straight leg, and swinging of the flexed knees from side to side with the feet kept on the floor. These should initially be done in the first half of range and are used to loosen movements in the spine, thereby reducing muscle tension. Heat usually works better than ice in reducing the patient's symptoms. Ultrasound and laser applications can be attempted as the structures surrounding these joints are superficial enough to allow physiological changes to be augmented by these modalities. Interferential and transcutaneous electrical nerve stimulation may help relieve the effects of muscle spasm.

Once the patient is coping with this exercise program without any undue discomfort, then local stretching of the tissues in the low back can be commenced using passive mobilizations of the pelvis to produce the equivalent of side flexion and rotation-type movements. The amplitude of movement and the degree of force applied are steadily increased as the patient demonstrates the ability to tolerate this type of maneuver. At this time the patient can also be instructed in postural correction, which requires good abdominal work, producing a pelvic tilt to decrease the lumbar lordosis. Double knee raises in the supine lying position with the knees fully flexed is often the exercise that initially is best tolerated. Lumbar traction is also worth a short trial at this stage and should be carried out in the position of pain relief, but must be discontinued if any typical symptoms are produced either during or following its application. Patients can usually move quite quickly onto a general flexibility exercise program, including all movements of the lumbar spine, pelvis, and thoracic spine, with the exception of extension.

Once the flexibility exercises are established and tolerated by the patient it should be possible to start strengthening exercises, initially in a lying position using weights or an exercise band, with the patient continuing the same routine at home. A general physical workout involving all four extremities and the trunk is often beneficial. These patients are generally older, and are often being told by others to ease up because they are getting older, when on the contrary they should be encouraged to do as much as they possibly can. They simply must be aware of the restrictions imposed by the condition, which will be evident by increase in their typical symptoms. It is often unnecessary to introduce extension as a flexibility exercise as the patient will tend to maintain an increased lumbar lordosis, particularly if overweight. However, extension can be used in early ranges in the resisted exercises to promote general back strength. A full resisted exercise program, carried out in a gym setting, should be relevant to the patient's desired lifestyle (not his age).

Restrictions The patient should be advised to avoid all extension activities, particularly where they may be prolonged or repetitive in nature. Walking should be restricted to short distances and stopped before pain is produced, with short rests taken in a sitting or standing, slightly slumped, position. Swimming is often not beneficial for these patients because of the degree of extension required to keep their heads above water, although patients may find relief of discomfort by floating on their backs in a warm pool. General arm and leg exercises done in the pool may help with overall fitness and will help prevent onset of symptoms, as the water supports the weight of the trunk.

People such as electricians, welders, and mechanics are particularly at risk of exacerbation of symptoms, as their work often necessitates either sustained or repetitive extension of the back. These people need to be taught correct rest and stretching procedures. Resting in a slumped sitting position can be augmented by flexion stretches, although these may prove difficult to carry out in a work situation. Lifting, pushing, and pulling activities are often no problem, but carrying heavy loads in the arms can produce symptoms because of the natural extension of the spine that is required to counteract the weight. Heavy loads should be divided into smaller loads whenever possible and carried close to the body.

Sacroiliac Joint Strain

Overview

This injury is most commonly associated with incorrect lifting techniques where either flexion or extension from flexion is combined with a rotary component during movement. In women during pregnancy or in the first 6 to 9 months afterwards, the degree of force required to produce an injury can be relatively trivial. The injury can also be caused by repeated flexion activities such as changing the baby or leaning over the crib, which may occur over a period of several weeks. This condition, when dealt with effectively, should not present a problem to the patient; however, if it is poorly treated or left untreated it can become a recurrent and functionally very limiting condition (12, 13, 18, 45, 46).

Subjective Findings

Onset   Onset is sudden in nature due to either overuse or trauma in patients typically 20 to 40 years of age. It is most commonly associated with combined lifting and twisting motions (14, 18, 19).

Duration   The condition is functionally quite limiting and often very painful. The patient therefore usually presents for treatment within 3 to 6 weeks following onset.

Frequency   This often presents as the first time that the patient has suffered these particular symptoms; however, it can also present as a series of recurrent episodes occurring every few months over a 1- to 2-year period. In the later case the history will indicate progressively less force required to trigger the symptoms in each subsequent episode.

Area of Symptoms   The patient can usually localize the symptoms to one side of the low back at the junction of the spine and pelvis. Very commonly symptoms are experienced in one buttock, and in some cases may be referred down the posterior of the thigh as far as the knee (Fig. 5.11) (4, 7, 12, 13).

Type of Symptoms   The patient usually describes a dull aching pain in the low back and buttock, with a sensation of heaviness or tiredness in the legs bilaterally. Certain movements may produce a sharp pain, most commonly felt in the buttock (7, 12, 18).

Miscellaneous   Pain may often be most marked on rising from sitting, particularly from a low seat such as a sofa, or when getting out of a car, where a rotation component is required during rising from flexion (12, 13, 17).

Objective Findings

Observation   Some flattening of the lumbar lordosis is usual. There may be apparent increased lordosis and the patient may favor the leg on the affected side when walking. Muscle spasm may be observed in the paravertebral muscles in the lumbar region on the affected side, in particular (12, 18, 23).

Active Movements   Mild pain and slight limitation of flexion of the lumbar spine is usually found on examination, with a greater degree of discomfort produced on rising from a flexed position. There is often more limitation of extension of the lumbar spine and with a sharper pain experienced in the sides of the low back or buttock on the movement of extension. Mild discomfort may also be experienced during side flexion,

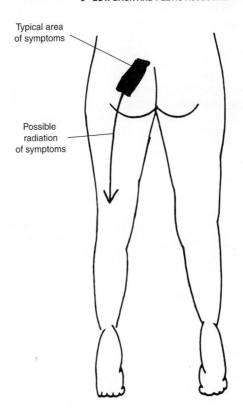

FIG. 5.11   Area of symptoms for left sacroiliac joint strain.

with pain felt on the same side as the movement tested; however, there is no particular limitation of range of side flexion and rotation of the spine is full and pain free bilaterally (12–14, 17, 46).

Passive Movements   Pain may be produced by overpressure on either flexion or extension of the lumbar spine and is felt near the sacroiliac joint (Fig. 5.2). Pain may also be experienced in this region if overpressure is applied to either rotation (4, 7, 13, 23).

Resisted Movements   Resisted movements of the low back and lower extremities should be pain free, although strongly resisted movement may produce pain on the side of the affected joint, as the stronger muscle action produces shearing stresses at the joint.

Palpation Tenderness is normally elicited approximately a thumbs breadth medially and inferior to the posterior superior iliac spine on the affected side. There may be also some degree of tenderness in the lumbar paravertebral muscles (Fig 5.3), but only if they are in spasm (18, 23, 24).

Specific Tests Compression and distraction testing of the sacroiliac joints will usually produce typical symptoms, although false positive and false negative results are quite common. On straight leg raise testing, pain felt in the low back after 70 degrees, found in conjunction with pain before 70 degrees on bilateral straight leg raise testing, suggests a lesion of the sacroiliac joints (12, 13, 22, 23, 26).

Treatment Ideas
(3, 4, 6, 7, 12–14, 17–19, 44, 49–52)

The patient usually finds the most effective rest position is in lying prone with two pillows placed under the pelvis, or lying on the non-affected side with the knees and hips flexed and a pillow placed between the knees. Ice or heat is often useful in decreasing pain, as is transcutaneous electrical nerve stimulation or interferential therapy. Interferential therapy can also be effective in helping to decrease muscle spasm. Active exercise should be started with single hip and knee flexion, initially using the leg on the opposite side to the painful joint. Dropping the knee of the affected leg out to the side when the hip and knee are flexed (combined lateral rotation and abduction of the hip), and swinging the flexed knees from side to side in the supine lying position through approximately 50% of range are effective active exercises that help prevent stiffening of the low back. Ultrasound in pulsed dosages initially may be helpful when given over the tender areas around the posterior superior iliac spine. At home the patient will often find relief from discomfort by lying flat on his back on the floor with his legs up on a sofa or coffee table.

As the patient's back pain decreases he can be progressed to pelvic tilting and light abdominal work, combined with hip abduction as tolerated. The use of modalities should be continued as long as the patient demonstrates pain, stiffness, or muscle spasm in the affected areas. Increased stretch can be applied to the lower extremity during exercise by using a towel around the thigh or by placing the hand on the knee or thigh to apply light overpressure at the end of each exercise. A particularly useful exercise is bilateral hip and knee flexion in the supine lying position with a large towel wrapped around the thigh so that the patient can use his hands and arms to supply the motive force for the exercise. Once the patient is feeling slightly more comfortable, back education can commence, with an emphasis placed on maintenance of posture and correct lifting and material-handling techniques.

As the patient begins to cope with active exercises, passive pelvic mobilizations, used to produce rotary and side flexion movements are usually well tolerated, particularly if small applitude movements are initially used. At this time active single hip extension in the prone lying position and bridging exercises for the pelvis in the supine lying position can be introduced to improve spinal/pelvic mobility. Once the rotary and side flexion mobilizations are well tolerated, then posterior/anterior glides of the sacrum can be attempted lying prone. At this time resisted abdominal work can also be progressed as tolerated. It is often useful to get the patient to stretch the low back at home by lying with his knees at the edge off the bed and his lower legs hanging off the side. This provides quite a strong tractional force on the sacroiliac joints and lumbar sacral region. Patients usually tolerate 15 to 20 seconds with the legs hanging, followed by 30 to 40 seconds rest repeated five or six times. This particular exercise can be progressed to the point where the patient is able to tolerate 30 seconds of stretch followed by 30 seconds of rest repeated five or six times.

The patient should be progressed onto general spinal flexibility exercises, with particular attention paid to stretching of the hamstrings because of their effect on the position of the pelvis. Patients are usually most compliant with a relatively short program of exercises involving 20- to 30-second stretches for each movement, repeating each movement only once or twice in each exercise session. Sessions can then be spread out so that the patient is completing them three or four times per day. Resisted exercises using dead weights and a resistance exercise band can be started once the symptoms of pain and stiffness in the low back are definitely resolving. At this time proprioceptive neuromuscular facilitation techniques used on the lower extremities can improve the rate at which the patient regains muscle strength in the affected region.

It is also worthwhile progressing the patient into a general resisted exercise program for the trunk and all four extremities in a gym setting, initially using low weights with relatively high repetitions. This can then be combined with sets using heavier weights and lower repetitions, so that both the endurance and power requirements of the musculature are met. Education should be continued throughout the treatment program and as the patient nears the end of treatment particular emphasis must be placed on correct lifting, carrying, pushing, and pulling techniques, as related to their normal level of daily activities.

Restrictions In the early stages the patient is best advised to avoid all rotation movements of the low back. Patients should also be advised to reduce the number of repetitions of back flexion, or time spent in a flexed position. Holding weight in the arms may also prove problematic, particularly if the hands are held away from the body. In the same way patients will have difficulty working with the arms above shoulder height, particularly with the arms stretched, as in work that requires placing objects on high shelves or in many tasks associated with welding or mechanical maintenance. The patient has to be advised to limit the amount of weight handled and to take appropriate rests as required to prevent exacerbation of symptoms. Whenever possible the patient should avoid sitting in low chairs, and may benefit from the use of a lumbar roll in sitting, particularly for driving. Finally, education for back care must stress the necessity for ongoing monitoring of personal activities, as recurrence of symptoms is common, but should be avoidable.

Lumbar Muscle Strain

Overview

This is a condition that is often diagnosed, but is seldom found present as a primary condition in its own right. It is more often combined with one of the other back conditions, which helps to confuse things nicely, as symptoms will often overlap. The patients themselves may be the commonest cause of misdiagnosis due to their typical comment that "I pulled a muscle in my back," which may inadvertently influence the examining therapist's assessment. When this condition is found in isolation it is relatively easy to treat compared to most back conditions, as the repair process appears to be more rapid in muscle than in other soft tissues such as ligaments or tendons (2, 4, 17, 21).

Subjective Findings

Onset This is always sudden due to trauma or overuse, in patients normally between 20 and 50 years of age (2, 5, 21).

Duration The patients are most commonly seen in the acute stage, with onset occurring a few days or 2 to 3 weeks prior to being seen.

Frequency This is usually the first time the patient will have suffered these types of symptoms as it is rarely recurrent as an individual pathological entity.

Area of Symptoms Symptoms are localized to the sides of the lumbar spine and possibly the region of the thoracolumbar junction. Symptoms will usually be more marked on one side compared to the other, but although the patient is able to describe a fairly local area of symptoms, it is often difficult for him to put a finger on the spot. Patients tend to indicate a fairly broad area of the back using the whole hand (Fig. 5.12) (5, 6, 16, 24).

Type of Symptoms The patient's main complaints are usually of sharp pain on movement and possibly a dull ache afterwards which is not usually much of a problem functionally.

Miscellaneous The most common cause of this condition is lifting with the weight held in both hands and held away from the body. Typically the patient describes a movement of extension of the back from the flexed position with some degree of rotation (4, 17, 21).

Objective Findings

Observation Spasm is often observable in the paravertebral muscles in the thoracolumbar region, often with more pronounced spasm on one

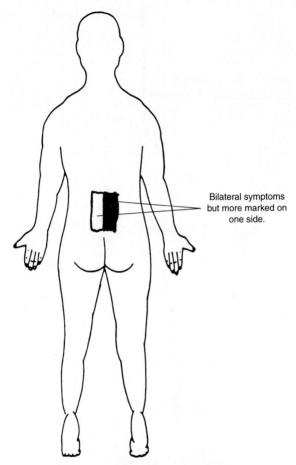

Bilateral symptoms but more marked on one side.

FIG. 5.12 Area of symptoms for lumbar muscle strain.

side compared to the other. This spasm will be more noticeable by the end of the physical examination. The muscle spasm usually produces some degree of flattening of the normal lumbar lordosis (4–6).

Active Movements Mild limitation of flexion of the lumbar spine will be found with the patient complaining of a pulling-type sensation in the back. Extension will be mildly limited, with pain at end range of movement. Rotations are normally of full range, and while pain is often experienced on both rotations, it is felt at the same side of the back for both movements. Side flexions are normally full and pain free, although there may be a mild pulling sensation on movement away from the painful side (2, 6, 8, 16, 17).

Passive Movements If it were possible to carry out truly passive movements for the affected region of the spine, they would be near full range and essentially pain free. In fact, it is impossible to produce a true passive movement because it is not possible to support the weight of the body segments while carrying out the movement. Therefore, overpressure at end of available range is the alternative test; applied to flexion, pain is usually produced in the typical pattern described in the history. Muscle spasm usually resists overpressure applied to either or both rotations. In general the findings on passive testing of side flexion movements are not relevant for establishing diagnosis in this condition (4–6, 23).

Resisted Movements Pain is produced on isometric contraction of the back muscles. This can be tested by having the patient lie comfortably in a prone position over pillows, and then gently resist isometric extension of the hip. This maneuver should produce pain in the affected muscles. Any strongly resisted movements of the legs are likely to produce back pain, but there should be no loss of strength noted during testing of resisted movements in the back or lower extremities.

Palpation Tenderness should be elicited on relatively superficial palpation of the affected muscles. This pain should be localized to a particular part of the muscle as compared to the general tenderness experienced by a patient when a muscle in spasm is palpated. There is also usually some discomfort produced by posterior/anterior pressure centrally over the spinous processes of the spinal segments lying at the same level as the injured part of the muscle (6, 8, 23, 24).

Treatment Ideas

If the patient is seen relatively quickly following injury, treatment is similar to that used for any other soft-tissue injury, comprising mainly ice and rest for 2 to 4 days. As soon as he is able, the patient should be encouraged to start gentle back exercises lying supine with single knee and hip flexion (taking the knee to the chest), dropping the flexed knee out sideways (abduction and lateral rotation of the hip), pelvic tilt with the knees bent, and swinging the legs from side to side with the hips and knees flexed and the feet resting on the bed. The patient should also be instructed to carry out active arm exercises, such as elevation through flexion or abduction in the supine lying position, as all of these movements help to prevent stiffness occurring in the muscles as healing takes place.

After the first few days of treatment the patient can be progressed to the use of thermal modalities, such as hot packs and ultrasound, prior to exercise. Ultrasound should be applied to the tender area of the muscle, initially, starting with pulsed doses and progressing to a constant treatment cycle. The patient can usually be progressed quite rapidly onto a general active exercise program for all movements of the shoulders, shoulder girdle, hip, and pelvis as an indirect means of producing muscle work and muscle stretch in the affected area of the spine. These exercises should be carried out initially in supine, side, and prone lying positions, and they can then be progressed to sitting or standing positions.

As the patient's pain level decreases active exercises for warm up can be used instead of thermal modalities, and the exercises can be progressed to general resisted work, with an exercise band or dead weights, with resistances increased steadily as tolerated by the patient. Back education should be an integral and ongoing part of the program from the early stages of treatment, with particular emphasis on proper lifting and material-handling techniques.

Latter Stages Patients should finally be progressed into a general gym workout with a full exercise regime for all the musculature of the trunk, upper extremities, and lower extremities. A program of stretching exercises should be spread throughout the workout. Further progression can be made into functional exercises involving lifting, carrying, pushing, and pulling activities, as well as working with the arms in different positions above the head and at various degrees of arm stretch, with the program specifically tailored to the patient's typical daily activities.

Restrictions In the first 1 to 2 weeks following injury the patient is best advised to avoid all bending and lifting activities, and they should not maintain either an extended or flexed position of the spine for any period of time. Once the patient has been shown how to lift weights correctly, he can begin to lift light weights during the treatment sessions. As the ability to cope with static positioning in the clinic setting is demonstrated, then the amount of time for which the patient is allowed to sustain a given position can be steadily increased as tolerance is demonstrated. However, the patient must be instructed to rest from each static position and stretch before any pain starts, rather than as a response to discomfort.

In work and daily activities one particular area of concern is the patient having to hold weight away from the body. This often happens in mothers with young babies and in jobs where the patient is required to place articles onto shelves, particularly if the shelving is deep. This is of even more concern when any twisting motion of the trunk is required while maneuvering the weight. As regards work activities the patient should be advised to use hoists and other aids to lifting wherever they are available. A back brace may be an effective method of reminding the patient to maintain both a proper posture and good body mechanics. However, it must be explained to the patient that a back brace does not, in effect, support either the spine or its musculature, which is a common misconception, but is rather a device to assist the patient in maintaining proper body mechanics during activities that might put them at particular risk of reinjury.

Low Back Postural Strain

Overview

This is not as common a problem in the low back as it is in the neck and upper back, but it is still fairly common. The patient is often unwilling to accept that the degree of discomfort being experienced is due to such a "trivial" cause as simply not maintaining a correct posture. In such cases, where resistance to diagnosis is met, the condition could be referred to as a lumbar soft-tissue dysfunction, which is essentially the same thing, with a far more impressive sounding title. Treatment is mainly aimed at counteracting and eventually eliminating the cause of the condition, which is poor postural habits (2, 11, 12, 47).

Subjective Findings

Onset Onset is gradual usually due to no cause, but occasionally associated with overuse, particularly the sustaining of one position for a period of time. It occurs mainly in those 20 to 40 years of age (11, 12, 18).

Duration Most patients suffer symptoms for several weeks before seeking help, although a particular episode can be so acutely painful that they may appear for treatment only a few days to 2 weeks after onset.

Frequency There is always a history of some degree of prior back problems with similar symptoms, although possibly not as severe. It is not uncommon for the patient to say that he has had this before, but it had never been as bad and it had always gone away in the past, although this time it has not. Therefore the history is one of recurrent episodes, of which this is the worst episode so far (11, 18).

Area of Symptoms Pain is experienced in the sides of the lumbar spine with referral across the low back at the level of the lumbosacral junction. As the condition becomes more chronic the pain will also spread over the lower thoracic spine, and even bilaterally into the scapula area (Fig. 5.13) (2, 4, 12).

Type of Symptoms Initial pain is usually an ache that becomes very persistent. The patient then often complains of muscle spasms or tightness or lumps in the muscles in their back. Common complaints are that there is something that feels like a golf ball in one of the muscles or the patient will state that an area of the back appears to swell (4, 11, 18).

Miscellaneous Common causes are sitting at a computer or working on a production line for extended periods of time. Patients will often demonstrate extension of the spine, as in standing and stretching or leaning back in a chair and stretching, and state that this is something they have to do regularly to try to relieve their symptoms after sitting or standing for a period of time. Further inquiry usually reveals that the offending position involves a degree of forward flexion of the spine.

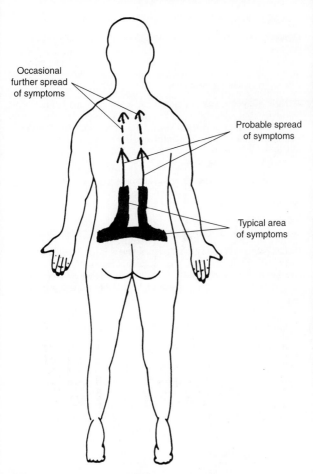

Occasional further spread of symptoms

Probable spread of symptoms

Typical area of symptoms

FIG. 5.13 Area of symptoms for low back postural strain (note possible spread of symptoms to shoulder girdle).

Objective Findings

Observation A degree of muscle spasm, or at least increased muscle tension, may be noted throughout the thoracolumbar region. Patients normally demonstrate a poor posture with a flattened lumbar lordosis, increased rounding of the shoulders, and increased thoracic kyphosis, with protrusion of the head (4, 11, 12).

Active Movements All movements in the spine are full range, although the patient may complain of tightness or pressure felt at end range of any or all of the movements. There is usually no specific pain produced on testing of movements and particularly not the sharp discomfort that the patient will develop after a period of sustained sitting or standing involving forward flexion of the spine (2, 11, 12).

Passive Movements Overpressure on any movement, particularly flexion or side flexion, will produce complaints of tightness, but no particular pain during testing.

Resisted Movements All isometric resisted movements of the spine, upper extremities, and lower extremities will be strong and pain free.

Palpation Mild poorly localized tenderness is usually elicited in the paravertebral muscles of the thoracolumbar region. Posterior/anterior pressure on the spinous processes will reveal decreased intervertebral mobility, often in several segments of the mid thoracic to lower lumbar spine (2, 12, 23, 24).

Treatment Ideas
(2, 4, 11, 12, 18, 31, 37, 49–52)

Before any other treatment is commenced the patient should be educated about the normal postural curves of the spine and the mechanical interrelationship of bone, disc, ligament, and muscle, as no treatment is going to work unless the patient is willing to change their postural habits. The patient should then start back stretches, lying on their back with a towel roll placed lengthways along the spine and with another small rolled towel placed in the cervical spine. The patient should be advised to lie in this position for 5 to 10 minutes two or three times per day, as a means of counteracting the flexion strain that is put on the body through typical daily activities. This simple stretching can be progressed by raising the arms overhead or out to the sides, as in a crucifix position. The patient will often gain the most benefit from this form of exercise if their back is heated thoroughly before beginning.

Patients will also need to be instructed in how to perform a sitting stretch, which can be used to prevent onset of discomfort in high-risk situation, such as when working at the computer. This stretch involves leaning back in the chair with hands on the head and elbows back, extending the whole spine. This stretch should be carried out for approximately 20 seconds every 20 minutes. The patient must be told not to wait for discomfort to start before using the stretch, but to use it to prevent discomfort from starting.

When the patient is comfortable with a regime of regularly repeated extension stretches throughout the day, then he can be instructed in the use of an exercise band for resisted horizontal abduction of the shoulders in sitting. The patient is instructed to maintain a correct posture by sitting upright and "thinking tall" while pumping a light resistance band for some 10 to 20 repetitions, depending on muscularity. This short burst of exercise should produce a satisfying tension in the muscles of the shoulder girdle and upper back, as well as in the shoulders and upper arms. Repeating this exercise once every hour throughout the workday is one means of preventing the "9–5 syndrome" of a posture becoming steadily more slumped throughout the day.

Further progression can be made by teaching the patient general resisted upper extremity exercises for shoulder flexion, extension, and abduction, with the arms kept straight. This will help to reinforce muscle strength in the postural muscles of the mid and upper back. Lower extremity exercises using a resistance band wrapped around the ankles with the patient in standing can be used for hip abduction, extension, and flexion. This can be progressed to static extension in the prone lying position, with a head and chest raise and a double-straight leg raise in the prone lying position, with each position held for 30 to 60 seconds at a time.

Abdominal work can also be encouraged with a pelvic tilt in supine lying and with the feet then held off the bed, or a head and chest raise in the supine lying position with the knees bent. This should be done in early range only and again held for 30 to 60 seconds at a time. All of the above exercises are used to promote strength in postural muscles and can only be effective if the patient is constantly aware of his posture, with an attempt to maintain good posture for as much of the day as possible. If not, the resisted exercises will only serve to reinforce a poor posture.

Where poor local intervertebral mobility is found on examination, manual mobilizations of the spine and pelvis can be used in conjunction with a general flexibility exercise program for the trunk and extremities. The more flexible the patient's spine, the more adaptable it will be to a new, and hopefully better, posture. Where mobilization proves difficult, the use of thermal modalities and interferential therapy to relax muscle can be effective in helping to gain further range of motion. Ultrasound and interferential are also useful in conjunction with ice postexercise to decrease discomfort arising from tender muscles.

When the patient is showing better postural awareness, neuromuscular electrical stimulation can be used on the postural muscles of the low back, with leg extension lying prone with weights suitable to the patient's physique. This should be combined with stronger abdominal work to strengthen the natural girdle that nature has provided for the low back. Back education remains an ongoing part of the treatment program. It has been shown that repeated explanation using different forms of presentation, such as slides, booklets, and videos can all be helpful in heightening awareness of cause and effect in this type of condition. A gym program of general strengthening exercises, with emphasis on strengthening of the postural muscles, can be used, and must be tailored to the patient's desired lifestyle.

It is important that the patient understands the serious consequences of a poor posture, such as possible disc lesions, as this is a high-risk group for that type of problem. However, as noted earlier, the patient is often unwilling to accept the seemingly innocuous explanation of poor posture as the cause of the condition, and will be equally as likely to belittle its consequences later in life. Exercise and postural awareness have to be an ongoing theme and must be linked to a general change in lifestyle. A major part of the therapist's work is to convince the patient of the value of this approach.

Restrictions The patient must be instructed not to remain in a slumped sitting position or in any forward flexed posture, such as standing working at a bench, unless the height of the workbench is such that the patient is able to carry out activities with a normal degree of lumbar lordosis. As a general rule of thumb, no position should be sustained for more than 20 minutes; at the end of that time the patient should carry out an extension stretch either sitting or standing. The patient should also alter his body posture by either standing, if he has been sitting for a time, or walking if he has been standing stooped for a time. If at all possible the patient's work conditions should be observed, or at the least discussed, and adaptations made to eliminate any repeated or sustained forward flexion of the spine. The patient must also be instructed to take regular stretch breaks throughout the day, which should include not only stretches done while at work, but also when sitting in front of the television at home.

Lumbar Facet Joint Irritation (with Radiculopathy)

Overview

There is a great deal of controversy about the roll of the facet joint in the production of symptoms in the back. In the case of this condition it may be safer to say that it seems to be related to the apophyseal joints and, possibly (although by no means definitely), to degenerative changes in the spine. The symptoms that arise appear to be due to pressure applied to the posterior spinal structures, as the main distinguishing features are back and leg symptoms caused mainly by activities that require extension of the lumbar spine. Treatment is aimed at relieving this pressure on a regular basis, then attempting to establish a degree of spinal mobility that is often found to be absent on initial examination (1, 3, 12, 13).

Subjective Findings

Onset Patients are typically over 50 years of age. Onset is gradual with no cause, or on rare occasions it may occur after overuse. The leg symptoms may occur suddenly due to no cause following a bout of backache (3, 12, 15).

Duration The patient will normally report 2 to 3 months of steadily increasing symptoms in the back, with the leg symptoms usually present for less than 6 weeks.

Frequency A history of many years of recurrent episodes of central back pain is not uncommon. Over time the symptoms will radiate towards the buttocks, although on many occasions this will be the first time that the patient has experienced symptoms in the leg (3, 7, 12, 15).

Area of Symptoms Symptoms are felt in the center of the low back, but will radiate into one or both buttocks and usually into only one leg. Leg symptoms will be experienced posteriorly in the thigh traveling about as far as the posterior aspect of the knee (Fig. 5.14) (12, 13, 15).

Type of Symptoms Patients usually complain of aching in the low back and buttocks, with sharp pain on certain movements, felt centrally in the lumbar spine. The leg pain is normally sharp in nature and may be combined with some aching. The patient often reports that sitting in a slightly slumped position will ease the immediate symptoms, but can cause stiffness after a period of time. Walking will typically produce the leg symptoms, which are then again relieved by a short period of sitting. This condition may also occur, although not very commonly, in pregnant women (1, 3, 12, 13).

Objective Findings

Observation Patients will typically have an increased lumbar lordosis. Muscle spasm may be observable in the lumbar and lower thoracic paravertebral musculature (7, 12, 19).

Active Movements Range of motion of flexion is normally good, with stiffness at end range of motion and possibly complaints of a pulling-type sensation in the low back, but no leg symptoms. Extension is usually quite limited and reproduces both the back and leg pain. Side flexion to one side may be limited, with pain at end range of motion, but as often as not both side flexions are pain free. Rotation is within normal limits, but the patient may complain of stiffness at end range of motion on turning to either side (3, 4, 7, 12, 19).

Passive Movements Overpressure applied at end range of extension will meet a solid resistance, with production of the patient's typical back and leg symptoms (3, 7, 12).

Resisted Movements No pain should be elicited on isometric resisted movements of the lower extremities or back, and the musculature is normally as strong as would be expected for the patient's age and overall physical condition.

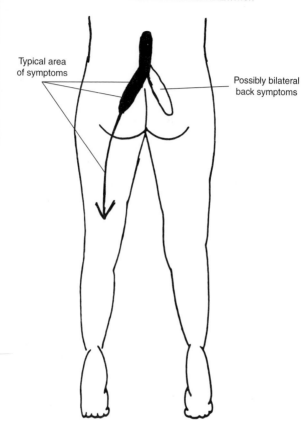

FIG. 5.14   Area of symptoms for lumbar facet joint irritation (with radiculopathy).

Palpation   Tenderness is usually elicited locally over one or two segments of the lumbar spine on posterior/anterior pressure, with noticeably decreased intervertebral mobility present throughout the lumbar spine (12, 13, 23, 24).

Specific Tests   Reflexes and skin sensation in the lower extremities are normal. Straight leg raising should be negative for sciatic stretch.

Treatment Ideas (1, 3, 4, 7, 12, 13, 15, 19, 49–52)

If flexion of the lumbar spine is shown to ease the patient's leg symptoms during the physical examination, then it should be used regularly both during treatment sessions and at home to relieve symptoms whenever possible, such as sitting for short periods after equally short walks. The patient can do this when outside by sitting on a seat (where available) with forearms resting on thighs or, if there is no seat available, standing and leaning against a wall or railings.

The patient should be instructed in the use of non weight-bearing exercises, initially single- and double-leg hip and knee flexions, to bring the knees to the chest. If the patient has difficulty achieving the movements actively, then a towel wrapped around the thigh can be used to allow use of the arms for assistance during the movement. Lying supine with the knees bent, and the knees and feet together with the feet on the floor, then swinging the legs gently from side to side will help to loosen the patient's pelvis and lower back without producing symptoms. The patient must be instructed not to carry the movement too far. Heat, transcutaneous electrical nerve stimulation, and interferential therapy usually help to ease local discomfort and are best given either in the half-lying position or in the side lying position.

As symptoms start to decrease, particularly in the leg, the non weight-bearing exercise program can be expanded to include dropping the leg out sideways with the hip flexed at 45 to 50 degrees and the knee to 90 degrees, thus producing abduction and lateral rotation of the hip. This should be carried to the point where the pelvis on the opposite side starts to rise from the bed. Hip abduction can be attempted lying supine and can be progressed to trunk rotation, side flexion, and further flexion stretches in the sitting position. Light abdominal exercises can also be started using a pelvic tilt to maintain a reduced lumbar lordosis throughout the required movements.

When the patient's leg pain has cleared, there will still be some back discomfort, so hip extension can be started but only if a painless range of motion is found to exist for this movement. Resisted exercises can be started for straight leg raising and hip abduction with either ankle weights or exercise bands. Abdominal work can be increased relative to the patient's overall desired level of physical conditioning. Flexion, rotation, and side flexion stretches can be taken to their full limits in both sitting and standing. Further trunk and extremity resisted exercises, with the patient maintaining the spine in a neutral position, should be progressed as symptoms allow. General trunk and lower extremity strengthening should be graduated to realize the patient's maximum potential and should be related to the required activities of daily living.

Restrictions Initially, walking must be kept to a subsymptom level through the use of regular rests. Swimming is often uncomfortable for the patient and likely to provoke both back and leg symptoms. The patient should be instructed never to sleep on his stomach or even to rest in that position. Any form of aggressive sports (requiring a high degree of twisting, bending, etc.) should be avoided in the early stages of the condition, as the facet joints could become inflamed and reactive.

Extension activities such as dusting, reaching into cupboards or up to shelves, hanging out washing, and changing light bulbs should be modified by the use of steps or stools. Welders and mechanics often have to maintain back extension for considerable periods of time; when they suffer from this type of condition these activities must be modified until the symptoms have cleared completely. Eventually the patient should be able to attempt all these tasks—they simply need to determine the right amount of rest breaks and stretches that are needed to prevent onset or exacerbation of symptoms.

Lumbar Facet Joint Strain

Overview

It is impossible to truly tell if the facet joints actually sustain injury in this condition, but all the movements that tend to produce the patient's typical symptoms are those that would reasonably be expected to do so if the facet joints were stretched or stressed. Also in this condition there is an absence of any more specific signs that would suggest another type of ligament or disc injury, or the effects of joint degeneration or irritation. The condition could also be described as a form of pseudolocking of the facet joints, as this is effectively achieved by the muscle spasm that accompanies onset of the condition (12, 13, 17).

Subjective Findings

Onset This is sudden due to trauma commonly associated with a lifting and twisting, or a pushing and pulling, activity, or there may be direct injury, as in a collision during contact sport. Patients are most often between 20 and 50 years of age.

Duration The patient usually presents for treatment within a matter of days or 2 to 3 weeks following onset, as initially the condition is quite disabling and functionally disruptive.

Frequency This is usually the first time the patient will have experienced these symptoms, although there may be one or two previous episodes several years apart, with no specific history of back problems in the intervening period.

Area of Symptoms Pain is felt centrally in the lumbar spine and to either one or both sides. The pain will quite often radiate over the iliac crest, again, either unilaterally or bilaterally (Fig. 5.15) (24).

Type of Symptoms Pain is sharp on movement, with a nagging ache that comes and goes. The patient will usually report muscle spasms occurring throughout the low back.

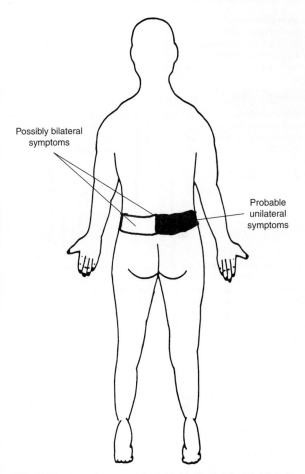

FIG. 5.15 Area of symptoms for right sided lumbar facet joint strain.

Miscellaneous   The patient should always be able to give the exact time of injury, as this is not a condition that develops over time, although the degree of discomfort experienced may increase over the first few hours immediately following injury. In general, flexion activities cause increased back pain in patients with this condition, which sitting may relieve.

Objective Findings

Observation   Muscle spasm is commonly observable in the lumbar paravertebral muscles, this may, in turn, cause flattening of the normal lumbar lordosis. There may also be some deviation of the lumbar spine away from the site of pain when the pain is predominately one sided (12, 13).

Active Movements   Both flexion and extension of the lumbar spine are limited and produce the patient's typical symptoms at end of available range of motion. Side flexion may be painful to either side, or may only be limited to the painful side when the pain is unilateral. Both rotations are normally of full range but may produce a pulling sensation in the painful area. This will be more marked on rotation to the affected side when the pain is unilateral (12, 13, 17).

Passive Movements   Muscle spasm is the common restricting factor on any overpressure at end range of either restricted or painful movements. If the pain is bilateral, overpressure at the end of any movement will normally produce some degree of discomfort.

Resisted Movements   Isometric contraction of the muscles of the low back, either tested directly or by testing movements of the lower extremities, will be pain free and will remain strong. However, strong resistance applied to any movement may produce low back pain due to indirect pressure applied to already irritated and sensitive tissues (13, 23).

Palpation   Diffuse tenderness is elicited over the lumbar spine, in the lumbar paravertebral musculature, and in many cases also over the iliac crests. There is usually no specific localized tender region. Often one or two spinal segments are stiff and produce discomfort, compared to the movements of other segments around them, on posterior/anterior pressure.

Treatment Ideas
(12, 13, 17, 48, 50–52)

If the patient is seen within a few days of injury, then ice and rest should be employed for 2 to 3 days, although the patient should be instructed not to remain in any one position for an extended period of time. After approximately 3 days, heat can be used instead of ice. Since all movements of the spine are usually uncomfortable to one degree or another, active exercises should be started with the least painful movement, which is normally rotation. This can be carried out either lying supine, with the hips and knees bent and the patient's feet on the treatment table with the patient swinging the knees side to side, or sitting, with the patient's arms stretched out in front and the hands clasped, swinging the arms side to side. These movements should be carried out within the patient's comfort zone, short of production of pain.

The exercises can be progressed to include hip abduction and single hip and knee flexion (taking one knee at a time to the chest). Both of these exercises should be carried through 50 to 75% of the available range of motion. Hip extension can be attempted in the side lying position; once completed comfortably it can be progressed to the prone lying position. Both interferential therapy and transcutaneous electrical nerve stimulation are useful for the relief of muscle spasm, as is massage. Ultrasound and laser are not normally effective in this condition, as there is no specific spot at which to apply treatment. From the early stages the patient should be educated about good body mechanics, particularly lifting and carrying, and the avoidance of rotation of the spine when maneuvering heavy loads.

Once the patient copes well with active leg and arm exercises, light resisted exercises can be commenced using dead weights and a resistance band. The movements of flexion, extension, and side flexion of the low back can be assimilated using flexion, extension, and abduction of the hips in lying. Active exercises can be progressed by completing them first in standing, then in sitting. The patient can then move on to general flexibility exercises for the low back, hips, and knees.

Further back education will be required as regards correct posture and lifestyle changes required to avoid recurrence of the back injury. If stiffness is encountered or complained of in or around the pelvic region or in the lumbar spine, then passive mobilizations may be used to augment the flexibility program. Once a good range of movement is achieved on both passive and active testing, the patient can move into further stretching exercises and weight training. A patient with a stiff back should never undertake any strength training, as this will simply cause a strong stiff back—a sure recipe for further injury.

Restrictions Initially the patient will limit himself due to discomfort when attempting activities such as lifting, carrying, pushing, stooping, or bending. Once the patient demonstrates the ability to cope with such activities, they should first be attempted in a slow, cautious manner with minimal weights. As noted earlier, sitting is not usually a problem, although the patient may stiffen if he remains in any one position for too long a period of time. This will also be true on waking first thing in the morning. At these times the patient will need to spend a few minutes loosening up prior to activity.

The patient should be instructed to avoid combined movements of either rotation or side flexion with flexion or extension of the lumbar spine. Any sustained activity with the back in a flexed or extended position will produce symptoms; the patient should therefore stop the activity, preferably before symptoms start, but at least as soon as they do. Walking is often a problem and should therefore be kept to short bursts, with regular rests in a sitting position as required to prevent exacerbation of symptoms. The patient can make a graduated return to all of these activities as the symptoms decrease and as he shows the ability to tolerate the specific activity in the clinic during treatment sessions.

Combined Disc/Facet Joint Problem

Overview

This is a mixed bag of symptoms that can be confusing, until it is noted that flexion tests produce fairly typical disc symptoms, while extension tests produce typical posterior spinal element symptoms. Treatment options often present a particular problem, as exercises that can help one set of symptoms often tend to exacerbate other symptoms. It is also common for patients to have a certain degree of chronic back problems, and their previous history may be of either a disc or facet joint problem. Patient may also become set in their ways as regards their approach to treatment or in self limitation of activities. These preconceived notions can sometimes be the greatest barrier to effective treatment, as patients may want to do the things that have always helped before (11–15, 32).

Subjective Findings

Onset Onset is almost always sudden in nature and may be for any of the three typical reasons, although no cause or trauma are less common than simple overuse. Patients are commonly between 35 and 55 years of age (3, 12, 15, 20).

Duration The patient normally presents with an acute episode of back pain within 1 to 6 weeks of onset, with an underlying longer-standing problem that will have lasted months or years.

Frequency There will always be a previous history of back problems that may be disc or facet joint related, either by the patient's history or previous diagnosis. The present symptoms may differ significantly in one way or another from the previous symptoms, but there will be a definite overlap (11, 12, 15, 16, 35, 42).

Area of Symptom These are found in the lumbar spine, buttock, and leg, and as far as the foot on occasion. Symptoms will also spread up the back into the thoracic spine and occasionally across the upper shoulder girdle (Fig. 5.16) (3, 12, 13, 24).

Type Of Symptoms The patient will present with a variety of symptoms, but will usually complain of a nagging ache in the low back or buttock, shooting pains and paraesthesia or dysaesthesia in the legs, and muscle spasms throughout the back (5, 6, 19, 20).

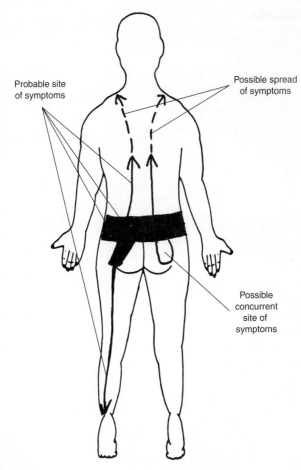

Probable site of symptoms

Possible spread of symptoms

Possible concurrent site of symptoms

FIG. 5.16 Area of symptoms for combined disc and facet joint problem in lumbar spine.

Miscellaneous   The patient will often complain that all activities increase symptoms in one way or another, which are only eased by lying down, usually on the side in a semi-fetal position.

Objective Findings

Observation   Marked muscle spasm should be visible in the thoracolumbar spine; there may be a lateral shift of the spine either towards or away from the painful side. Flattening of the lumbar lordosis may also be present due to the muscle spasm (11, 19, 20).

Active Movements   Normally all movements are limited except rotation. Flexion and extension will not necessarily be limited to the same degree, but will produce typical symptoms, with extension causing central sharp back pain and possibly some leg discomfort, and flexion producing a pulling sensation in the back and pain into the buttocks and leg. Side flexions will normally produce an unpleasant pulling sensation in the back, with a varying degree of either back or leg pain (4, 5, 11, 14, 20).

Passive Movements   Overpressure on extension will produce spasm and local back pain with or without leg symptoms. Overpressure on flexion will produce back and leg pain with either spasm or a strong pulling sensation produced in the low back at the end of available range of motion (3, 6, 12, 13, 23).

Resisted Movements   Muscle strength will be normal throughout the back and lower extremities. Any strongly resisted isometric movement of the back or legs will normally produce some degree of back discomfort, but not of any great intensity.

Palpation   Palpation will elicit all kinds of tenderness along the lumbar spine, over the posterior sacroiliac joint region, and in the muscles of the lower half of the body, but it will be very difficult to isolate or localize any tender spots. There is normally very poor lumbar and lumbar–sacral intervertebral mobility found on applying posterior/anterior pressure to the lumbar spinous processes or the body of the sacrum. The patient may experience some loss of skin sensation in the area of a specific dermatome in one of the lower extremities (12, 13, 23, 24).

Specific Tests   The patient may have a positive sciatic stretch on straight leg raise testing or a positive femoral stretch test. Reflexes are usually normal at the knee and ankle, although there may be muscle weakness present in a specific myotomal distribution (22, 23).

Treatment Ideas
(1, 2, 4, 7, 8, 11–13, 15–17, 20, 30, 34, 37, 38, 49–52)

Since side lying is usually the only position that the patient can adopt comfortably, it is often the best starting position for treatment. With the patient in this position the use of heat, ice, ultrasound, interferential therapy, or transcutaneous electrical nerve stimulation may all help to relieve discomfort to some degree. At the same time exercises can be done in this neutral back position using the upper leg, taken into a degree of hip and knee flexion and then extension, moving within the middle range of motion, with the patient taking regular rests with a pillow placed between their knees. Progression of exercise can be made by the patient lifting his leg off the pillow (hip abduction). This can be attempted on both sides, although it may only be carried out successfully on one. The patient is then instructed to continue the exercise on this one side only, until able to sustain movement without any marked degree of discomfort on the other side.

The exercise program should work towards a flexion or extension bias, depending on which movement provokes symptoms the least. However, it is advisable to continue with some degree of exercise for all other movements as the patient is able. Combined hip abduction and lateral rotation done with the knees bent and the patient lying supine, and mid-range swinging of the knees from side-to-side with the hips and knees flexed and the feet on the bed, are often tolerated quite well. Back-care education should be started immediately, with a thorough explanation of the causes of the patient's symptoms and the reasons why the patient should follow a policy of moderation in all movements and activities.

With the patient once again in the side lying position manual mobilizations of the pelvis and lumbar spine, initially of low amplitude and done in short bursts, may help to both relax the patient and gain some degree of flexibility in the spine. The use of physical agents and electrical modalities both pre and post exercise are usually essential from the point of view of patient comfort. Once the patient is able to lie comfortably on his back, or to sustain the half-sitting position, he should start attempting light resisted exercises for the upper extremities, initially in early ranges. This can usually be done comfortably and will help to work some of the musculature of the trunk, albeit indirectly. Muscle stimulation for the muscles of the mid and low back with the patient lying in a comfortable position will help to prepare the patient for further advances in exercise.

As pain levels decrease and the patient shows better tolerance for exercise, he can be progressed to isometric leg work, with concurrent muscle stimulation for the muscles in the low back. Patients may at this time be able to tolerate upper extremity work in a gym, using weight-training equipment with light weights and low repetitions, as long as they are able to maintain a fairly neutral position of the spine. At this time the program should be working towards general spinal flexibility, however, the patient will still require rests in a neutral spinal position at frequent intervals. It is important to maintain balance between flexion- and extension-type exercises while progressing all other movements.

The patient will normally be left with a certain degree of loss of range of motion either into flexion or extension; pushing beyond this point will aggravate symptoms very quickly. At this time the patient has to be clearly advised about the need for a prolonged and sustained program of mobilizing exercises, which the patient should be able to progress by himself at home. The aim of the exercise program is to recover the lost range of motion, which normally relates to the underlying chronic condition, rather than to the present acute episode. A full gym exercise program, including the use of a step machine, exercise bike, treadmill, as well as weight-training equipment, should be used to stimulate recovery of full spinal function related to the patient's typical level of daily activities. Continued back education should restress points of posture and body mechanics using various forms of teaching aides if available. These patients will often benefit from regular review in the clinic on a monthly or bimonthly basis in order to monitor any changes in their underlying back conditions.

Restrictions The patient must be advised in the beginning not to sustain any one position for any period of time, even if it is comfortable. All pain-producing activities should be altered by attempting them in a different position or for a shorter period of time, or by using pacing strategies, such as only vacuuming one room at a time. Where a specific task or position produces pain, the patient must stop the activity, relieve the symptoms, then continue, but rest again as often as required. These restrictions must be explained carefully to the patient, otherwise there is a tendency to stop attempting all and any activities. This will ultimately produce more profound stiffness and weakness in the spine and a general deconditioning of musculature.

Driving can be attempted using a lumbar roll on an intermittent basis (15 minutes use of the roll followed by 15 minutes without it). All activities should be interspersed with short rests in the comfortable side-lying position. Lifting using correct body mechanics should be possible with light weights (less than 10 lb.). Maintaining a flexed or extended back position should only be attempted for a few minutes at a time, but an effort must be made to eliminate these activities from the patient's daily routine, rather than attempting to increase the patient's tolerance for them. Return to full activities is normally a very slow process—regular setbacks should be expected. The patient needs to be aware of this uneven recovery process so as not to become too disheartened.

Spinal Stenosis

Overview

This condition is produced by narrowing of the spinal canal in the lumbar region. The patient's symptoms are worsened by extension activities because the spinal canal narrows during extension. These symptoms are then eased by some degree of flexion of the spine. The condition can either be congenital or acquired. The congenital type is due to developmental anomalies in the spine that may occur in conditions such as achondroplasia. The acquired type may be related to disc degeneration and facet joint bony hypertrophy. In some cases this may also produce narrowing of the neural foraminae, leading to nerve root symptoms that will occur unilaterally, although most commonly the symptoms in this condition are bilateral. Although this is a bony deformity, patients often get a lot of relief from symptoms with a properly designed exercise program (3, 6, 14–16, 20, 21).

Subjective Findings

Onset Patients are usually over 50 years of age and give a history of a gradual onset of symptoms occurring for no known reason (14, 15, 19).

Duration Patients will have had symptoms for at least 3 to 6 months and often as long as 2 or more years, as initial symptoms can be quite innocuous in nature.

Frequency There will be a history of recurrent episodes of symptoms over months to years, with steadily increasing intensity of symptoms spreading over a greater area, starting in the back and then moving into the lower extremities (2, 3, 13, 16).

Area of Symptoms Initially the patient's symptoms are localized to the back and are very minor. The pain in the back remains as symptoms spread, usually into both legs, but occasionally into only one (which would suggest involvement of a single nerve root). The distribution in the legs when symptoms are bilateral is not within a specific nerve root distribution (Fig. 5.17) (1, 3, 6, 23).

Type of Symptoms Initial symptoms are tightness and sharp pain in the back, which progresses to an aching pain, paraesthesia, anaesthesia, and often a sensation of heaviness in one, or more commonly both, legs (1, 2, 16).

Miscellaneous Symptoms occur most commonly after the patient has walked a specific distance, although they may also occur after a period of time spent in the standing position. The distance or time does not change dramatically from week to week, although over a period of months the patient will usually find that he is walking less far or standing for a shorter period of time. Symptoms caused by these activities are then relieved, although not immediately, by sitting in a slumped position or by standing leaning forward and supported on the elbows, such as in leaning on a shopping cart or a fence. The symptoms can also be relieved by lying down (4, 5, 13, 14, 16).

Objective Findings

Observation The patient may present with a moderately increased lumbar lordosis, but as often as not the appearance of the patient's back is unremarkable on examination.

Active Movements Extension of the lumbar spine will be moderately limited and will produce back pain, although not necessarily leg symptoms. Leg symptoms are more likely to arise if extension is tested in standing as compared to lying. Flexion of the spine is usually unlimited

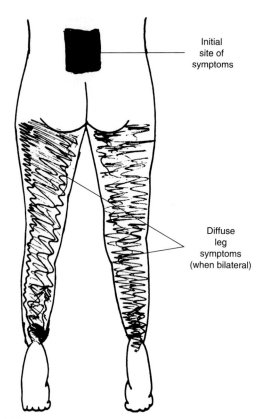

Initial
site of
symptoms

Diffuse
leg
symptoms
(when bilateral)

FIG. 5.17   Area of symptoms for spinal stenosis (symptoms may be unilateral in which case symptoms should be within the distribution of a particular nerve root).

and if symptoms are present in the leg they will normally decrease slightly with back flexion, but not dramatically. Side flexions of the spine and rotations to either side will be within normal limits and will have no effect on the symptoms (3–5, 10, 19, 20).

Passive Movements   A solid block should be found on attempted overpressure at end range of extension of the lumbar spine with sharp pain produced in the low back and possibly some leg paraesthesia. Overpressure on all other movements is unlikely to affect the symptoms (3, 4, 13).

Resisted Movements As long as the position in which the patient is tested is comfortable, then isometric resisted testing will reveal normal strength and produce no symptoms in either the back or leg. In patients who have suffered this condition for an extended period of time there will be a general decrease in activity levels; therefore, some general deconditioning of the muscles of the trunk and lower extremities may be encountered.

Palpation There will be very poor intervertebral mobility in both the lumbar and thoracic spine as tested by posterior/anterior pressure applied to the spinous processes. This maneuver may also produce local discomfort over one or more segments of the spine, particularly in the lower lumbar region (3, 19, 23, 24).

Specific Tests Radiological findings may show narrowing of the spinal canal, particularly on computerized tomography scanning.

Treatment Ideas
(1–6, 8, 13–16, 19–21)

The application of thermal modalities such as heat packs may help to loosen a stiff back, but in general modalities are not useful in this condition. The patient will usually have already learned to rest either in supine lying, slumped sitting, or slumped standing position in order to relieve the leg symptoms when they arise. Initial active exercise should be taken through the available pain-free range, with a strong bias towards flexion exercises. Single- and double-knee hip flexion (taking the knees to the chest) is often well tolerated. If the patient has difficulty (due to leg weakness) in completing this type of exercise, then a towel wrapped around the thigh can be used so that the patient can assist the leg movement using the upper extremities. Hip rotation and abduction with the knees bent, straight leg raising, hamstring stretches, and light abdominal work with pelvic tilting, all done lying supine, may help regain flexibility of the spine and pelvis and should not produce any symptoms. Extension of the spine in any form should be avoided at this stage.

Resisted abdominal work can be progressed through head and chest raises in the supine lying position and the patient will usually tolerate sit ups quite well. Resisted arm and leg exercises in a lying position using weights or an exercise band can be used to reinforce a reduction of the lumbar lordosis where applicable. Flexion, side flexion, and rotation exercises can be done sitting. Flexion stretches, used to ease pressure on the facet joints and open up the spinal canal, can be progressed by having the patient lean forward while sitting to place the hands as far back between the feet as can be managed comfortably. Local spinal and pelvic mobilizations to achieve rotary and side flexion movements of the pelvis and spine are also usually well tolerated by the patient and help to produce better local flexibility in the lumbar/pelvic region.

For aerobic activity in patients with de-conditioning the use of an exercise bike is beneficial, as it allows the patient to exercise in a slightly forward-flexed position. Patients often respond well to endurance-type work with light weights and high repetitions of exercises as long as they are able to maintain a posture that produces some flattening of the lumbar lordosis during the exercises. Any onset of leg symptoms during a treatment program should be relieved by a 5-minute period sitting in a slumped position with the forearms resting on the knees.

Restrictions In back-pain patients with this condition, it is useful to teach the patient to slump in a chair with flattening, rather than flexion, of the lumbar spine. Given the type of condition and the age of the patient, he will often stiffen up quite easily, so it is important to promote regular changes in position. Walking, and probably standing, will have clearly defined limits; the patient should be advised to stop those particular activities before the symptoms start and to rest in a slightly slumped position for a few minutes before continuing. Patients should be advised not to lie on their stomach to sleep or for any other activity, although they will probably have already found this to be difficult.

Swimming will tend to provoke both back and legs symptoms because in most swimming strokes extension in the lumbar and cervical regions is necessary so that the swimmer can continue to breath. If patients are very keen on aquatic activities, this author advises them to swim mainly on their backs or in short bursts, interspersing these activities with exercises such as walking sideways or backwards in the swimming pool, or doing arm exercises while floating on their backs. As a patient progresses through the exercise program, he will usually find that he can steadily extend the time over which specific activities are carried out, but should be advised to always stop short of the point where leg symptoms begin.

Chronic Spinal Instability

Overview

Lack of flexibility is a common presenting factor in many back conditions, however, on this occasion the patients are, in a sense, too flexible. Essentially the patient presents as a person with a great deal of mobility in their spine, good strength, and very little to find on physical testing, yet still complaining of recurrent episodes of back pain (16, 19, 21, 48).

Subjective Findings

Onset Onset is commonly gradual with no known cause or on very rare occasions following injury. The patient is usually young, being between 15 and 35 years of age (13, 14, 16).

Duration The patient is usually able to suffer the symptoms for weeks or even months before seeking help, unless these affect a particular sporting activity, in which case a patient is likely to present for treatment a little more quickly.

Frequency The typical history is recurrent symptoms over a period of 1 to 2 years or more, with the patient offering comments such as "I have suffered back pain off and on for as long as I can remember."

Area of Symptoms Symptoms are distributed throughout the lower back, with the patient often demonstrating the location by placing both hands over the lumbar region. On rare occasions symptoms can spread into the buttocks or the lateral aspect of the hips bilaterally (Fig. 5.18) (3, 14, 16, 19).

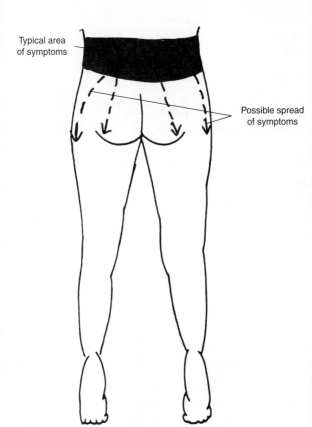

FIG. 5.18 Area of symptoms for chronic spinal instability.

Type of Symptoms   The patient will complain of a diffuse ache or burning sensation, which occurs most particularly after strenuous or unaccustomed activity (19, 21).

Miscellaneous   Most commonly patients are fit, active, and sports oriented, or were sports oriented, but are now restricted by the back pain.

Objective Findings

Observation   The appearance of the back is normal, although on rare occasions there may be an increased lumbar lordosis, particularly in the case of young gymnasts or dancers. There is never any flattening of the normal lumbar lordosis (13, 14, 16).

Active Movements   The patient will often demonstrate exceptional range of motion in all directions on testing of the lumbar spine, usually with no discomfort either during or at end range of motion (3, 19, 21).

Passive Movements   As in active movements there will be an unusually large degree of movement available, with no discomfort produced, even when overpressure is given at the ends of the already excessive ranges of motion.

Resisted Movements   Isometric testing will reveal good strength and no discomfort in all muscle groups of the trunk and lower extremities.

Palpation   A marked degree of intervertebral mobility will be found on posterior and anterior pressure throughout the spine, usually with no complaints of tenderness or discomfort on testing (13, 14, 19, 23, 24).

Specific Tests   Patients often show hypermobility when peripheral joints are tested, particularly hyperextension of the elbows, fingers, and knees.

Treatment Ideas
(3, 13, 14, 16, 19, 21, 30, 38, 49–51)

Initial active exercises can be carried out in lying, sitting, and standing positions with the patient taking the joints of the trunk and extremities through "normal" range of motion with a high rate of repetitions, but with no overpressure at end range. These exercises can be progressed to gentle, prolonged, and painless stretches held for 15 to 30 seconds for each movement. At this time postural correction, mainly in the form of pelvic tilting in lying, sitting, and standing positions can be commenced.

Pelvic stability exercises are then started, such as lying prone with the knees flexed at 90 degrees and letting one foot drop out to the side. The movement should then be held at the point at which the contralateral side of the pelvis starts to rise from the bed. This position should be held for 5 to 10 seconds, and the exercises are repeated several times for each leg. The foot is then dropped in towards the other leg; on this movement the ipsilateral pelvis will start to rise at end range of motion. The movement is then held at this point, with the patient instructed to keep the pelvis flat on the bed. These exercises can be progressed by the use of weights on the legs. The patient should be told that all exercises must be done slowly and smoothly, and taken only to the point of what would be considered normal range of motion. If the exercises produce local discomfort there may be tightness at one segment of the lumbar spine or in one sacroiliac joint compared to the other. In this case local passive mobilizations of the spine and pelvis may prove helpful.

Isometric resisted exercises for the lower extremities can be performed in the first 20 to 30% of range using quite heavy weights or a strong resistance band, which can help to tighten up the muscles around the back and pelvis. Neuromuscular electrical stimulation can be applied to the back extensors during the exercises, but the patient must maintain a slightly flattened lumbar lordosis while the stimulation is applied. When the patient begins to experience decreased discomfort from day to day, he can be progressed to gym exercise with weight training, again working within what would be considered normal ranges of motion, with an emphasis on pelvic tilt and abdominal work. The overall gym program should be related to the patient's desired level of daily activities.

Restrictions If specific sports, recreation, or work activities are producing symptoms on a regular basis, then the patient will require approximately 1 month of rest from the activities to allow the exercise program to take effect. The patient can then return gradually through light training, to heavy training, to competitive sports, or in a graduated fashion towards work activities that were previously uncomfortable. Other than that there are no particular restrictions related to this condition. Restriction on activities will become more stringent if the patient is pregnant, as there may then be a risk of sustaining a ligament strain in the low back, and for up to 1-year postpartum due to the ligament laxity associated with childbirth.

REFERENCES

1. Skinner H.B. (ed): Current Diagnosis and Treatment in Orthopaedics. Appleton and Lange, Norwalk, CT, 1995
2. Crowther C.L.: Primary Orthopaedic Care. Mosby, St. Louis, 1999
3. Salter R.B.: Textbook of Disorders and Injuries of the Muscular Skeletal System (3rd ed). Williams and Wilkins, Baltimore, 1999
4. Braddom R.L. (ed): Physical Medicine and Rehabilitation. W.B. Saunders, Philadelphia, 1996
5. Dandy D.J., Edwards D.J.: Essential Orthopaedics and Trauma (3rd ed). Churchill Livingston, New York, 1998
6. Mercier, L.R.: Practical Orthopaedics (4th ed). Mosby Yearbook, St. Louis, 1991
7. Payton O.D. (ed): Manual of Physical Therapy. Churchill Livingston, New York, 1989
8. Snider R.K. (ed): Essential of Musculoskeletal Care. American Academy of Orthopaedic Surgeons, Rosemont, IL, 1997
9. Donatelli R.A., Wooden M.J. (eds): Orthopaedic Physical Therapy (2nd ed). Churchill Livingston, New York, 1994

10. Goldie B.S.: Orthopaedic Diagnosis and Management: A Guide to the Care of Orthopaedic Patients (2nd ed). ISIS Medical Media, Oxford, U.K., 1998

11. McKenzie R. The Lumbar Spine: Mechanical Diagnosis and Therapy. Spinal Publications, Waikanae, New Zealand, 1981

12. Mertagh J., Kenna C.J.: Back Pain and Spinal Manipulation (2nd ed). Butterworth Heinemann, Oxford, U.K., 1997

13. Corrigan B., Maitland G.D.: Vertical Musculoskeletal Disorders. Butterworth, Oxford, U.K., 1998

14. Kesson M.P., Atkins E.: Orthopaedic Medicine: A Practical Approach. Butterworth Heinemann, Oxford, U.K., 1998

15. Hadler N.M.: Occupational Musculoskeletal Disorders (2nd ed). Lippincott Williams and Wilkins, Philadelphia, 1999

16. Apley A.G., Solomon L.: Apley's System of Orthopaedics and Fractures (6th ed). Butterworth, London, 1983

17. Prentice W.E.: Rehabilitation Techniques in Sports Medicine. WCB/McGraw Hill, New York, 1999

18. Anderson B.C.: Office Orthopaedics for Primary Care: Diagnosis and Treatment (2nd ed). W.B. Saunders, Philadelphia, 1999

19. Corrigan B., Maitland G.D.: Practical Orthopaedic Medicine. Butterworth, London, 1983

20. Cyriax J.: Textbook of Orthopaedic Medicine: Vol.1, Diagnosis of Soft Tissue Lesions (8th Ed). Bailliere Tindall, Eastbourne, U.K., 1982

21. Malone T.R., McPoil T.G., Nitz A.J. (eds): Orthopaedic and Sports Physical Therapy (3rd ed). Mosby St. Louis, 1997

22. Konin J.G., Wilksten D.L., Isear J.A.: Special Tests for Orthopaedic Examination. Slack, New Jersey, 1997

23. Magee D.J.: Orthopaedic Physical Assessment (2nd ed). W.B. Saunders, Philadelphia, 1992

24. Field D.: Anatomy: Palpation and Surface Markings (2nd ed). Butterworth Heinemann, Oxford, U.K., 1997

25. Gross J, Feeto J., Rosen E.: Musculoskeletal Examination. Blackwell Science, Cambridge, MA, 1996

26. Donatelli R.A., Wooden M.J. (Eds): Orthopaedic Physical Therapy (2nd ed). Churchill Livingston, New York, 1994

27. Fritz J.M.: Use of a Classification Approach to the Treatment of Three Patients with Low Back Syndrome. Phys. Ther., 78 (7):766–777, 1998

28. McGill S.M.: Low Back Exercise: Evidence For Improving Exercise Regimes. Phys. Ther., 78 (7):754–765, 1998

29. Maher C., Latimer J., Refshauge K.: Prescription of Activity For Low Back Pain: What Works?. Aus. J. Physiother., 45:121–132, 1999

30. De Rosa C.P., Porterfield J.A.: A Physical Therapy Model For Treatment of Low Back Pain. Phys. Ther., 72:261–272, 1992

31. Quebec Task Force on Spinal Disorders: Scientific Approach to the Assessment and Management of Activity Related Spinal Disorders. Spine, 12:75, 1987

32. Wisneski R.J., et al.: Lumbar Disc Disease. In: Herkowitz H.N., et al., eds., The Spine, p. 613–679. WB Saunders, Philadelphia, 1999

33. Cole A.J., Herring S.A.: The Low Back Pain Handbook: A Practical Guide for the Primary Care Clinician. Hanley and Belfus, Philadelphia, 1997

34. Sofa A., et al.: Centralization of Low Back Pain and Perceived Functional Outcome. J. Orthop. Sports Phys. Ther., 27 (3):205–212, 1998

35. Vocalic N., Strand D. Gunter P., Swenson O.: Diagnosis and Prognosis in Lumbar Disc Herniation. Clin. Orthop., 361:116–122, 1999

36. Kawakami M., et al.: Possible Mechanisms of Painful Radiculopathy in Lumbar Disc Herniation. Clin. Orthop., 351:241–251, 1998

37. Kerssens J.J., Sluijs E.M., Veraak P.F.M.: Back Care Instruction In Physical Therapy: A Trend Analysis of Individualized Back Care Programs. Phys. Ther., 79 (3):286–295, 1999

38. Vandervalt R.W.A., Dekker J., Vanbaar M.E.: Physical Therapy For Patients with Back Pain: A Description. Physiother., 81:345–351, 1995

39. Onel D., et al.: Computed Tomographic Investigation of the Effect of Traction on Lumbar Disc Herniation. Spine, 14:82–90, 1989

40. Bringkman P., Porter R.W.: Laboratory Model of Lumbar Disc Protrusion: Fissure and Fragment. Spine 19:228–235, 1994

41. Aspden R.M., Porter R.W.: Localized Stresses in the Intervertible Disc Resulting from a Loose Fragment: A Theory for Fissure and Fragments. Spine 24:2214–2218, 1999

42. Mignucci L.A., Bell G.R.: In: Differential Diagnosis of Sciatica. In Herkowitz H.N., et al eds., The Spine p. 89–107, WB Saunders, Philadelphia, 1999

43. Zdeblick T.A.: Discogenic Back Pain. In The Spine, Herkowitz H.N., et al., eds., p. 749–765, WB Saunders, Philadelphia, 1999

44. Cibulka M.T.: Treatment of the SI Joint Component to Low Back Pain: A Case Report. Phys. Ther., 72:917–922, 1992

45. Walker J.M.: The Sacroiliac Joint: A Critical Review. Phys. Ther., 72 903–916, 1992

46. Mooney V: Sacroiliac Joint Dysfunction. The Spine, In Herkowitz H.N., et al., eds., p. 767–778, WB Saunders, Philadelphia, 1999

47. Franklin M.E., Conner-Kerr T.: An Analysis of Posture and Back Pain In the First to Third Trimesters of Pregnancy. J. Orthop. Sports Phys. Ther., 28 (3): 133–138, 1998

48. Fritz J.M., Erhard R.E., Hagen B.F.: Segmental Instability of the Lumbar Spine. Phys. Ther., 78 (8):889–896, 1998

The following tables contain test movements for examination of the hip and knee. The starting positions and a description of each movement are given. These would be considered the optimal test positions in each case, which would have to be modified for individual patients who are unable to achieve or sustain a described position.

Active Movements of the Hip Joint

Name of Movement	Starting Position	Movement
Flexion	The movement is tested in supine or side lying. The patient's leg is placed in the neutral position (i.e., with the toes pointing upwards and the leg out straight, in supine).	The patient is instructed to take the knee towards the chest allowing the knee to flex as necessary. Average range of motion: 120–130°
Extension	The movement is tested in prone lying or side lying with the leg straight. The therapist stabilizes the pelvis to minimize back extension.	The patient is instructed to take the thigh backwards (i.e., raise the leg off the bed). Average range of motion: 30°
Abduction	The movement is tested in supine lying or side lying with the hip in the neutral position.	The patient is instructed to take the leg out sideways away from the other leg. The hips should remain in the neutral position between flexion and extension during movement and the patient's toes should continue to point upwards when supine to avoid rotation of the hip. Average range of motion: 45–50°
Adduction	The movement is tested in supine lying with the hip flexed enough to allow the leg to be carried over the opposite leg. If the patient has large thighs the test movement can be	The patient is instructed to carry the raised leg over the other leg while keeping it straight. In the modified test the patient takes the test leg towards the other abducted leg. The

Active Movements of the Hip Joint (*continued*)

Name of Movement	Starting Position	Movement
	modified, starting with the other leg fully abducted.	therapist can also passively place the other leg in flexion while the patient tries to draw the tested leg under it. Average range of motion: 30°
Lateral Rotation	1. The patient is placed in supine lying with the legs straight and in the neutral position (i.e., toes pointing towards the ceiling). 2. With the patient in supine lying with the hip and knee flexed to 90°. 3. With the patient in prone lying and the knee flexed to 90°.	1. The patient is instructed to roll the leg outward so that the toes point away from the other leg. 2. The patient is instructed to take the foot in towards the opposite leg (i.e., as if to rest the heel on the opposite thigh). 3. The patient is instructed to take the foot in towards the other leg (i.e., heel towards the back of the other knee). Average range of motion: 45°
Medial Rotation	1. The patient is placed in supine lying with the leg straight and the toes pointing up towards the ceiling. 2. With the patient in supine lying with the hip and knee flexed to 90°. 3. With the patient in prone lying with the knee flexed to 90°.	1. The patient is instructed to roll the legs inwards so that the toes are pointing towards the opposite leg. 2. The patient is instructed to take the foot out and away from the opposite leg. 3. The patient is instructed to let the foot drop outwards away from the other leg. Average range of motion: 45°.

Passive Movements of the Hip

Name of Movement	Starting Position	Movement
Flexion	With the patient in supine lying cup the patient's heel in one hand and place the other hand under the patient's thigh.	The patient's thigh is carried up towards the abdomen while the knee is flexed as required to achieve full range of motion.
Extension	With the patient in prone lying and the hip in the neutral position, place one hand on the buttock of the side to be tested. To fix the pelvis. Place the other hand on the anterior of the patient's thigh.	The patient's thigh is raised off the treatment table while downward pressure is applied to the buttock.
Lateral Rotation	1. With the patient in supine lying with the legs straight and the toes pointing up, one hand on the anterior of the patient's thigh and the other hand on their shin. 2. With the patient in supine lying with the hip and knee flexed to 90°, grip the patient's heel with one hand and support the calf with the other hand.	1. The patient's leg is rolled over so that the foot and knee turn outwards. 2. The patient's lower leg and foot are carried in towards the opposite leg.
Medial Rotation	1. With the patient in supine lying with the legs straight and the toes pointing up to the ceiling, place one hand on the anterior of the patient's thigh and the other hand on the shin. 2. With the patient in supine lying with the hip and knee flexed to 90°, grip the patient's heel with one hand and support the calf with the other.	1. The patient's leg is rolled over so that the foot and knee are turned in towards the opposite leg. 2. The patient's lower leg and foot are carried out away from the opposite leg.

Passive Movements of the Hip (*continued*)

Name of Movement	Starting Position	Movement
Abduction	With the patient in supine lying with the legs straight and the toes pointed up, support the patient's leg under the heel and the knee.	The patient's leg is drawn out sideways away from the other leg. Avoid any flexion, extension, or rotation of the hip during the movement.
Adduction	With the patient in supine lying with the legs straight and the toes pointed up, support the patient's leg under the heel and the knee.	The patient's leg is carried into sufficient flexion at the hip to allow it to clear the opposite leg. The leg is then carried across the opposite leg. Patients with large thighs or patients who have difficulty with flexion are tested by taking the opposite leg into abduction and then drawing the test leg towards it.

Resisted Movements of the Hip

Name of Movement	Starting Position	Movement
Flexion	1. With the patient in supine lying with the leg straight and the toes pointed upwards, place one hand on the anterior of the patient's thigh. 2. With the patient sitting over the edge of the treatment table with the hips flexed to 90°, place one hand on the anterior of the patient's thigh.	1. Instruct the patient to try and raise the leg off the bed while you resist the movement, or have the patient raise the leg 10–20° off the treatment table, then try to push the leg back onto the bed as the patient resists the movement. 2. The patient is instructed to raise the thigh off the treatment table while you resist the movement, or have the patient raise the thigh off the treatment table. Try to push the thigh back onto the table while the patient resists the movement.
Extension	The movement is tested with the patient in prone lying with the foot off the end of the treatment table. Place one hand on the posterior aspect of the patient's thigh.	The patient is instructed to raise the leg off the bed while the movement is resisted, or have the patient raise the leg off the treatment table and then try to push the leg back onto the table while the patient resists the movement.
Abduction	The movement is tested with the patient in supine lying. Place one hand on the lateral aspect of the thigh and the other hand at the lateral aspect of the knee.	The patient is instructed to try and draw the leg outwards away from the other leg as the movement is resisted, or instruct the patient to maintain the leg position while you try to push the leg in towards the opposite leg.

Resisted Movements of the Hip (*continued*)

Name of Movement	Starting Position	Movement
Adduction	The movement is tested in supine lying, with the leg straight and the toes pointing upwards. One hand is placed on the medial aspect of the thigh and the other hand on the medial aspect of the knee.	The patient is instructed to hold the leg still while you try to draw it away from the other leg, or hold the leg still while the patient tries to draw the leg in towards the other leg.
Lateral Rotation	1. With the patient in prone lying and the knees flexed to 90°, place both hands on the medial aspect of the patient's lower leg. 2. With the patient sitting with his legs over the edge of the treatment table, and the hips and knees flexed to 90°. Place one hand on the medial aspect of the lower leg.	1. Apply pressure to the lower leg to pull the foot out away from the opposite leg as the patient maintains the position. 2. Apply pressure to the lower leg to push the foot out, up, and away from the opposite foot while the patient resists the movement.
Medial Rotation	1. With the patient in prone lying and the knees flexed to 90°, place one hand on the lateral aspect of the patient's lower leg. 2. With the patient sitting with the legs over the edge of treatment table with the hips and knees flexed to 90°, place one hand on the lateral aspect of the lower leg.	1. Apply pressure to the lower leg to push it in towards the opposite leg. 2. Apply pressure to the lower leg to push the foot in towards opposite leg.

Active Movements of the Knee Joint

Name of Movement	Starting Position	Movement
Flexion	1. The movement is tested in supine lying, with the leg straight and the toes pointed upwards. 2. With the patient sitting over the edge of the treatment table with the leg held out straight at the knee.	1. The patient is instructed to slide the heel up the table towards the buttock. 2. The patient is instructed to bend the knee, taking the foot down and under the treatment table and bending the knee as much as possible. Average range of motion: 130–135°
Extension	1. In the supine lying position with the knee bent as far as possible. 2. The patient sits over the edge of the treatment table with the knee bent as fully as possible.	1. The patient is instructed to straighten the leg, sliding the heel down the bed. 2. The patient is instructed to straighten the knee, raising the foot as far as possible while keeping the thigh in contact with the treatment table.
Lateral Rotation	The patient sits over the edge of a treatment table with the knee flexed to 90° and the foot clear of the floor.	The patient is instructed to turn the foot outwards, taking the toes away from the opposite leg and the heel towards the opposite leg. Average range of motion: 30–40°
Medial Rotation	The patient sits over the edge of a treatment table with the knee flexed to 90° and the foot clear of the floor.	The patient is instructed to turn the foot so that the toes point towards the opposite leg and the heel away from it. Average range of motion: 20–30°

In practice, the movements of flexion and extension are tested simultaneously with the patient alternately bending and straightening their knee. Average ranges are given as 0–130/135°, with zero ° being the knee fully extended.

Passive Movements of the Knee

Name of Movement	Starting Position	Movement
Flexion	1. The patient is placed in supine lying with the legs straight and the toes pointed upwards. Support the patient's heel with one hand with the other hand placed on the posterior of the patient's thigh. 2. The patient is seated over the edge of the treatment table with the foot clear of the ground. Place one hand on the anterior of the patient's lower leg.	1. The patient's heel is brought up towards their posterior thigh while the knee is allowed to flex (half way through the movement, transfer the hand from the posterior of the patient's thigh to the anterior of the knee). 2. Pressure is applied to the anterior of the patient's lower leg to push the foot under the treatment table, bending the knee as far as possible.
Extension	1. The patient is in supine lying with the leg straight and the toes pointed upwards. Cup the patient's heel with one hand with the other hand placed over the anterior thigh just above the knee. 2. With the patient sitting over the edge of the treatment table cup the patient's heel with one hand and place the other hand over the anterior thigh just above the knee.	1. Downward pressure is applied to the anterior of the patient's thigh while the heel is raised off the bed. 2. Pressure is applied to the patient's anterior thigh while the foot is raised to straighten the knee. The posterior thigh must be kept in contact with the bed.
Lateral Rotation	The movement is tested with the patient sitting over the edge of the treatment table with the foot clear of the ground and the knee flexed to 90°.	The patient's foot is turned so that the toes face away from the opposite leg and the heel points towards it (rotating the tibia on the femur).

(continued)

Passive Movements of the Knee (*continued*)

Name of Movement	Starting Position	Movement
Lateral Rotation (continued)	Place one hand on the lateral aspect of their heel and the other hand on the medial aspect of the forefoot.	
Medial Rotation	The movement is tested with the patient sitting over the edge of the treatment table with the foot clear of the floor. Grip the medial aspect of the patient's heel with one hand and the lateral aspect of the forefoot with the other hand.	The patient's foot is turned so that the toes are pointed towards the opposite leg and the heel points away from it.

Passive Movements of the Patella

Name of Movement	Starting Position	Movement
Inferior Glide	Place one hand so that the web between the index finger and thumb is over the superior pole of the patella.	Pressure is applied to the superior pole of the patella to push the patella down towards the foot.
Medial Glide	Both thumbs are placed over the lateral border of the patella.	Pressure is applied to the lateral border of the patella to push it medially.
Lateral Glide	Both thumbs are placed over the medial border of patella.	Pressure is applied to the medial border of the patella to push it laterally.

All movements of the patella are tested with the patient's leg supported on the treatment table with the knee straight and the toes pointing upwards.

Resisted Movements of the Knee

Name of Movement	Starting Position	Movement
Flexion	The patient sits with the legs over the edge of a treatment table with the knees flexed to 90° and the foot unsupported. One hand is placed over the anterior of the patient's lower leg.	1. Attempt to bend the patient's knee while the patient resists the movement. 2. The patient is instructed to try and straighten the knee while the movement is resisted.
Extension	The patient sits over the edge of the treatment table and one hand cups the patient's heel posteriorly.	1. Attempt to straighten the knee while the patient resists the movement. 2. The patient is instructed to try and bend the knee while the movement is resisted.
Lateral Rotation	The patient sits with the legs over the side of the treatment table and the foot unsupported. Grasp the medial aspect of the heel and the lateral aspect of the forefoot.	Attempt to turn the patient's foot so that the toes are pointing towards the opposite leg and the heel points away from it, while the patient resists the movement.
Medial Rotation	The patient sits over the edge of a treatment table with the knees bent and the foot unsupported. Grip the lateral aspect of the heel and the medial aspect of the forefoot.	Attempt to turn the patient's foot so that the toes point away from the opposite leg and the heel points towards it while the patient resists the movement.

Examination Findings Related to Specific Conditions

	Onset				
Sudden Due to Trauma	Gradual Due to Trauma	Gradual with No Cause	Sudden Due to Overuse	Gradual Due to Overuse
Groin Strain	OA Hip	OA Hip	Trochanteric Bursitis	Trochanteric Bursitis
Hamstring Muscle Tear	OA Knee	OA Knee		Adductor Tendonitis
Quadriceps Muscle Tear		Piriformis Syndrome		Psoas Bursitis
Quadriceps Tendon Tear		Patella Femoral Syndrome		Iliotibial Band Syndrome
Knee Ligament Strain				Hamstring Tendonitis
				Patella Femoral Syndrome

Typical Age Ranges				
15–45 Years	20–40 Years	20–50 Years	25–55 Years	50+ Years
Trochanteric Bursitis	Adductor Tendonitis	Collateral Knee Ligament Strain	Piriformis Syndrome	OA Hip
Hamstring Muscle Tear	Psoas Bursitis	Patella Femoral Syndrome	Iliotibial Band Syndrome	OA Knee
Patella Femoral Syndrome	Groin Strain			Quadriceps Tendon Tear
	Hamstring Tendonitis			
	Quadriceps Muscle Tear			

			Duration				
1 Day to 1 Week	2 Days to 2 Weeks	1 to 3 Weeks	3 to 6 Weeks	6 Weeks to 3 Months	2 to 3 Months	3 to 6 Months	Longer Than 1 Year
Quadriceps Tendon Tear Hamstring Tear Groin Strain	Groin Strain Hamstring Muscle Tear Quadriceps Muscle Tear Knee Ligament Strain	Adductor Tendonitis of the Hip Hamstring Tendonitis	Adductor Tendonitis of the Hip Psoas Bursitis Iliotibial Band Syndrome Hamstring Tendonitis	Piriformis Syndrome Patella Femoral Syndrome	Trochanteric Bursitis	OA Hip OA Knee	OA Hip OA Knee

		Frequency		
First Time with These Symptoms	Previously Similar Symptoms, but the First Time This Bad	One Long Episode with Exacerbations and Remissions	Recurrent (Seasonal) Problem	Recurrent Episodes of 1 to 2 Years
Adductor Tendonitis Psoas Bursitis Groin Strain Iliotibial Band Syndrome Hamstring Muscle Tear Quadriceps Muscle Tear Quadriceps Tendon Tear Knee Ligament Strain	Patella Femoral Syndrome Iliotibial Band Syndrome Hamstring Tendonitis	Trochanteric Bursitis OA Hip OA Knee	Adductor Tendonitis of the Hip Groin Strain Iliotibial Band Syndrome Hamstring Muscle Tear	Piriformis Syndrome Knee Ligament Strain

(continued)

Examination Findings Related to Specific Conditions (continued)

Area of Symptoms

	Lateral Aspect of Hip	Anterior Hip	Buttock and Back of Thigh	Anteromedial Thigh	Medial Aspect of Thigh	Back of Leg	Lateral Aspect of Thigh
	Trochanteric Bursitis	OA Hip Psoas Bursitis	Piriformis Syndrome Hamstring Muscle Tear Hamstring Tendonitis	OA Hip Psoas Bursitis Groin Strain	Adductor Tendonitis Groin Strain	Piriformis Syndrome	Iliotibial Band Syndrome Trochanteric Bursitis

	Posterior Thigh	Anterior Thigh	Anterior Knee	Posterior Knee	Lateral Aspect of the Knee	Medial Aspect of Knee	Generally around the Knee
	Piriformis Syndrome Hamstring Muscle Tear	OA Hip Quadriceps Muscle Tear Quadriceps Tendon Tear Patella Femoral Syndrome	Quadriceps Tendon Tear Knee Ligament Tear	Hamstring Muscle Tear Hamstring Tendon Tear	Iliotibial Band Syndrome Lateral Collateral Ligament Tear	Medial Collateral Ligament Tear	OA Knee Knee Ligament Tear

Type of Symptoms

Sharp Pain on Movement	Pain following Activity	Ache at Rest	Pain after Rest	Nagging Ache	Pain with Stiffness	Painful Pulling Sensation	Paraesthesia and Numbness in Leg
Groin Strain Hamstring Muscle Tear Quadriceps Muscle Tear Quadriceps Tendon Tear Knee Ligament Strain	Trochanteric Bursitis Psoas Bursitis Iliotibial Band Syndrome Hamstring Tendonitis Knee Ligament Tear Patella Femoral Tear	Quadriceps Muscle Tear Hamstring Muscle Tear Knee Ligament Strain	OA Hip OA Knee	Adductor Tendonitis Psoas Bursitis Iliotibial Band Syndrome Hamstring Muscle Tear Patella Femoral Syndrome	OA Hip OA Knee	Adductor Tendonitis Hamstring Tendonitis	Piriformis Syndrome

(continued)

Examination Findings Related to Specific Conditions (continued)

	Observation				
Nothing Unusual to Observe	Altered Gait	Wasting of Muscles of Thigh	Bruising at Medial Thigh	Bruising at Anterior Thigh/Knee	Bruising Posterior Thigh or Knee
Trochanteric Bursitis	OA Hip	OA Hip	Groin Strain	Quadriceps Muscle Tear	Hamstring Muscle Tear
Adductor Tendonitis	OA Knee	OA Knee		Quadriceps Tendon Tear	
Psoas Bursitis	Quadriceps Muscle Tear				
Piriformis Syndrome	Knee Ligament Strain				
Iliotibial Band Syndrome	Groin Strain				
Hamstring Tendonitis					
Patella Femoral Syndrome					

Swelling around Lateral Epicondyle of Femur	Swelling Anterior Thigh	Swelling at Knee	Swelling at Posterior Thigh	Soft Tissue Thickening at Knee
Iliotibial Band Syndrome	Quadriceps Muscle Tear	Collateral Ligament Tear	Hamstring Muscle Tear	OA Knee
	Quadriceps Tendon Tear			Patella Femoral Syndrome (Chronic)

Active Movements

Pain on Hip Abduction with Rotation	Hip Medial Rotation and Extension Most Limited	Abduction of Hip Only Limited Movement	Hip Extension Only Limited Movement	Abduction of Hip Painful	Pain on Hip Extension	Hip Extension and Abduction Painful	Hip Medial Rotation Painful
Trochanteric Bursitis	OA Hip	Adductor Tendonitis Groin Strain	Psoas Bursitis Groin Strain	Trochanteric Bursitis Adductor Tendonitis	OA Hip Psoas Bursitis	Groin Strain	OA Hip

Hip Lateral Rotation Limited and Painful	Straight Leg Raising Limited and Painful	Knee Flexion Limited	Knee Extension Limited	Mild Loss of Both Flexion and Extension at the Knee	Pain on Knee Flexion from Extension	Increased Limitation of Knee Flexion with Hip Extension	All Movements of Hip and Knee Pain Free and Full Range
Groin Strain	Piriformis Syndrome Hamstring Muscle Tear Hamstring Tendonitis	Quadriceps Muscle Tear Quadriceps Tendon Tear	Quadriceps Tendon Tear Hamstring Muscle Tear	Knee Ligament Tear OA Knee	Iliotibial Band Syndrome	Quadriceps Muscle Tear Quadriceps Tendon Tear	Patella Femoral Syndrome Piriformis Syndrome Trochanteric Bursitis

(continued)

Examination Findings Related to Specific Conditions (*continued*)

Passive Movements

Pain at End Range Hip Extension	Pain at End Range Hip Flexion	Pain at End Range Hip Abduction	Pain at End Range Hip Lateral Rotation	Pain at End Range Hip Medial Rotation	Stiff End Feel to All Hip Movements
Psoas Bursitis	Groin Strain	Adductor Tendonitis	Groin Strain	OA Hip	OA Hip
Groin Strain		Groin Strain	Piriformis Syndrome		
Hamstring Muscle Tear			Trochanteric Bursitis		

Pain on Hip Lateral Rotation with Abduction	Pain on Straight Leg Raise	Pain on Hip Extension with Knee Flexion	Pain at End Range Knee Flexion	Pain at End Range Knee Extension
Trochanteric Bursitis	Hamstring Muscle Tear	Quadriceps Muscle Tear (Rectus Femoris)	Quadriceps Muscle Tear	Knee Ligament Tear
Iliotibial Band Syndrome	Hamstring Tendonitis	Quadriceps Tendon Tear	Quadriceps Tendon Tear	OA Knee
	Piriformis Syndrome		Knee Ligament Strain	
			Patella Femoral Syndrome	
			OA Knee	

Resisted Movements

Pain on Hip Abduction	Pain on Hip Adduction	Pain on Hip Medial Rotation	Pain on Hip Lateral Rotation	Pain on Hip Flexion	Pain on Hip Extension	Weak Hip Abduction
Trochanteric Bursitis	Adductor Tendonitis Groin Strain	Trochanteric Bursitis	Piriformis Syndrome	Psoas Bursitis Quadriceps Muscle Tear	Hamstring Muscle Tear	OA Hip

Pain on Knee Flexion	Pain on Knee Extension	Pain on Knee Rotation	Weak Knee Flexion	Weak Knee Extension	General Weakness Hip and Knee	All Movements Pain Free and of Good Strength
Hamstring Muscle Tear Hamstring Tendonitis	Quadriceps Muscle Tear Quadriceps Tendon Tear	Hamstring Muscle Tear Hamstring Tendonitis Knee Ligament Tear	Hamstring Muscle Tear	Quadriceps Muscle Tear Quadriceps Tendon Tear	OA Knee OA Hip	Iliotibial Band Syndrome Patella Femoral Syndrome

(continued)

Examination Findings Related to Specific Conditions (*continued*)

Palpation

Tender Lateral Hip	Tender Anterior Hip	Tender Proximal/Medial Thigh	Tenderness in Buttock	Tender Posterior Thigh	Tender Anterior Thigh	Tender Lateral Epicondyle of Femur
Trochanteric Bursitis	OA Hip Psoas Bursitis Groin Strain	Adductor Tendonitis Groin Strain	Piriformis Syndrome Hamstring Tendonitis	Hamstring Muscle Tear	Quadriceps Muscle Tear	Iliotibial Band Syndrome

Tender Posterior Knee	Tender Anterior Knee	Tender Knee Joint Line	Tender Medial Aspect Knee	Tender Lateral Aspect Knee	Soft Tissue Thickening around Knee
Hamstring Tendonitis OA Knee	Quadriceps Tendon Tear Patella Femoral Syndrome	Knee Ligament Strain OA Knee	Knee Ligament Strain OA Knee	Iliotibial Band Syndrome Knee Ligament Strain OA Knee	OA Knee Patella Femoral Syndrome

PALPATION OF THE HIP AND KNEE

In this section a description is given of the method of palpating each structure referred to in relation to the following conditions:

- Trochanteric bursitis
- Osteoarthritis of the hip
- Adductor tendonitis of the hip
- Psoas bursitis
- Groin strain
- Piriformis syndrome
- Iliotibial band friction syndrome
- Hamstring muscle tear
- Hamstring tendonitis
- Quadriceps muscle tear
- Quadriceps tendon tear
- Collateral ligament strain of knee
- Patella femoral syndrome
- Osteoarthritis of the knee

Hip Area

Greater Trochanter

With the patient in the side lying position and the upper leg extended, run the palm of your hand over the lateral aspect of the patient's thigh at the hip. This will reveal a hard bony surface just below the rounded contour of the hip, which is the greater trochanter. Further palpation one-fingers breadth proximal to the greater trochanter will be on the site of the trochanteric bursa (Fig. 6.1 and 6.2)

Ischial Tuberosity

With the patient in the prone lying position take your hand around on a line from the greater trochanter going over the medial side of the buttock, then move approximately 5 cm (2 inches) distal to that point. Firm pressure into the flesh of the buttock at that point will reveal the presence of a rounded protuberance, the ischial tuberosity (Fig. 6.2). The easiest manner in which to identify this structure is to have the patient sit upright on your hands, as in this position the body weight is taken through the ischial tuberosities, making their presence more noticeable.

Hip Joint

The anterior of the hip joint lies approximately a fingers breadth below a line drawn between the anterior superior iliac spine and the pubic tubercle. Another way to identify this area is to find the femoral triangle, which can be done by putting the patient in the supine lying position with the knee and hip flexed and the foot of the leg to be tested resting on the opposite thigh. In this position the borders of the femoral triangle are visible: the medial border of the sartorious muscle laterally, the lateral border of the adductor longus muscle medially, and the base of the triangle formed by the

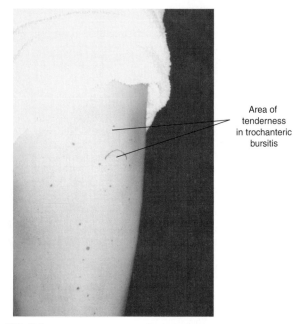

Area of
tenderness
in trochanteric
bursitis

FIG. 6.1   Line indicates the upper extent of the right greater trochanter and demonstrating the area of tenderness possible with a trochanteric bursitis.

inguinal ligament. Just distal to the base of the triangle lies the anterior hip joint line. This is a naturally tender area, so palpation must be carried out gently. The iliopsoas is also found in this area lying superficial to the joint line (Fig. 6.3).

Adductor Tendons of the Thigh

With the patient in the supine lying position and the knees slightly flexed, the adductor muscle mass is easily palpated and identified at the medial aspect of the upper half of the thigh (Fig. 6.4). This can be more clearly identified if the muscle is put into a gentle isometric contraction, in which case the tendons can be traced towards their origin in the groin.

Piriformis Muscles

The piriformis muscle lies along a line drawn from the greater trochanter to the middle half of a line drawn between the posterior superior iliac spine and the ischial tuberosity.

Ischial tuberosity

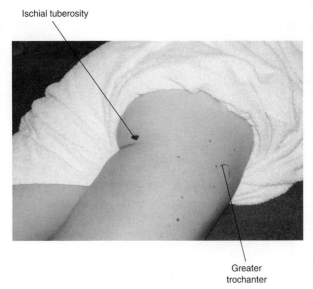

Greater
trochanter

FIG. 6.2   Surface marking of the ischial tuberosity and the right greater trochanter.

Hamstring Muscles

The bulk of the hamstring muscles can be identified easily in the posterior aspect of the upper two thirds of the thigh, and are most easily palpated when the knee is flexed isometrically against gentle resistance. The cordlike tendons of the hamstrings can be seen and palpated at the posterior aspect of the knee. The biceps femoris tendon lies laterally and the tendons of the semimembranosus and semitendinosus medially (Fig. 6.5). Their proximal attachment is into the ischial tuberosity (Fig. 6.2).

Knee Area

Patella

With the knee flexed at 90 degrees the patella is easily palpated at the anterior aspect of the knee (Fig. 6.6) and in this position the margins of the patella should be palpated. With the patient's knee fully extended the patella can be pushed laterally so that the lateral undersurface of the bone can be palpated. This maneuver can then be repeated on the medial side

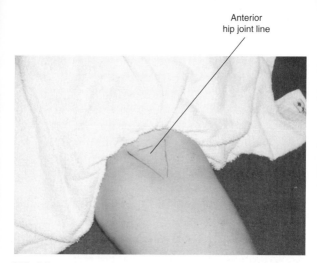

FIG. 6.3 Surface marking of the left femoral triangle demonstrating the position of the anterior hip joint line.

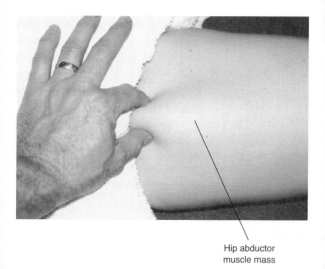

FIG. 6.4 The adductor muscle mass of the left thigh. The examiner's finger and thumb are gripping the adductor tendons.

Hamstring muscle
mass

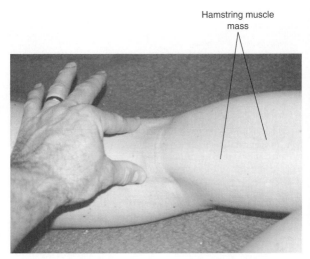

FIG. 6.5 The hamstring muscles of the left thigh. The examiner's index finger is on the tendon of the biceps femoris. The thumb is over the tendons of the semitendinosus and semimembranosus

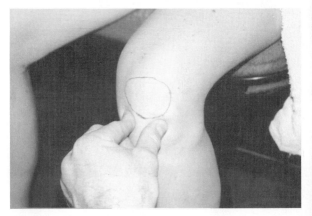

FIG. 6.6 Surface marking of the margins of the left patella. The examiner's index finger and thumb are placed in the depressions at the sides of the patella tendon marking the area of the joint line.

and in this way approximately half of the articular surface of the patella can be palpated.

Lateral Epicondyle of the Femur

With the patient's knee flexed to 90 degrees run your hand down the lateral aspect of the knee and the lateral epicondyle is then easily identified as a prominent bony point approximately at the level of the middle of the patella (Fig. 6.7).

Medial Epicondyle of the Femur

Run your hand down the lower part of the medial aspect of the thigh. The bony rounded protuberance first encountered is the medial condyle and the small bony protuberance is the medial epicondyle. Again this is approximately level with the midpatella when the knee is flexed to 90 degrees (Fig. 6.8).

Tibial Tubercle

If you take you hand downwards across the patella you will encounter a bony protuberance on the anterior of the tibia, called the tibial tubercle. This is more prominent when the knee is flexed at 90 degrees (Fig. 6.9).

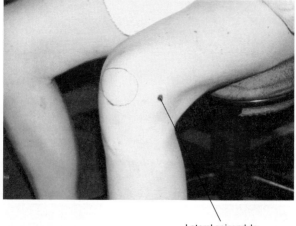

Lateral epicondyle
of femur

FIG. 6.7 Surface marking of the lateral epicondyle of the left femur and its position relative to the patella.

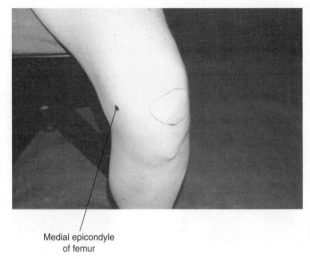

Medial epicondyle
of femur

FIG. 6.8 Surface marking of the medial epicondyle of the left femur and its position relative to the patella.

Patella Tendon

This can be felt in the space between the patella and the tibial tubercle and can be felt to tighten on contraction of the quadriceps muscle (Fig. 6.9).

Knee Joint Line

This is most easily identified with the patient in the sitting position with the lower leg hanging over the edge of the treatment table and the foot clear of the floor. The joint line lies at the halfway point of the patella tendon where there is a depression just at the sides of the tendon. When your fingers are placed in this depression the tibial condyles can be felt just below and the femoral condyles just above (Fig. 6.6). If the patient's lower leg is allowed to swing slightly it is easier to identify the joint as the tibia moves on the femur. It is then possible to trace the joint line around approximately to the halfway point, both medially and laterally, before it is covered by soft tissue (Fig. 6.9). It is impossible to palpate the knee joint line posteriorly.

Head of The Fibula

With the knee maintained in the flexed position a bony protuberance is visible and palpable at the lateral aspect of the lower leg, approximately

Patella tendon

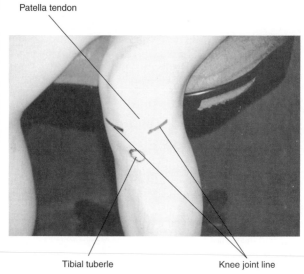

Tibial tuberle   Knee joint line

FIG. 6.9 The position of the tibial tubercle and patella tendon at the left knee. The two lines mark the palpable portions of the left knee joint line.

a thumbs breadth below the knee joint line. This is the head of the fibula (Fig. 6.10).

Medial Collateral Ligament

This ligament can be palpated throughout its extent between the medial epicondyle of the femur and the antero-medial aspect of the tibia just below the tibial condyle (Fig. 6.11).

Lateral Collateral Ligament

This ligament can be palpated throughout its extent from the lateral epicondyle of the femur to the head of the fibula (Fig. 6.10).

Quadriceps Muscles

These are easily identified at the anterior of the thigh; particularly noticeable are the rectus femoris muscle centrally in the thigh extending from the hip to the knee, and the bulk of the vastus medialis oblique just medial and proximal to the patella (Fig. 6.12).

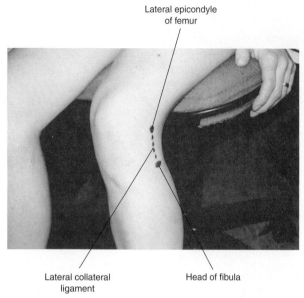

Lateral epicondyle
of femur

Lateral collateral
ligament

Head of fibula

FIG. 6.10   The position of the lateral collateral ligament at the left knee relative to the lateral epicondyle of the femur and the head of the fibula.

Quadriceps Tendon

This runs from the end of the quadriceps muscle bulk in the thigh into the upper patella (Fig. 6.12) and is most easily palpated and identified when the muscles are alternately contracted and relaxed.

SPECIFIC TESTS OF THE HIP AND KNEE (1–3)

Hip Region

Thompson's Test for Hip Flexion Contracture

The patient is placed in the supine lying position and is instructed to draw one knee onto the chest and hold it there with both hands while at the same time keeping the other leg straight, with the posterior thigh in contact with the treatment table. If the straight leg rises at the thigh or if there is a noticeable increase in lumbar lordosis as the patient tries to keep the leg

Medial epicondyle

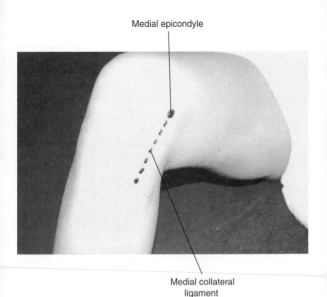

Medial collateral
ligament

FIG. 6.11   Position of the medial collateral ligament of the right knee relative to the medial epicondyle of the femur and the medial surface of the tibia.

down, then the test is considered positive for hip flexion contracture. The degree of contracture is demonstrated, and can be measured, by the amount of hip flexion occurring in the straight leg, which is the side that is being tested.

Trendellenburg Sign

With the patient suitably unclothed so that it is possible to observe the position of the pelvis at the iliac crests, instruct him to stand on one leg. This should cause the pelvis on the non-weight-bearing side to rise. If the pelvis drops then the test is considered positive for weakness in the abductor muscles of the standing leg.

Leg Length

To measure leg length, place the patient in the supine lying position with the leg straight and in a neutral position (i.e., no abduction or rotation). If the patient is unable to maintain this position with the affected leg then the

Vastus lateralis   Rectus femoris

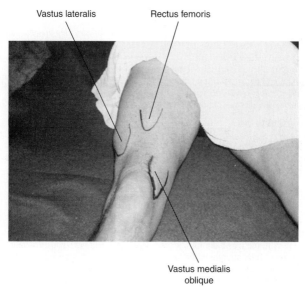

Vastus medialis
oblique

FIG. 6.12 The right quadriceps with surface markings of the bulk of
the vastus lateralis, rectus femoris and vastus medialis oblique.

unaffected leg must be placed in a position similar to the test leg or a false
reading will result. Each leg is measured in turn from the anterior superior
iliac spine (ASIS) to the tip of the medial malleolus and then from the ASIS
to the lateral malleolus. A difference of approximately a quarter of an inch
between the two legs is considered normal, because it is questionable if this
degree of shortening will produce symptoms as this variation can be found
in the normal population.

Sign of the Buttock

This is a test that is carried out in conjunction with the straight leg raising tests. If during straight leg raising, limitation of movement is present,
then the patient's knee is flexed. If further hip flexion cannot then be
gained it indicates that the patient has a lesion in the buttock, rather than
a hip, sciatic nerve, or hamstring problem. The most benign cause would
be a gluteal bursitis, but possibilities causing greater concern are a neo-
plasm or abscess in the buttock. Any patient showing this sign should be
checked thoroughly. If any doubt exists as to the cause of the discomfort
then the patient should be referred to a specialist.

Piriformis Test

With the patient in the side lying position and the affected leg uppermost, the knee is flexed between 60 and 70 degrees. The knee is then allowed to hang off the side of the bed and pressure is applied with one hand on the outside of the knee, pushing it towards the floor, while the other hand stabilizes the pelvis. Pain felt in the buttock suggests tightness in the piriformis muscle. If the sciatic nerve is pinched by the piriformis muscle then leg symptoms should also be produced by this maneuver.

Hamstring Tension

There are two ways of testing the amount of play in the hamstring muscles. The first is with the patient in the long sitting position on the treatment table with one knee flexed towards the chest and held there with the hand of that side. With the other hand the patient reaches down the straight leg to try and touch his toes. The patient must not be allowed to bend the leg. The normal patient should be able to reach at least as far as the dorsal surface of the foot, and in most cases the toes. Patients with tight hamstrings may only be able to reach halfway down the shin.

The second method of testing hamstring tension is with the patient sitting with the legs hanging over the edge of the bed. The patient is then asked to fully straighten the knee. If the patient has to lean back on the bed, placing his hands behind him (tripod sign), it is considered a positive indication of tight hamstring muscles.

The Knee Region

Noble Compression Test

With the patient in the supine lying position and the knee flexed to 90 degrees, pressure is applied with the thumb at and just above the lateral epicondyle. The patient is then asked to slowly straighten the knee. Pain occurring at the lateral epicondyle at approximately 30 degrees of flexion is positive for iliotibial band friction syndrome.

Ligament Stress Tests

Medial Collateral Ligament (Valgus Strain)

The patient is placed in the supine lying position with the hips slightly abducted. If the right leg is being tested then hold the right lower leg between your right arm and your side and then flex the knee to about 30 degrees. Place your left hand on the lateral aspect of the knee to hold it steady while abducting the lower leg. The test is then repeated with the knee fully extended. Pain produced at the medial side of the knee when the knee is flexed but not when it is extended, suggests a medial collateral ligament problem. Discomfort, which is also present with the knee tested in the extended position, suggests the possibility of an anterior cruciate or medial capsular injury.

Lateral Collateral Ligament (Varus Strain)

The leg is held in the same position as that described for the medial collateral ligament stress test, but one hand is placed on the medial aspect of the knee to stabilize it as the lower leg is pushed into adduction. Pain with the knee flexed at 30 degrees but not during extension suggests lateral collateral ligament injury. If pain is also present with the knee extended then anterior cruciate and lateral capsular injury should be considered. In practice valgus and varus strains are applied alternately to each knee.

The following tests for problems affecting the cruciate ligaments or menisci are included so that these conditions can be ruled out during assessment. Patients who demonstrate positive signs on the tests should have an orthopaedic consult. If treatment is then required either pre or post surgery the treatment protocol is similar to that given for patella femoral syndrome. If the patient will undergo reconstructive surgery, many orthopaedic surgeons will have their own written protocols for rehabilitation.

Anterior Drawer Test

With the patient in the supine lying position and the hip flexed at 45 degrees and the knee at 90 degrees, sit on the dorsum of the patient's foot and grip the back of the upper calf just below the knee with both hands. Then pull forwards and push backwards repeatedly on the tibia in order to assess the degree of laxity present compared to the other knee, or compared to what would be considered normal for the patient's sex and age. If a mild degree of laxity exists there may be a problem with the medial and lateral capsular ligaments. If there is a greater degree of laxity then the anterior cruciate is also likely to be insufficient. If instability is noted on the movement of posterior gliding of the tibia then the posterior cruciate and posterior capsular ligaments are possibly at fault. It is very hard to truly ascertain the degree of posterior laxity present in a knee unless it is obviously marked in comparison to the other side.

Appley's Compression Test

With the patient in the prone lying position and the knee flexed to 90 degrees, grasp the lower leg around the ankle and pushes the tibia down towards the bed to approximate the knee joint surfaces. While maintaining this compression force, rotate the lower leg medially and laterally. Then place your knee at the posterior aspect of the patient's thigh just above their knee. Again, gripping the patient's leg around the ankle, pull up on the tibia to distract the joints surfaces. Repeat the rotation movements with the distraction force maintained. A complaint of pain or clicking on compression and rotation suggests a problem with the menisci. Discomfort on distraction and rotation suggests a ligament problem.

McMurray's Test

With the patient in the supine lying position and the hip and knee flexed, cup the patient's heel in one hand and place your other hand on the patient's knee with the finger and thumb palpating the knee joint line. Then laterally rotate and abduct the lower leg to test for the medial meniscus. While maintaining this position of the lower leg, the knee is then extended through full range. A painful click is positive for a medial meniscus tear. To test for the lateral meniscus, the lower leg is initially placed in a medially rotated position and the knee is then flexed and extended several times.

Springy Block

With the patient in the supine lying position and the knee fully flexed cup the patient's heel in one hand and passively extend the knee. If end range of extension is marked by a springy block (which feels like trying to pinch a thick piece of rubber), there may be a tear of the meniscus.

Clark's Sign

With the patient's knee extended and resting on the treatment table, place your hand so that the web space between the thumb and index finger lies over the upper pole of the patella. Then push the patella downwards towards the foot and instruct the patient to contract the quadriceps muscle. It is wise to instruct the patient to attempt a gradual quadriceps contraction as pressure is applied to the patella since this test can be extremely painful. If pain is produced on testing then the results are considered positive for chondromalacia of the patella.

Q Angle (Patella-Femoral Angle)

This is a means of determining the angle that occurs between the quadriceps and the patella. A line is drawn from the anterior superior iliac spine to the mid point of the patella (it is best to use a meter ruler to connect the two points and then mark a short line on the skin for about 10 cm above the patella). A second line is drawn from the tibial tubercle through the mid patella and then continued on for 10 cm proximal to the patella. The angle that is formed between these two lines is known as the Q angle. If it is less than 15 degrees or greater than 17 degrees in the female, or less than 10 degrees or greater than 13 degrees in the male, then the patient is considered at a higher risk for possible patella-femoral joint problems.

McConnell Test

With the patient in the sitting position, an isometric quadriceps contraction is tested with the femur laterally rotated and the knee in full extension. This is then repeated with the knee in 30 degrees, 60 degrees, 90 degrees and 120 degrees, of flexion. If pain is felt on an isometric contraction at any one of the angles the knee is returned to the extended position. Then glide the patella medially and maintain this position while returning the patient's knee to the point of flexion that was previously painful on testing. Isometric testing is then repeated; if the pain decreases on the repeated test then the discomfort is considered to originate in the patella-femoral joint.

HIP AND KNEE CONDITIONS

Trochanteric Bursitis

Overview

This is usually an overuse type of injury that is most commonly found in runners and dancers. The trochanteric bursa separates the tensor fascia lata from the greater trochanter and the tendon of the gluteus medius muscle. Another smaller bursa lies between the gluteus medius tendon and the greater trochanter. Repetitive activities, particularly in subjects with a tight tensor fascia lata, and hence iliotibial band, will produce excessive friction, which in turn initiates and then sustains an inflammatory reaction (1, 3, 7).

Subjective Findings

Onset Patients are normally between 15 and 50 years of age. Onset is gradual after overuse, or may be due to no cause when found in the middle-aged female. The condition may be found in conjunction with episodes of back pain (3, 7, 8).

Duration Initially the condition tends to be irritating, rather than functionally limiting, so normally the patient will have suffered symptoms for 2 to 3 months before seeking treatment. This, however, can vary depending upon the level of sporting activity or recreational activity enjoyed by the patient and can lead to two disparate presentations. In the one case, patients present early because they are concerned about effects on their performance and are hoping for a speedy recovery. In the other case there can be a prolonged period of symptom build up in patients who are unwilling to give up their sport or recreational activities, and who therefore put off seeking advice until they find they are unable to participate in the their chosen activity (2, 5, 8).

Frequency This is typically a chronic condition with one long persistent episode featuring periods of exacerbation and remission usually associated with specific activity. Typically it is the first time the patient has had these symptoms, as recurrence of symptoms once the condition has cleared is not common. However, there may be a typical picture of pain on activity, forcing rest during which time symptoms abate. Symptoms then recur as soon at the activity is attempted again, no matter how long the rest period (8, 17, 20).

Area of Symptoms These are normally well localized to the lateral aspect of the hip, particularly in the early stages of the condition. However, over time symptoms can spread, particularly if the patient persists in the activity that produces discomfort, in which case symptoms may also be found in the lateral or posterolateral aspects of the thigh (Fig. 6.13) (8, 15, 20).

Type of Symptoms The patient normally complains of a nagging ache following activity, and if the activity is continued or there is an attempt to stretch once the pain has become apparent, then sharper pain can be brought on. The patient may also complain of tenderness to touch in the areas described above (1, 3, 20).

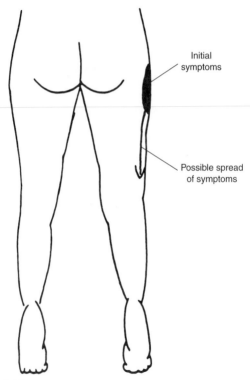

Initial symptoms

Possible spread of symptoms

FIG. 6.13   Area of symptoms for trochanteric bursitis of the right hip.

Miscellaneous Patients often state that they have a lot of discomfort on attempting steps or stairs when the symptoms are present, but they have no particular difficulty with day-to-day activities when the condition is more quiescent. In many patients (be they runners, dancers, or simply patients who like to walk a lot) onset and continuation of symptoms is usually related to one specific activity.

Objective Findings

Observation There is normally nothing unusual to be observed in the area of the hip or thigh (2, 3, 18).

Active Movements There is usually no limitation of movements in the hip, pelvis, or knee, but pain may be produced at end range of movement on abduction of the hip when this is combined with medial or lateral rotation (9, 10, 23).

Passive Movements The patient's discomfort is produced at end range of lateral rotation of the hip when this movement is tested while the hip and knee are flexed at 90 degrees. A painful stretching sensation will also be produced if the straight leg is carried into adduction, flexion, and lateral rotation at the hip (10, 22, 23).

Resisted Movements Mild discomfort is normally produced on either abduction or medial rotation of the hip and will be particularly noticeable when these two movements are combined. All movements of the hip and knee will show normal strength (2, 10, 11).

Palpation Tenderness is usually well localized over the region of the greater trochanter, particularly at its most proximal point (Fig. 6.1). In some cases tenderness is also elicited just above the greater trochanter when there is a concomitant tendonitis present (1, 22, 26).

Specific Tests X-ray examinations of the hip are normal in most cases, although occasionally they may reveal calcification of the tendons in the area, particularly in older patients.

Treatment Ideas
(1, 3, 5, 6, 8, 11, 13, 15, 16, 19, 20, 23)

Initial Treatment Initial treatment must include rest from the causative activity. This may be quite difficult to achieve, as patients commonly present for treatment precisely because they do not want to stop the activity that is causing their discomfort. It is not unusual for a patient to present for treatment only 1 to 2 weeks before a regional or national final in their particular sport. Where the competition is of major importance it may be best to assist the patient to compete, as the patient is unlikely to produce damage to (although there will be irritation of) the affected tissues. However at some point the patient will have to take a complete rest from both competition and practice if he wants to recover from the condition. At the time that activities are stopped, the pathology and chronicity of the condition needs to be clearly explained to the patient.

A trial of intensive icing (at least 10–15 minutes every hour for 4 or 5 hours per day) should be started as soon as cessation of activity is commenced. This can be continued for 2 to 3 days. At the end of that period of time the patient is progressed to the use of heat with gentle passive or assisted stretches of the hip. These stretches should focus on the movements of adduction and lateral rotation of the hip, initially individually, then in combination. In the initial stages of treatment heat and stretching exercises should be followed by the application of ice; in these early stages passive longitudinal distraction of the hip may prove helpful, particularly in the older patient suffering from concurrent back problems.

As the patient's level of discomfort starts to decrease, active hip exercises can be commenced in early ranges for flexion, extension, and both rotations. The application of thermal modalities, such as ultrasound, to the tender area may help with stretching and interferential or TENS may help decrease discomfort. When the patient experiences no discomfort with these active exercises, they can be progressed to hip abduction and adduction, again initially in early ranges and then progressing to full range. At this time the patient continues with the adduction and lateral rotation stretches and each treatment session should finish with the application of ice.

Further progression can be made by including resisted hip exercises in the treatment program, again commencing with flexion and extension, and progressing to abduction and adduction. Each set of resisted exercises should be followed by prolonged gentle stretches into adduction and lateral rotation. The period of time for which each stretch is held should be steadily extended while the number of stretches attempted is slowly decreased. When the patient is able to work through the resisted exercises and the associated stretches without discomfort, then he can be progressed to weight-bearing exercises. This can include work on a static bicycle, a step machine, step-ups (both forward and laterally), and wall squats. These exercises should be progressed from double-leg work to single-leg work, such as balance exercises and hopping, as soon as the patient demonstrates the ability to cope with the exercises without exacerbating the condition. All exercise sessions should include non-weight-bearing and weight-bearing hip stretches repeated regularly throughout the exercises program. It may also be advisable to continue with the use of ice post-exercise, even after symptoms are no longer apparent. It will be necessary to progress the patient onto heavy resisted exercises relevant to particular sport or recreational activities. These must be tolerated by the patient over an extended period of time before allowing an attempt to return to practice or competition at the level that previously produced symptoms.

In recalcitrant cases, particularly those that do not respond to a regime of ice and rest, even when applied over an extended period of time, consideration should be given to referral to the general practitioner or orthopaedic specialist for injection of local anesthetic and corticosteroids. The patient will then still need a program of stretching and strengthening exercises as described above before returning to the previous levels of activity.

Restrictions It is essential that the patient stops the pain-producing activity for whatever period of time is required to achieve a satisfactory result. It is also important for the patient to return to this activity in a graduated manner once the symptoms are resolving. To a lesser extent, activities such as steps and stairs, walking, or simply prolonged standing need to be restricted if they prove to be any problem. Short breaks taken in the sitting or lying position and pacing of the above activities should be a satisfactory means of preventing any exacerbation of symptoms. If the patient is required to stand for a prolonged period of time, then he should be encouraged to place the foot of the affected leg on a low support (6 to 8 inches high) at regular intervals throughout the period of time for which he is required to carry out the activity.

Osteoarthritis of the Hip

Overview

This is possibly the most common hip disease seen in clinical practice. It is poorly named, as there is no inflammation as such in the affected joint. It is mainly a degenerative disease and is now believed to be associated with either previous trauma to the joint or underlying anatomical abnormalities in the majority of cases; however, onset of symptoms normally occurs long after the fact. The degeneration of bone and cartilage that occurs within the joint are not the actual cause of pain as these structures contain no sensory nerve endings. It is periarticular structures that are stressed and deformed, and therefore produce the discomfort felt by the patient. Physical treatment has good results in the early stages, whereas surgery is the more effective intervention later in the condition (3, 9, 18).

Subjective Findings

Onset This is gradual after trauma or due to no cause. The patient is typically over 50 years of age, although onset may be earlier if it is a sequel to a congenital problem such as Legg-Perthes disease (2, 3, 20).

Duration The patient will normally have a history of symptoms present over a period of months or years as the condition is chronic in both nature and pathology (13, 14, 18).

Frequency The patient's history will indicate one long ongoing episode with steadily increasing symptoms over the years. There will be periods of marked increase in symptoms related to increase in the amount of normal weight-bearing activities or on attempting unaccustomed weight-bearing activities (13, 14, 18).

Area of Symptoms The patient will normally suffer symptoms in the anterior of the hip in the region of the groin, with radiation of symptoms along the anterior and anteromedial aspects of the thigh (Fig. 6.14). The patient may also suffer symptoms in his back, particularly if he limps constantly in order to favor the affected hip (2, 3, 18).

Type of Symptoms Pain is the initial and main complaint. It is first felt in the hip anteriorly and then spreads into the leg and possibly the low back. In time the patient will also complain of stiffness and then from day-to-day either pain or stiffness will be the main complaint. In the later stages stiffness is a constant problem and the degree of pain varies from day-to-day (2, 6, 8).

Miscellaneous One of the first things to be affected with this condition is the patient's ability to walk as hip extension is required through nearly full range on every step taken. The patient will also report a particular problem with steps and stairs early in the onset of this condition (3, 9, 11).

Objective Findings

Observation The patient usually presents with a limp. It may also be noted during examination, that the patient, either standing or lying, is holding the hip slightly flexed, abducted, and laterally rotated. Some wasting of the muscles in the buttock and thigh may also be observed (10, 17, 22).

Active Movements Medial rotation is usually the first movement to be lost or limited; subsequently, extension also becomes limited, followed by abduction. As the condition progresses all movements of the hip may eventually be affected, but this typical pattern of restriction is a pattern that should exist throughout the course of the condition. Testing of active movements may not be particularly painful at the time of assessment, but the patient will usually complain of increased pain and stiffness following the assessment (15, 17, 18).

Passive Movements The pattern of restriction of movement is the same as that described in active testing. In the earlier stages of the condition there is a stiff soft tissue end feel to all restricted movements, whereas in the later stages of the condition many of the movements present with a bony block at end range of motion (15, 22, 24).

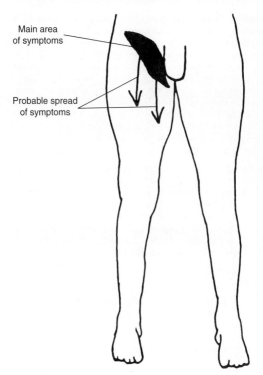

Main area
of symptoms

Probable spread
of symptoms

FIG. 6.14   Area of symptoms for osteoarthritis of the right hip.

Resisted Movements Over time weakness develops in most movements of the hip, with abduction the most commonly and most obviously affected. Generalized weakness of the musculature around the hip in many cases may be due to inactivity and stiffness, rather than to any particular pathology of the musculature itself. Pain is not normally a feature of resisted muscle testing in this condition on lightly applied isometric resistance. However, stronger resistance may produce pain due to the stresses placed on stiff and sore muscles or periarticular structures, not because of any muscle pathology (2, 9, 17).

Palpation Tenderness is often elicited on deep palpation at the anterior of the hip joint (Fig. 6.3). This has to be checked against the other side, as palpation in this area is often uncomfortable anyway. It should be noted that with arthritis of the hip joint there is no tenderness at the lateral aspect of the hip. However, because of loss of muscle action and joint range of motion, and with the patient limping, an unnatural strain is placed on the abductor muscles of the hip, which may produce either a tendonitis or trochanteric bursitis. In these cases tenderness will be elicited over the lateral aspect of the hip, but at the same time the typical signs and symptoms of a trochanteric bursitis or gluteal tendonitis should also be present. In this case the two conditions are separate and should be treated as such (22, 26).

Specific Tests Thomas' test may demonstrate a hip flexion deformity in the affected leg. The presence of a Trendelenburg gait may be noted and there may be some degree of leg length discrepancy. X rays can, on occasion, confirm the presence of this condition, but limitations of movement and function will often appear ahead of any observable radiological changes. The degree of findings on x-ray examination do not always relate well to the degree of either discomfort experienced or limitation of movements found on examination (17, 22, 27).

Treatment Ideas
(1–3, 5, 6, 8, 11, 15, 17, 19, 20, 23)

The patient should be advised to rest from weight-bearing activities or to do them in short bursts, organizing their activities so that they can pace themselves through the day (i.e., going up the stairs once to do two or three tasks, rather than going up and down the stairs two or three times). Use of a cane will help to take weight off the affected leg when used in the opposite hand. Patients who purchase a cane for themselves will almost invariably put it in the hand on the side of the affected leg and will ambulate by putting the same arm and leg forward together. This in fact means that they are taking more weight on the affected leg as they lean to that side to take weight on the cane. They are also walking not as a human does but as a camel with the two limbs on the same side moving forward together.

The patient should be started on active non-weight–bearing exercises so as to maintain range of motion, with particular emphasis placed on the movements of extension, medial rotation, and abduction. These exercises are most beneficial if done in warm water. Sling suspension, if available, can also produce good results. The use of heating agents may relieve discomfort through pain gating and will therefore allow more freedom of movement; however, modalities such as hot packs do not produce deep enough penetration of the heat to actually affect the joint. When the patient is comfortable with the active exercises, gentle passive stretches may be attempted, in particular distraction of the hip joint. This should be carried out with the leg resting in a pain-free position and traction is then applied longitudinally through the leg by use of both hands gripping the patient's foot and heel. If the patient experiences discomfort in the ankle the grip can be moved up to the lower leg. If thermal agents are used the best time to apply them is just prior to this type of stretching.

Resisted non-weight–bearing exercises can be attempted, initially isometrically against a strap or by the application of heavy weights (20 or more lbs.) to the thigh, with the patient instructed to attempt to lift the leg but not to such a degree that movement actually occurs. Isotonic strengthening exercises can be used for the quadriceps and hamstrings. Hip exercises should progress to isotonic resisted exercises once isometric exercises are tolerated well. It is often beneficial to finish treatment sessions with heat and joint distraction, although some patients benefit from ice at the end of a session of exercises.

If the patient finds particular relief from the distraction techniques, he can be taught to stretch the hip by extending the leg lying supine over the edge of a bed at home. The bed has to be high enough so that the foot does not touch the floor; if it is too low the patient should place pillows under his body to achieve the correct height. The leg is then allowed to hang over the edge of the bed with the knee flexed and the foot off the ground. If this initially proves too strong a stretch for the patient, pillows can be placed under the foot so that it is slightly supported, decreasing the degree of stretch applied. This exercise should be carried out for short periods of time (15–20 seconds) and should be preceded and accompanied by the application of heat to relax the muscles and decrease pain.

Proprioceptive neuromuscular facilitation techniques are useful, particularly when carried through the middle half of range. In this way good resistance is applied to the movements without excessive stretch being applied to painful tissues. The distraction techniques used on the hip can be progressed to the point where the leg is stretched with the hip in an extended, medially rotated, and abducted position. Patients often benefit from introduction to a fitness program with exercises done in water (aquafit). On the other hand, weight-bearing exercises are never really a treatment option for this condition.

Restrictions As stated above the patient should be advised to limit weight-bearing activities, doing short bursts of activities as tolerated before onset of pain and in this way they may condition themselves to greater functional tolerances. When patients' force themselves to the point of pain and then insist on continuing with an activity while in pain, their functional capabilities will steadily decline. Patients' should be advised not to use either the full squat position or kneeling, particularly kneeling back on the heels, and in these patients it may be better to advise them to bend their back to pick up light weights rather than bending their hips or knees, as the risk of injury to their back is usually less than the risk of exacerbation of the hip condition. If the patient has a problem with only one hip joint then the golfers lift, where the patient stands on the unaffected leg raising the other leg behind them as they bend to pick up an object, will spare both their back and the painful hip.

Adductor Tendonitis of the Hip

Overview

This is an overuse injury that was originally described in horse riders, and has become less common since the advent of motor transport. It is found in athletes, particularly those with good thigh muscle development, where it may occur due to inadequate stretching during the period that the muscles were being so thoroughly strengthened. The condition usually responds both well and quickly to physical treatment (15).

Onset   This is gradual due to overuse and most commonly found in athletes from 20 to 40 years of age (15, 17).

Duration   Patients normally present for treatment within 1 to 3 weeks of onset, as the condition often limits their athletic endeavors. In less active patients it could be 3 to 6 weeks before they become concerned enough to seek attention.

Frequency   This is typically the first occasion on which the patient has experienced these symptoms; however, it can become a recurrent seasonal problem if left untreated or if initially inadequately treated (15).

Area of Symptoms   Symptoms are usually well localized to the proximal musculo-tendinous or tendo-periosteal junction of the abductor muscles at the medial aspect of the upper thigh. In particularly acute cases, generalized discomfort may spread down the medial aspect of the thigh almost as far as the knee (Fig. 6.15) (17, 23).

Type of Symptoms   Patients usually complain of a nagging ache, an unpleasant pulling sensation, or a painful tightness on activities that stretch the affected muscles or that require prolonged action of the muscle (such as riding a horse) (15, 17, 23).

Objective Findings

Observation   There is usually nothing out of the ordinary to be observed in the affected area (15, 23).

Active Movements   Mild limitation of hip abduction is usually present, with pain produced at end range of motion and localized to the medial aspect of the thigh proximally. Pain may also be produced at the end range of hip adduction; however, there will be no limitation of this movement (17, 23).

Passive Movements   Pain will be experienced at end range of abduction, which is usually slightly limited compared to the other hip. Pain

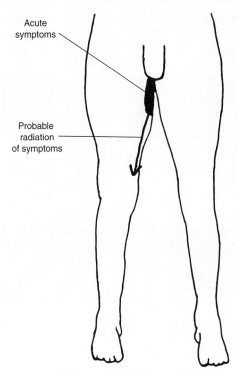

Acute
symptoms

Probable
radiation
of symptoms

FIG. 6.15   Area of symptoms for adductor tendonitis at the right hip.

will again be felt in the proximal and medial aspect of the thigh. All other movements will be of full range and pain free.

Resisted Movements   Pain is produced at the site of the lesion on isometric adduction of the hip. This movement will be particularly painful if the patient is asked to adduct the leg from the fully abducted position (15, 17, 23).

Palpation   Tenderness is localized to the proximal and medial thigh over the adductor tendons and will be palpable from the medial muscle mass in the thigh up into the groin (Fig. 6.4) (22, 23, 26).

Specific Tests X-ray examination may show calcification of the offending tendon, but this is rare and does not affect treatment planning.

Treatment Ideas

Advise the patient to try ice and rest for a period of 2 to 3 days, icing the painful area for 10 to 15 minutes every 1 to 2 hours throughout the day. For the average patient this usually proves impossible due to work and other commitments, so the best course of action is to ice every hour in the evenings, 3 or 4 hours consecutively, so that the icing has a cumulative effect. Once the patient has attempted a few days of this protocol, instruct him to try application of heat and gentle passive stretching of the affected tendon. This can be initially carried out with a straight leg raise in the side lying position with the patient abducting the affected leg so that the abductor muscles have to work against the resistance of gravity. The patient must be instructed to avoid the natural tendency of trying to jerk the leg up in an attempt to gain further range.

Stretch can also be applied with the patient lying supine and the hip and knee flexed with the foot resting on the bed. The patient is then instructed to let the knee drop out sideways, hence abducting and laterally rotating the hip. The stretch should initially be held for 10 to 15 seconds at a time and should steadily progress to 30 to 60 seconds, with the patient advised to rest for a similar amount of time between stretches. The use of interferential therapy applied to the thigh musculature prior to stretching can help the patient gain range without undue discomfort. Thermal doses of ultrasound or the use of laser over the site of the lesion may also improve the quality of stretch applied to the injured tissues. Patients should continue with active exercises for all other movements of the hip and knee. If the patient is an athlete he should also continue strengthening exercises for all other unaffected muscle groups.

When the patient is comfortable with the active stretching regime, he can be progressed onto light resisted work for the adductor muscles, followed by gentle stretches, initially non-weight–bearing, then progressed to weight-bearing. Standing stretches should first be attempted with the patient holding onto either wall bars or the wall to stabilize himself, then progressed to free standing. When the patient is comfortable with these stretches, contract–relax techniques can be used to achieve a greater degree of stretch, which the patient can be taught to continue at home.

In the more recalcitrant cases where a degree of discomfort remains on either activity or stretching, a short course of transverse friction massage may prove effective in resolving residual discomfort and tightness. When the patient is coping well with weight-bearing stretches, the resisted exercises can be progressed to a full weight-bearing gym workout at the normal training levels applicable to the individual patient. Stretching must still be maintained before, during, and after resisted exercise training. The patient can only return to competition after having demonstrated the ability to deal with explosive activities, involving the affected muscle group, in the clinical setting. By this time the patient should have no discomfort at the end of a treatment session. If otherwise, when returning to competitive activities, the chance of recurrence is high.

Restrictions Any activities that require stretching or forceful contraction of the adductor muscles (riding a horse, throwing a javelin, etc.) should not be attempted until the patient is progressing well on the exercise program. Other than these types of explosive athletic events, the activities of daily living are not a problem in the majority of cases. The patient is therefore only required to demonstrate a modicum of common sense in order to avoid exacerbation of their symptoms.

Psoas Bursitis

Overview

The tendon of the iliopsoas is attached to the greater trochanter of the femur and is separated from the hip joint capsule by a large bursa. On repeated overstretching or straining of the joint, particularly if coupled with powerful contraction of the muscles (as in explosive type events such as sprinting), the bursa can become inflamed, swollen, and painful (15, 17).

Onset This is normally gradual due to overuse and is found mainly in patients from 20 to 40 years of age (15, 23).

Duration The patient will not normally present for treatment until 3 to 6 weeks after onset, as initial symptoms are usually not severe or particularly functionally limiting.

Frequency This is usually the first and only time the patient will suffer from this condition.

Area of Symptoms Symptoms are normally experienced in the anterior of the hip joint region, in the groin, and at the anterior of the upper thigh (Fig. 6.16) (15, 17, 26).

Type of Symptoms The patient will complain of a persistent ache that is worse during or following particular activities (15, 17, 28).

Objective Findings

Observation In very rare or very acute cases there can be some mild swelling noted at the anterior of the hip joint. However, in the majority of cases there is nothing to be observed in the area of symptoms (6, 13, 17, 23).

Active Movements There is normally mild limitation of hip extension with pain experienced at end range of motion. Pain will also be produced at end range of flexion of the hip, particularly if the patient is trying hard to gain further movement. However, there should be no restriction of range of hip flexion and all other movements of the hip and knee are of full range and pain-free (15, 17, 19, 24).

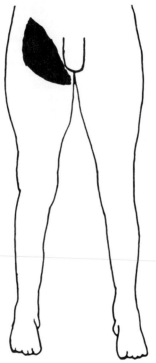

FIG. 6.16   Area of symptoms for Psoas bursitis at the right hip.

Passive Movements Passive extension of the hip is painful and normally produces muscle tension at end range of motion. This pain is not increased when hip extension is combined with knee flexion (thus ruling out the rectus femoris muscle) (17, 19, 24).

Resisted Movements Pain is normally experienced on isometric contraction of the hip flexors. This is worse if the muscle is tested in inner range, as will happen when the patient in the sitting position holds the hip fully flexed as force is applied and then tries to extend the hip.

Palpation Tenderness is elicited on palpation over the anterior of the hip joint (Fig. 6.3). This discomfort must be produced by less pressure than that which is required to reach the anterior of the hip joint itself, and also in comparison to the other side, as there is a degree of tenderness on palpation in this area in the normal population. Repeated attempts to discover tenderness in this area will inevitably be successful, as the neurovascular bundle in the femoral triangle becomes sensitive due to the repeated prodding and poking (15, 17, 22, 26).

Treatment Ideas
(6, 11, 13, 15, 17, 19, 23, 24)

The patient is advised to avoid any known causative activities. They should be encouraged to continue stretching all other muscle groups in the region of the hip and knee, which can be coupled with passive stretching (distraction) of the hip longitudinally. This is best done with the patient lying supine with the hips slightly abducted and laterally rotated.

The patient is progressed onto passive stretches of the iliopsoas muscles, which are done initially in the side lying position with a pillow placed between the patient's knees. The stretches should be maintained for 10 to 15 seconds and increased gradually to 30 to 60 seconds. Active flexion exercises for the hip can be started in early to mid range and then progressed to inner range as soon as this proves to be painless. Heat should be applied prior to stretching, as its relaxation effect is beneficial for the patient. Ice can be applied after exercise, combined with transcutaneous electrical nerve stimulation if there is any marked degree of discomfort. Pulsed dosages of ultrasound and interferential therapy may help to relieve discomfort at this time.

At home the patient can be advised to lie with his leg extended over the edge of a bed and the knee flexed, with the foot lightly resting on the ground in order to apply gentle traction forces to the affected tendon. Contract–relax or hold–relax techniques can be employed to gain further stretch of the affected musculature, techniques the patient can be taught to use at home. The patient can then progress the stretching exercises on the bed to the point where the foot is clear of the floor, applying the full weight of the leg to the anterior region of the hip. In the clinic, the patient can undergo the same stretching routine and light to moderate ankle weights can be used to increased the degree of stretch. Again, these techniques can be followed by the application of ice so as to prevent undue reaction to the stretching.

As the patient's pain level decreases and he is able to cope with active and assisted stretching, he should be progressed to a weight-bearing stretching routine combined with a lower extremity workout in the gym. The weight-bearing stretches should be carried out both during and after the exercise session, and the patient should continue to use contract–relax and hold–relax techniques with the stretches. Explosive activities such as short runs, lateral bounding, and quick stop-and-start activities are all useful in preparing the patient for competitive activities. Athletes should only be returned to competition when able to complete a full exercise session in the clinic without any discomfort.

Restrictions All explosive-type movements involving use of the hip flexor muscles should initially be avoided. Once the patient is able to tolerate weight-bearing stretches of the affected muscle, without any pain during or after stretching, there can be a gradual return to those activities that previously produced symptoms. However, any risk of collision or contact in sports should be avoided until the therapist is sure the condition has cleared completely.

Groin Strain

Overview

Most commonly this injury involves the adductor muscles or flexor muscles of the hip, but can also occur in any of several muscles found in the anteromedial aspect of the upper leg. Effective early treatment will allow for speedy return to activity and will decrease the likelihood of chronic complications (11, 16).

Subjective Findings

Onset This is sudden due to trauma, which is usually some form of extension and lateral rotation strain of the hip. It can also occur when a forceful adduction, flexion, and medial rotation movement is strongly resisted. The patient is normally under 40 years of age (13, 16, 19).

Duration Patients are normally seen within a matter of days or at most 1 to 2 weeks following injury, as the condition is very painful. If related to sport or recreational activity it is also very functionally disabling.

Frequency This will probably be the first time the patient has suffered the condition, but on occasion it can become a chronic problem, particularly if it is not dealt with effectively the first time, and even more so in the well-developed athlete with poor flexibility (11, 16, 19).

Area of Symptoms These are usually well localized to the medial and proximal aspect of the thigh at either the myotendinous or tendoperiostal junctions of the affected muscles (Fig. 6.17) (11, 13, 16, 26).

Type of Symptoms Pain is sharp on use of the affected muscle, with a steady ill-defined ache at rest (11, 16).

Miscellaneous There are many varying degrees of strain to be encountered, from mildly annoying to totally disabling. The degree of injury sustained usually relates well to the degree of force applied at the time of injury.

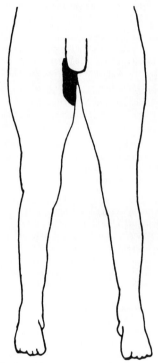

FIG. 6.17   Area of symptoms for groin strain at right thigh.

Objective Findings

Observation Bruising is often evident in the first 7 to 10 days following the injury, but other than that there is normally nothing out of the ordinary to be observed in the area (11, 19).

Active Movements Depending on the specific muscles injured, either hip abduction, hip extension, or both will be limited, with pain produced at end of available range. Lateral rotation may also at times be mildly limited and painful. Active adduction and flexion are normally of full range, but may be painful either during the movement or at end range of motion, particularly if the patient makes a strong effort to take the leg into further range (11, 16, 24).

Passive Movements Pain localized to the site of injury will be felt at end range of either adduction, extension, or on both movements, and quite often on lateral rotation as well. The end feel will be one of muscle spasm resisting the movements of abduction and extension (11, 16, 24).

Resisted Movements Pain may be experienced on isometric resisted hip adduction, hip flexion, or both. More marked discomfort will be elicited if these movements are tested at the end range of abduction and extension, respectively (13, 16).

Palpation Sharp well-defined tenderness will be elicited over the adductor tendons at the proximal and medial aspect of the thigh (Fig. 6.4) or over the anterior of the hip joint (Fig. 6.3). In severe cases both areas may be tender (11, 16, 22, 26).

Specific Tests If resisted hip adduction is more painful when tested in the supine lying position with the leg straight, then the injury is more likely to be in the adductor muscles. If resisted hip adduction is more painful when tested with the hip and knee flexed, then the injury is more likely to be to the hip flexors. In severe cases both of these movements may prove painful, indicating a tear of both muscle groups (19, 22, 24).

Treatment Ideas
(11, 13, 16, 19)

If the patient is seen in the early days following injury, then ice and relative rest must be advised. The patient can continue with active movements of the hip through all pain-free ranges. If the patient is an athlete then he should also be encouraged to continue with strengthening exercises for the unaffected leg, trunk, and upper extremities. Interferential therapy can help to decrease muscle spasm in the affected area. After 3 to 4 days the patient can progress to gentle stretches of the injured leg into both abduction and extension. This is done initially in the side lying position, and then in the prone lying position so that the stretch is applied by muscle action and not by gravity, thus eliminating the effect of the weight of the leg being applied to injured tissues.

Once icing has been attempted for a few days the patient can be progressed to the use of heat prior to exercise, which will help to relieve pain and promote muscle relaxation. Active movements of the hips should be progressed to include all movements and resisted exercises can be attempted for all movements that are actively full-range and pain- free. Thermal doses of ultrasound or the use of laser to the injured muscle may promote repair. Muscle stimulation can be applied to the injured muscle, with the patient contracting the muscle group isometrically along with the muscle stimulation. This can then be progressed to active movements combined with the muscle stimulation.

Further progression can be made to isometric resisted hip flexion and adduction exercises, followed by stretches for the injured muscles. The patient can also be instructed to hold the leg in extension or abduction against the contraction produced by the muscle stimulator. The use of ice is warranted at the end of treatment sessions, as this tends to limit post-exercise pain. Proprioceptive neuromuscular facilitation techniques for combined movements of flexion and adduction of the hip can then be started and the patient can attempt active movements of abduction and extension of the hip against contraction of the adductor muscles, as provided by the muscle stimulator. Weight-bearing hip and knee exercises can then be commenced with gentle, prolonged weight-bearing stretches for the adductor and flexor muscles of the hip.

The patient is finally progressed to a general lower extremity workout in the gym, combined with weight-bearing exercises such as step-ups, work on a balance board, lateral step-ups, and lateral gliding or bounding. The patient must be advised to continue with a thorough stretching regime both during and after exercise. The patient can also be progressed to plyometric exercises and sports-specific training. Patients should eventually reach the point where they are able to contract the affected muscles while at the same time stretching them quite forcefully.

Restrictions No activity that requires forceful gripping with the thighs or stretching of the hip flexor or adductor muscle should be attempted until the patient is able to sustain weight-bearing stretches without discomfort. No contact sports or explosive activities, such as sprints, should be allowed until the patient is able to mimic these movements in the clinical setting without pain. The patient is advised to avoid side-stepping-type moves; a return to this type of activity should only be attempted when the patient has demonstrated the ability to tolerate the required stresses and strains in the clinical setting. This can take from 2 to 6 weeks, depending on the severity of the initial injury.

Piriformis Syndrome

Overview

Sciatica-type symptoms can be produced by compression of the sciatic nerve as it passes through the piriformis muscles (as it does in approximately 15% of the population). The patient presents with sciatica but no history of back pain. This is a history that can be found in patients with a back problem that is producing sciatic-type leg symptoms. In those cases if treatment fails it is worth attempting stretching of the piriformis muscle if it appears to be tight (20, 21).

Subjective Findings

Onset This is gradual with no known cause and occurs most commonly in patients from 25 to 55 years of age (3, 5, 21).

Duration The patient will have suffered symptoms for at least several weeks, if not months. This is partly due to the insidious nature of onset and also partly due to the fact that this condition is normally confused with a back problem. It is often therefore treated incorrectly, and thus unsuccessfully, for some time before being correctly identified (13, 21).

Frequency This will, in all likelihood, be the first time that the patient has experienced these particular symptoms, although there may have been a few previous episodes over a period of 1 to 2 years, with increasing spread of symptoms into the leg. It is important to check the patient's back pain history very carefully, as it may provide useful clues that will help to differentiate between this condition and other conditions that might produce nerve root irritation in the sciatic distribution.

Area of Symptoms Symptoms are felt in the buttock and in the area of sciatic nerve distribution in the leg (the back of the thigh), as well as the posterior or lateral aspect of the lower leg (Fig. 6.18) (3, 19, 20).

Type of Symptoms Pain is the main presenting symptom, although the patient can also have paraesthesia or numbness in the leg. There should be no back pain, even if there is pain or discomfort in the buttock (13, 20, 21).

Miscellaneous Coughing and straining should not produce the leg symptoms. There is also not the typical history associated with discogenic type pain, where flexion activities such as sitting, are incriminated as the main pain-producing movements. However, forward flexion of the lumbar spine with the leg straight might produce the patient's discomfort because of stretch of the nerve at the point of entrapment in the muscle.

Objective Findings

Observation There will be nothing out of the ordinary to be observed in the back, buttock, or legs (3, 5, 13).

Active Movements There is usually no limitation of movement, however, the patient may get some discomfort in the buttock at end-range of internal rotation of the hip. Active straight leg raising may produce the patient's typical leg symptoms (5, 19, 20).

Passive Movements Pain is experienced at end range of internal rotation of the hip and muscle spasm may be found to resist this movement at the end of range. Passive straight leg raising may produce buttock and leg pain, which is tested in the supine lying position with the patient's knee flexed initially, so that the hip is flexed. Then, while the hip is kept flexed, extend the knee slowly (19, 20, 22).

Resisted Movements Good strength levels should be present on all movements of the hip and knee; however, pain may be produced on isometric resisted external rotation of the hip, particularly if this movement is tested lying prone with the knee flexed to 90 degrees (5, 19, 22).

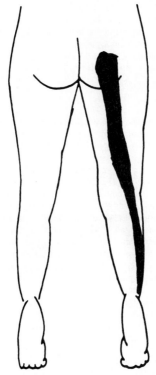

FIG. 6.18 Area of symptoms for piriformis syndrome at the right hip.

Palpation Some ill-defined discomfort may be produced on deep palpation of the buttock, but this must be compared carefully with the other side as the depth of palpation required may produce pain in the normal subject. The patient must be able to make a definite differentiation between the levels of discomfort in the two buttocks for the finding to be considered positive (3, 5, 22, 26).

Specific Tests With the patient in the side lying position on the unaffected side, the hip of the affected leg is flexed between 60 and 70 degrees. The knee of that leg is then allowed to lie over the edge of the treatment table and pressure is applied to the outside of the knee with one hand while the other hand stabilizes the pelvis. Pain should then be produced in the buttock if the piriformis muscle is tight, and leg symptoms will be produced if the sciatic nerve is trapped by the muscle. Resisted external rotation attempted from the same position may also produce symptoms in the buttock and leg. The patient should be tested for the sign of the buttock as described in the section under specific tests for the hip and knee (21, 22, 27).

Treatment Ideas
(3, 5, 13, 19, 20, 21)

Any activity that is known to produce the patient's typical symptoms should be avoided for a few days and ice should be applied to the buttock, preferably in several doses approximately 1 hour apart and repeated three or four times during the day. Modalities such as interferential therapy and transcutaneous electrical nerve stimulation can help to decrease localized discomfort in the buttock. The patient can then be progressed onto heat applied to the area of the buttock in order to promote muscle relaxation. Gentle stretches can be started for the hamstring and gluteal muscles.

Specific piriformis muscle stretches can be performed, the simplest of which is carried out in long sitting with the affected leg crossed over the thigh of the unaffected leg. The patient then applies pressure on the outer aspect of the knee to take the knee towards the chest (i.e., into flexion and medial rotation). A program of general lower extremity stretches should also be provided for the patient, as tightness in the piriformis muscle is usually associated with a general lack of flexibility in the trunk and extremities.

The patient can be further progressed to light to moderate resisted exercises for all movements of the hip, which should then be followed by appropriate stretches for each muscle group. Proprioceptive neuromuscular facilitation techniques in the patterns of hip lateral rotation combined with other hip movements can be used, followed by the application of contract–relax techniques to gain further stretch of the muscle. Patients can be taught to apply contract–relax techniques for themselves at home by first applying a flexion and medial rotation stretch to the affected hip, then maintaining a low-intensity isometric contraction of the lateral rotators, which in turn is followed by further stretch into medial rotation.

As their symptoms ease the patient can be placed on a gym program for general lower extremity exercises. The patient must continue with the stretching exercises, particularly during and after the exercise program, as the affected musculature will then be warm, and hence more pliable. Applying gentle, painless, and prolonged stretches to the muscles as they cool down after exercise can often produce good long-term effects. The patient must be advised to continue with the stretching routine (specifically the early piriformis muscle stretches) at regular intervals for an indefinite period, even after the signs and symptoms have cleared.

Restrictions Any specific activities that have been identified as producing the patient's typical discomfort should be avoided. Return to those activities should be made in a graduated manner as symptoms ease. These activities tend to be very specific to an individual patient, therefore, no general guideline would be of any value.

Iliotibial Band Friction Syndrome

Overview

As the knee is flexed and extended, the tendon of insertion of the iliotibial band glides anteriorly and posteriorly over the lateral epicondyle of the femur. An inflammatory reaction can be produced in this area by excess friction due to a sudden increase in running distances, a change to running up and down hills, or onto banked or uneven surfaces. Subjects with an already tight iliotibial band appear to be more likely to suffer from this condition.

Subjective Findings

Onset This is gradual after overuse and is most commonly found in runners, particularly when they have increased their training or returned to training after injury, or at the beginning of a new season. Patients are typically between 25 and 55 years of age (4, 5, 16).

Duration Patients will usually have suffered from symptoms for approximately 3 to 6 weeks before seeking treatment, depending on the level of their running activities, their training schedule, and their degree of determination to continue with the activity relative to either sporting endeavor or maintaining general health.

Frequency This is commonly the first time that the patient has had these symptoms, although there may have been mild episodes before, but usually only of very short duration (16, 19).

Area of Symptoms Symptoms are well localized to the lateral aspect of the thigh just above the knee, although with time they can also spread down the lateral aspect of the knee to the proximal and lateral aspect of the tibia (Fig. 6.19). This condition can occasionally be associated with discomfort at the lateral aspect of the hip and over the iliac crest on the affected side (4, 6, 18, 19).

Type of Symptoms The patient will complain of an initial ache in the knee after activity. As the condition progresses the pain will come on during running, at which time the patient will complain of a burning sensation at the side of the knee with occasional sharp twinges of pain followed by a steady ache after the activity (4, 6, 19).

Miscellaneous The patient will often state that running downhill, on uneven surfaces, or on banked surfaces will bring on the symptoms more rapidly. The patient may have a history of hip pain and trochanteric bursitis. The condition may also be associated with leg length discrepancy,

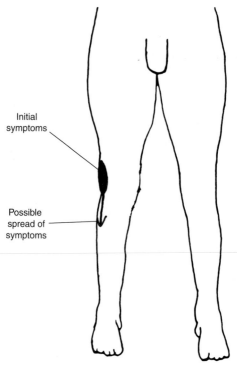

Initial
symptoms

Possible
spread of
symptoms

FIG. 6.19 Area of symptoms for iliotibial band friction syndrome at the
right knee.

tight quadriceps or hamstring muscles, or excessive pronation at the foot
and ankle.

Objective Findings

Observation Occasionally an area of swelling may be found in the affected leg over the lateral epicondyle of the femur (Fig. 6.7). The tendon
of insertion of the iliotibial band is often well defined in distance runners,
and may be clearly indicated as the source of discomfort. The patient may
also demonstrate knee deformities such as genu varum or genu recurvatum (4, 18, 19).

Active Movements Active range of motion of the knee should be within normal limits, although pain may be experienced in the final ranges of extension of the knee as this movement is taken from the flexed knee position. This discomfort normally occurs at the point at which the knee is flexed to approximately 30 degrees. Pain may also be produced at the lateral aspect of the hip at end range of abduction of the hip (12, 16, 18, 22).

Passive Movements The same pattern of discomfort will be found at the knee on testing of passive movements as found on active testing. Combined adduction and lateral rotation of the hip carried out passively may produce lateral hip pain, but passive abduction of the hip will be pain free (12, 16).

Resisted Movements There is normally good strength and no discomfort elicited on isometric resisted testing of all movements of the hip and knee (4, 16).

Palpation Tenderness is often elicited on palpation of the tendon of insertion of the iliotibial band at the point at which it passes over the lateral epicondyle of the femur. Crepitus (clicking or creaking) may be felt if a finger is placed on the tendon during the movements of flexion and extension when taken from full extension to 40 degrees of flexion (5, 22, 26).

Specific Tests With the patient lying supine and the knee flexed to 90 degrees, pressure is applied with the thumb over the lateral epicondyle and over an area approximately one centimeter above it. The knee is then straightened to approximately 30 degrees of flexion, at which point the patient should report their typical pain (noble compression test) (22).

Treatment Ideas
(3–6, 16, 18, 19)

The patient must be advised to rest from running and to ice the affected knee vigorously. This can be a problem as patients will often seek treatment when their symptoms are preventing a required progression in training, or in to higher levels of competition; they are therefore unhappy to take a step backwards. However, if the patient is allowed to attempt even modified running activities the condition is unlikely to resolve. The patient may be able to continue with weight training, swimming, or any other activity that does not produce the typical pain so as to maintain muscle strength and cardiovascular fitness, but there should be no compromise as regards taking a rest from running.

When the patient has gained relief from discomfort with rest and ice, he can be started on the use of heat and non-weight–bearing stretches of the iliotibial band. These can be done both passively and actively, requiring combined movements of adduction and lateral rotation at the hip. They should be combined with general lower extremity stretches for the hip flexors, hamstrings, quadriceps, calf muscles, and the anterior tibial muscles. Local applications of pulsed ultrasound or laser often prove helpful and can be progressed to thermal dose levels.

Strengthening exercises can be used and followed by a stretching routine, which in turn is followed by icing. As the patient is able to progress through exercises without discomfort, weight-bearing lower extremity stretches can be combined with proprioceptive neuromuscular facilitation techniques for combined hip adduction and medial rotation. Hold-relax and contract-relax techniques will further progress stretching of the iliotibial band. Specific iliotibial band stretches should be taught in weight bearing, with the patient maintaining prolonged (30–60 seconds) stretches, which should be interspersed throughout the exercise program. If at this time the symptoms prove recalcitrant, two or three sessions of deep transverse friction massage over the iliotibial band at the lateral epicondyle, may trigger a positive response and allow further progression of treatment.

Once the patient is able to cope with resisted exercises and stretches with no discomfort occurring, he can be progressed onto a lower extremity workout in a gym with weight-bearing activities such as crossovers, squats, step ups, lateral step ups, and running on a treadmill, with stretches carried out before, during, and after the exercise program. Running may then be started, initially on flat surfaces, and the patient should be instructed to try a shorter stride length. Progression can be made to running on hills, but must be made in gradual increments and limited by any onset of symptoms. If the patient has to run on the side of the road, he should alternate sides during running to equalize stresses between the two legs. The patient must also be instructed to follow a thorough warm-up and stretching routine before any run, or for that matter before any repetitive lower extremity activities.

Restrictions   As noted earlier, the major restriction is on running which is of primary importance for initial control of symptoms. Any repetitive flexion and extension of the knee, particularly involving the last 40 degrees of extension from flexion, should also be avoided. This may involve the use of pedals for controlling vehicles or machinery, cycling, or partial squatting to lift weights, and so on. Even when the patient is able to return to running, he should avoid hills and uneven terrain. In the very acute stages if static standing is proving problematic, the patient can be instructed to use a small step or stool (6–8 inches high) and to stand with the foot of the affected leg resting on the step to alleviate pressure on the knee during static standing.

Hamstring Muscle Tear

Overview

This is a common injury among athletes involved in explosive events such as sprinting, or in a more sedentary person trying a strenuous activity without preparation, such as sprinting to catch the last bus before it leaves. Often patients who present with this problem have generally tight muscles in their lower extremities. There may also be an imbalance between quadriceps and hamstrings muscle strength. The hamstring muscles should have approximately 65% of the strength of the quadriceps in order to maintain proper biomechanics in the leg. This condition needs to be treated both early and aggressively, as otherwise it easily becomes an annoying and disabling recurrent problem, particularly in the athlete (3–5).

Onset This is sudden due to trauma, normally involving an explosive leg action, and occurs most commonly in the patient, 15 to 45 years of age (4, 5).

Duration The patient usually presents for treatment within days of onset, as the condition is very painful and functionally limiting, although a minor tear may be ignored for 1 or 2 weeks until it affects a particular function.

Frequency This will either be the first time that the patient has had these symptoms or it may be a recurrent problem, particularly in the keen but unprepared athlete (the "weekend warrior") who may have a history of minor recurrent strains preceding this current larger tear (16, 19).

Area of Symptoms This will depend on the site of injury. The commonest sites are at the proximal and posterior aspect of the thigh or in the buttock at the insertion of the hamstring tendon into the ischial tuberosity. The next likeliest site of injury is at the posterior aspect of the knee and distal thigh, over the distal myotendinous junction. Finally, symptoms may be found in the mid- to upper aspect of the posterior thigh over the bulk of the hamstring muscles (Fig. 6.20) (5, 11, 15, 16).

Type of Symptoms Pain is sharp on use of the muscle or on stretch of the muscle. There will also be an ill-defined ache throughout the extent of the posterior of the thigh at all other times.

Miscellaneous The patient may complain of discomfort in the posterior of the thigh when sitting, particularly on a hard chair, as the seat of the chair presses into the site of injury. Patients are often found to have a general lack of flexibility either in the muscles of the lower extremity or a general tendency toward soft-tissue restrictions in the trunk and extremities (16, 19).

Objective Findings

Observation In moderate to severe injuries bruising will be visible, usually within 1 to 3 days of injury and occurring below the site of injury, as the blood tracks between the layers of fascia. In severe cases there may also be some swelling visible at the site of injury, particularly when the patient is in the prone lying position with the hamstrings relaxed by having the lower leg placed on a pillow so that the knee is slightly flexed (3, 4, 22).

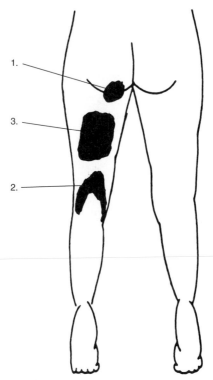

FIG. 6.20   Common sites of symptoms following a hamstring muscle tear at either: 1–the proximal myotendinous or tendoperiosteal junction, 2–at the distal tendoperiosteal junction or 3–in the belly of the muscle.

Active Movements   Movements of the hip and knee should be of full range, although pain may be experienced during knee flexion. Combined hip flexion with knee extension, as in a straight leg raise, will be limited to some degree or another, depending on the severity of the injury, and will produce the patient's typical discomfort at the end of available range of motion. The patient may also experience some discomfort on either active hip extension or at end range of active knee flexion, simply through use of the injured muscle (3–5).

Passive Movements The pattern of movement limitation will be the same as that found on active testing, although passive extension of the hip or flexion of the knee should be completely pain free. Passive straight leg raising will produce discomfort at the site of injury and spread of discomfort throughout the muscle if overpressure is applied (5, 15).

Resisted Movements Pain is experienced on isometric resisted hamstring contraction. In moderate to severe cases the patient may be unable to sustain the contraction against resistance, which will give the appearance of weakness in the muscle. Pain is produced most noticeably on isometric knee flexion when taken from the point of full hamstring stretch (i.e., with the knee extended and the hip flexed). Isometric resisted hip extension may also produce discomfort at the site of the lesion. All other movements of the hip and knee will be of normal strength and pain free (5, 15, 19).

Palpation Tenderness is marked over the site of injury. This is best elicited initially using the whole hand. Once the area of tenderness is found the fingers can be used to localize the exact site of the lesion (11, 16, 26).

Treatment Ideas
(3–5, 11, 15, 16, 19, 20)

If the patient is seen in the first few days following injury, then the principles of ice, rest, compression, and elevation should be followed for a period of 2 to 3 days. At the same time active exercises should be continued in pain-free ranges for all unaffected movements of the hip and knee. After the trial of ice and rest, heat can be used in conjunction with active exercises for all movements of the hip and knee, carried to the point of onset of discomfort where applicable, but not into pain. Pulsed ultrasound, interferential therapy, and transcutaneous electrical nerve stimulation can all help to decrease symptoms and improve the patient's tolerance for exercise. Ice should be applied at the end of the treatment session.

Resisted exercises can be started for all hip and knee movements with isometric resisted exercises for extension of the hip and flexion of the knee. At this time gentle hamstring stretches should also be attempted, which should be both prolonged (15–30 seconds) and painless. Weight-bearing exercises can be used to maintain muscle strength in the unaffected muscle groups, such as step ups, lateral step ups, and 30% squats, combined with active non–weight–bearing hamstring stretches and general lower extremity stretches carried out both during and after the exercise regime. At this time thermal doses of ultrasound or laser can be applied to the area of injury in the posterior thigh.

Further progression starts with weight-bearing stretches for the hamstrings; progression of the weight-bearing exercises can be made using an exercise bicycle or step machine. Neuromuscular electrical stimulation to the injured muscles to facilitate active exercises can be progressed to the point where the patient is stretching against the muscle contraction produced by the stimulator. Hold–relax and contract–relax proprioceptive neuromuscular facilitation techniques can be used to gain further stretch of the hamstring muscles, and simple contract–relax and stretch techniques can be taught to the patient for use at home.

The patient is progressed to plyometrics such as jump-downs and lateral bounding and lateral gliding exercises. These should be combined with a general exercise program for the lower extremities, including both power and endurance work and a continuing program of stretches performed before, during, and after the other exercises. The final gym workout will need to be sports specific. The patient needs to work out to the point where he is able to sustain explosive types of lower extremity activities, such as short burst sprints and vertical jumps, with no discomfort in the thigh, before returning to competitive activities.

Restrictions The patient should be restricted from participation in any running, jumping, or other explosive type of activities in the initial stages following injury. The patient should also walk with crutches or a cane as necessary to maintain a correct gait pattern. Heavy lifting from the squat position should be avoided, as should sitting on hard surfaces, which may well be self-limited due to discomfort. In the case of a moderate injury the patient will be out of competition for approximately 2 to 3 weeks. For more severe injuries this time period may be increased to 6 weeks to 3 months. The patient will be out of training for approximately half that time period. There must be no attempt to return to explosive activities, particularly in a competitive setting, until the patient is fully pain free on stretch testing within the controlled environment of the clinic.

Hamstring Tendonitis

Overview

An unaccustomed degree of running over long distances may produce overuse tendonitis of the hamstrings. This can occur either at the muscles proximal or its distal attachments. The condition often indicates an excessive degree of tension in the hamstring muscles and it can also predispose the patient to a hamstring tear (13, 15).

Subjective Findings

Onset This is normally gradual after overuse and is particularly associated with running up hills. The patient is typically under 40 years of age.

Duration Depending on the athletic demands and aspirations of the patient, he may present for treatment at any time from a few days to a few weeks after initial onset of symptoms.

Frequency This is usually the first time the patient will have experienced these particular symptoms, although there may have been previous episodes of minor hamstring problems.

Area of Symptoms Two separate and distinct areas may be affected, either in the buttock around the area of the ischial tuberosity or at the posterior of the knee joint over the tibial or fibular attachments of the hamstrings (Fig. 6.21) (15, 17, 19).

Type of Symptoms Initially the patient will complain of an ache after or towards the end of a particular activity. If the patient persists with that particular activity then it may become more of a burning pain. The patient may also complain of tightness or pulling in the affected area while participating in weight-bearing activities (15, 17, 23).

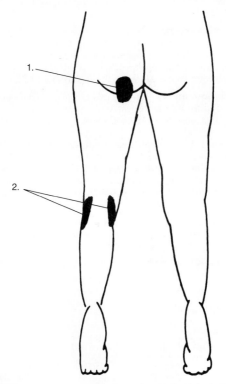

FIG. 6.21 Area of symptoms for hamstring tendonitis in the left leg at either: 1–the proximal attachment or 2–the distal attachment of the muscles.

Miscellaneous A general lack of flexibility may be found in the lower extremities.

Objective Findings

Observation There will be nothing out of the ordinary to observe in the area of the hip, thigh or knee (15, 17).

Active Movements Individual active movements of the hip and knee will usually be of full range with no discomfort present on testing. However, combined movements of hip flexion with knee extension, such as a straight leg raise, will normally produce some discomfort at the site of the lesion, either at the posterior of the hip or the posterior of the knee (13, 17, 23, 25).

Passive Movements Tightness of the hamstrings may be noted bilaterally on passive straight leg raising, with discomfort felt at the site of the lesion on overpressure applied at end range of motion when the knee is extended with the hip flexed. This discomfort should be relieved immediately if the knee is allowed to flex slightly (13, 17, 23).

Resisted Movements Pain is usually experienced on resisted knee flexion, particularly if the movement is tested several times in succession. Pain present on isometric resisted rotation of the knee may differentiate between a lesion affecting the biceps femoris muscle, when pain will be felt at the lateral aspect of the knee, and the semitendinosis and semi-membranosus muscles, when the discomfort is felt on the medial side of the knee. When the lesion lies at the proximal attachment of the muscles there will be no differentiation discernible at the buttock on similar testing, however, resisted hip extension may produced ischial pain when the lesion is more proximal (13, 22, 25).

Palpation Tenderness will be elicited on palpation of the affected tendon either in the buttock or at the posterior of the knee either medially or laterally (Fig. 6.2) (Fig. 6.5) (15, 22, 26,).

Specific Tests Where the patient's discomfort is experienced at the posterior aspect of the knee, non-weight–bearing and weight-bearing isometric and isotonic resisted contraction of the gastrocnemius muscle should be tested to rule out involvement of the calf muscle at its proximal attachments.

Treatment Ideas
(13, 15, 17, 19, 23, 25)

One to two days of ice and rest from activity may help to resolve any acute symptoms. Massage is also effective, particularly when the patient presents with generalized increased tension in the muscles of the lower extremities. Active exercises should be used for all movements of the hip and knee, but should only be carried to the point of tension, as compared to discomfort, for movements involving the hamstring muscles. After this initial trial of ice therapy the patient can use heat applied to the entire length of the muscle, not simply to the area of the lesion. This is followed by gentle hamstring stretches, initially, non-weight–bearing but assisted by the use of a towel wrapped around the patient's thigh, so that the leg can be pulled into further hip flexion while keeping the knee straight.

Application of ultrasound or laser can be given to the affected area. The use of heat should be continued and active stretches should be followed by light resisted hamstring work, which in turn should be followed by more stretches. These stretches should be prolonged in nature (30–60 seconds with an equal amount of rest), or shorter stretches (10–15 seconds) can be used, repeated 30–40 times in succession, in order to gain flexibility in the muscle.

Proprioceptive neuromuscular facilitation techniques can be used for both strengthening and stretching with specific hold–relax and contract–relax techniques taught to the patient for continued use at home. These exercises should be combined with a program of general weight-bearing lower extremity stretches. It is important at this time to check that there is the correct ratio between quadriceps and hamstrings muscle strength (hamstrings at 65% of the strength of the quadriceps). If there is any noticeable deviation from this ratio then the specific muscles should be strengthened accordingly.

The patient is finally progressed onto a general lower extremity workout of resisted exercises on weight training equipment with the use of an exercise bike, step machine, or both. Plyometrics should be attempted, with general lower extremity stretches before, during, and after the exercise regime. Running activities should be steadily progressed, starting with straight-line running on a flat surface, progressing to hills and turns, as well as running sideways and backwards. The patient often benefits from the application of ice after these activities, even if no immediate symptoms are produced.

Restrictions In the early stages the only restriction necessary is to limit the amount of running that the patient attempts to a level that does not produce symptoms. An excessive degree of stair climbing or squatting and lifting may produce symptoms, in which case they should be avoided or reduced in duration as required. These activities can be resumed in a graduated manner as the patient is able to tolerate them, although general stretching exercises for the hip and knee musculature should be continued well after the time at which symptoms are no longer produced on activity.

Quadriceps Muscle Tear

Overview

This condition occurs most commonly in younger patients and is due to a powerful contraction of the quadriceps muscle group against resistance.

The muscle most commonly affected is the rectus femoris because of its two-joint action. The movement during which this occurs is one of flexion of the hip with extension of the knee, such as in kicking a football, with a force then applied to the lower leg, driving the knee into flexion. It is initially a very painful and disabling condition, but responds well and quickly to physical treatment (18, 19, 24).

Onset Onset is sudden due to trauma in patients under the age of 40 years. The patient will give a history of forceful hip flexion and knee extension against resistance, such as in kicking the ground instead of kicking the ball (4, 18).

Duration The patient usually presents for treatment within a matter of days, or at most 1 to 2 weeks, as the condition is both painful and very limiting functionally.

Frequency It is very uncommon to find this occurring on more than one occasion in one individual.

Area of Symptoms The patient can usually localize his symptoms to the distal half or third of the anterior aspect of the thigh (Fig. 6.22) (3, 4, 26).

Type of Symptoms Sharp localized pain is present at the time of injury and also on subsequent contraction or stretching of the quadriceps muscle. A poorly defined ache is usually present at rest.

Miscellaneous The three vasti muscles are seldom involved, if these are the only ones that are involved, and the rectus femoris is spared, then the condition is nowhere near as painful or disabling (4, 8, 19).

Objective Findings

Observation There is usually a mild degree of swelling at the site of injury. If the muscle is torn, bruising may be observed in the anterior thigh and around the knee (5, 18, 19).

Active Movements There is usually mild limitation of flexion of the knee with discomfort at end range of motion that is felt at the site of injury. Knee flexion is more limited if tested with the hip taken into extension. Knee extension is full with discomfort at end range, as the quadriceps muscles contract more strongly as the patient tries to gain further range. All hip movements will be full range and pain free (18, 24).

Passive Movements All passive movements of the hip and knee should be full range, although stiffness and some muscle guarding may be found at end range of flexion of the knee. Flexion of the knee with the patient in the prone lying position may be slightly restricted and will always be uncomfortable, with the pain felt at the site of injury. The patient will normally resist attempts to flex the knee beyond the end of available range. Marked pain will be produced at the site of injury if the hip is passively extended while the knee is held in the flexed position (5, 18).

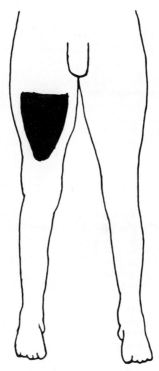

FIG. 6.22 Area of symptoms for a muscle tear in the right quadriceps.

Resisted Movements Pain will be felt at the site of injury on isometric resisted knee extension, and possibly on isometric resisted hip flexion if the rectus femoris muscle is involved. The patient will experience most discomfort on extension of the knee when this is tested with the knee in a fully flexed position. Quadriceps muscle strength will be diminished somewhat, usually due to pain rather than to intrinsic weakness of the muscle, because as noted above the vasti are normally spared and therefore the majority of the power of the muscle is still present (5, 16, 24).

Palpation Tenderness will be elicited over the site of injury, which is usually at the distal myotendinous junction of the rectus femoris muscle (4, 18, 22, 26).

Treatment Ideas
(3–5, 18, 19, 24)

For the first 2 to 3 days immediately following injury the patient should be treated with ice, compression, elevation, and rest. Active movements of the hip and knee should be continued in all pain-free ranges, with the movements taken to the point of onset of tightness, rather than pain, at the site of injury for the movements of hip extension and knee flexion. By the fourth day following injury the patient can be started on the use of thermal modalities, with light quadriceps stretching achieved actively lying prone using knee flexion. Resisted exercises can be continued for all other movements of the hip and knee. Isometric quadriceps contractions should be carried out by the patient regularly throughout the day.

Ultrasound and laser can be used at the site of injury with interferential to the quadriceps muscle bulk to promote relaxation and increased blood flow. If the patient has difficulty in producing an active isometric contraction of the quadriceps, then neuromuscular electrical stimulation can be very effective. Stretching exercises for the quadriceps muscles can be progressed by the use of hip extension combined with knee flexion carried out lying prone. Light resisted quadriceps work can be commenced with the application of ice to the site of the injury at the end of the treatment session. Proprioceptive neuromuscular facilitation techniques for combined hip flexion and knee extension can be used to progress strengthening and the patient can also be put on a program of general lower extremity stretches.

When the patient demonstrates full range of knee flexion and no discomfort when knee flexion is combined with hip extension, then he can be progressed to resisted weight-bearing exercises such as squats, wall squats (initially starting at 60 degrees and progressing to 90 degrees), and step ups. Stretching exercises for the lower extremities, particularly for the quadriceps, should be carried out before, during, and after the exercise program. The use of neuromuscular electrical stimulation can be progressed by having the patient flex the knee against the artificially generated quadriceps muscle contraction, thus recreating, in slow motion and under controlled circumstances, the mechanism of injury.

The patient is finally progressed into a general lower extremity workout program on weight-training equipment. Plyometrics such as jump downs should be commenced with explosive activities such as short sprints, stopping and turning, lateral gliding, and lateral bounding incorporated into the exercise program. This will help to strengthen and test the quadriceps prior to the patient returning to practice, competition, or simply the activity that produced the injury.

Restrictions   In the initial stages following injury it is very difficult for the patient to attempt any activities that may produce further injury. However, the patient must be advised against any explosive action of the quadriceps muscle, such as sprinting and jumping, and should also avoid any quick stop-and-start type of activities. Once active stretches become relatively pain-free the patient can return to light jogging and straight-line running. From that point the patient can build up to a return to light training, then normal training if applicable. Once the patient is pain-free on all exercises in the clinic and in practice sessions he can return to competition. The patient can be out of competitive activities from 2 to 12 weeks, depending on the severity of the injury.

Quadriceps Tendon Tear

Overview

The quadriceps tendon is susceptible to injury in slips and falls, particularly in older patients and if the knee is forcibly flexed as the quadriceps muscles are contracting. The tear occurs at the distal myotendinous or tendoperiosteal junction of the quadriceps, and may even extend into the expansion of the quadriceps tendon at the margins of the patella (5, 18).

Onset This is always sudden due to trauma and commonly occurs in patients over the age of 50. It is much more common in men than women (3, 19, 23, 24).

Duration The patient presents for treatment within days of onset of the condition, as it is both very painful and disabling as regards effect on normal daily activities.

Frequency This will always be the first and only time that the patient has suffered from these symptoms.

Area of Symptoms Symptoms are well localized to the distal third of the anterior of the thigh and possibly also around the margins of the patella if the quadriceps expansion is involved in the injury (Fig. 6.23) (5, 19, 23, 26).

Type of Symptoms The patient will complain of sharp pain on all weight-bearing activities or on any use of the knee. This is particularly noticeable on going up and down stairs or on walking up or down hills (5, 19, 23, 26).

Miscellaneous The patient will often be unable to either squat or rise from a squat position. Patients who suffer a complete rupture of the tendon will require surgical intervention, with a cast necessary after surgery. Once the patient comes out of the cast, treatment is the same as that described for a partial tear.

Objective Findings

Observation There is commonly bruising observable at the distal aspect of the thigh and occasionally laterally around the knee. There is often a mild to moderate degree of swelling observed in the area of the quadriceps tendon just proximal to the knee (3, 5).

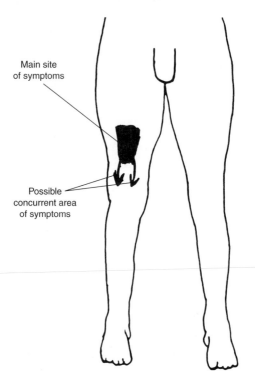

Main site
of symptoms

Possible
concurrent area
of symptoms

FIG. 6.23   Area of symptoms for a right quadriceps tendon tear.

Active Movements   There will be painful limitation of active knee flexion and the patient is usually unable to fully extend the knee partially due to pain and partially due to muscle weakness. There is often an observable lag in the quadriceps muscle on the straight leg raise test, where the knee flexes slightly as the patient raises the leg while trying to keep the knee straight (5, 10, 19, 23).

Passive Movements   Pain will be produced at the site of the injury at end range of knee flexion. This pain will increase if the patient's knee flexion is tested while lying prone, and it will increase even more if the hip is then simultaneously extended. In fact, the patient may well be unable to tolerate extension of the hip while the knee is flexed. Muscle spasm or voluntary muscle guarding will usually prevent any overpressure into knee flexion. All other passive movements of the hip and knee will be of full range and pain free (5, 18, 19).

Resisted Movements Pain and weakness will be noted on isometric knee extension, with the patient unable to sustain an isometric quadriceps contraction against resistance. If marked weakness of knee extension is present, but painless, then a complete tear of the quadriceps tendon should be suspected. The patient would then require referral to an orthopaedic surgeon.

Palpation There may be a palpable gap in the proximal part of the quadriceps tendon. Palpation over the site of injury will produce complaints of marked tenderness (5, 19, 24).

Treatment Ideas
(3, 5, 18, 19, 23, 24)

If seen immediately after injury, the patient should be advised to rest the leg and apply ice for approximately 15 minutes ever 2 hours. Active hip and knee movements should be continued in all pain-free ranges, with knee flexion taken to the point where pressure is felt at the site of the injury, but no pain. Four days postinjury the patient can start using heat, with active exercises for all movements of the hip and knee. The movements should be carried to the point of discomfort if applicable, but not pushed into pain at any time.

Resisted exercises can be introduced for all those movements of the hip and knee that are painless on active testing. Isometric quadriceps exercises can be combined with neuromuscular electrical stimulation and can be progressed to inner range quadriceps work over a towel roll. Application of ultrasound and laser may promote repair in the injured tissues, while interferential therapy may produce muscle relaxation and decrease discomfort. Ice and transcutaneous electrical nerve stimulation can be used to relieve postexercise discomfort.

Exercises are progressed to light resisted quadriceps work initially with inner range quadriceps followed by straight leg raising, as long as the patient can carry out the movement without any quadriceps lag. Further progress is made to extension of the knee from flexion, as with the patient sitting with his leg over the edge of a treatment table and straightening the knee. Active and passive knee flexion stretches can then be introduced, with steadily increasing amounts of hip extension, as tolerated by the patient. At this time muscle stimulation can be combined with active quadriceps contraction through full range of movement.

Proprioceptive neuromuscular facilitation techniques can be used for strengthening of the quadriceps with combined knee extension and hip flexion, strengthening the rectus femoris muscle in particular. Hold–relax and contract–relax techniques can be used to progress stretching of the quadriceps muscle, as can neuromuscular stimulation, with the patient stretching into knee flexion against the quadriceps contraction produced by the stimulation.

Gym exercises should be designed for all movements of the hip, knee, and ankle, including weight-bearing exercises such as step-ups and wall squats (starting at 30–40% range of motion and progressing gradually to 100%). The patient can then progress to more dynamic exercises for running, jumping, stepping, and so on, as related to the desired level of daily activities. Final degrees of stretch of the quadriceps muscle can be achieved using a neuromuscular stimulator with the patient completing a weight-bearing squat while the muscle is contracting. The patient can then be progressed to single-knee exercises, including work on a balance board for proprioceptive reeducation.

Restrictions   The condition is initially very self-limiting, the patient should use either crutches or a cane for walking to preserve a good gait pattern and to prevent injury through any inadvertent slip or fall. Pushing or pulling of heavy weights, and squatting to lift and carrying heavy weights, particularly up and down stairs, should be avoided. Climbing steps and stairs should be done in such a way as to favor the affected leg by taking one step at a time, always leading with the unaffected leg when going up and the affected leg when going down. Ladders, jumping, and walking over uneven surfaces should be avoided in the initial stages, and may only be attempted once the patient is able to tolerate active quadriceps stretches without any major discomfort.

Jumping from even small heights should be avoided until the condition has cleared. Walking up hills should be paced, with rests taken in either standing or sitting as required. The patient can return gradually to all of the above activities when able to tolerate the stresses and strains while in the protected environment of the clinical setting. All weight-bearing activities should first be attempted with minimal weight and then with a gradual increase in weight as tolerated.

Collateral Ligament Strain of Knee

Overview

This is the most common knee injury seen in orthopaedics and one of the most common of all soft-tissue injuries. There are three different degrees of the injury typically described. The first degree is a strain of the ligaments, in which the tissue is overstretched rather than torn. The second degree is a partial tear of the tissue, while a third-degree injury is complete rupture of the ligament.

Signs of a complete rupture are intense initial pain lasting for a matter of minutes, after which the discomfort eases quite quickly, but the knee will feel unstable on attempted weight-bearing. There is more swelling following a second-degree injury than after a third-degree strain. The capsule of the joint is torn in a third-degree injury, which therefore releases the edematous material; however, there will still be signs of loss of stability of the joint. These may not be as noticeable a few hours after injury because the swelling that stays in the joint will splint it, as will the attending muscle spasm. Complete rupture of a ligament will usually either require surgical intervention or a long period with the joint immobilized in a cast. In clinical practice the therapist is usually concerned with primary treatment of first- or second-degree injuries, both of which do well with conservative treatment (5, 15, 16, 18).

Onset Onset is sudden due to trauma and most commonly occurs when stress is applied to the flexed knee combined with a movement of rotation. The flexion produces relaxation of the capsule and ligaments, thus allowing the rotation to occur. Injury can occur with a straight leg through hyperextension or through force applied to either side of the knee. The injury may occur at any age, but is most common in patients from 20 to 50 years of age (1, 3, 5, 19).

Duration Patients typically present for treatment within a day to 1 or 2 weeks following injury.

Frequency Typically this will be the first time the patient has suffered this particular injury; however, depending on the type of sport the patient is involved in and the level of competition, it is possible, particularly in contact sports, for one player to sustain two or three injuries over a period of time (15, 19).

Area of Symptoms These are usually fairly well localized to either the medial or lateral sides of the knee, and may on occasion also be associated with pain to one or both sides of the patella, the anterior of the patella, or to one or both sides of the patella ligament (Fig. 6.24) (4, 5, 8, 15).

Type of Symptoms The patient will typically state that he heard a "pop" at the time of injury. Pain is sharp, particularly on activities that stress the knee, such as full squats or rotation of the flexed knee. There is usually also a general aching discomfort to one side of the knee at rest, especially following activity (1, 4, 5, 19, 20).

Miscellaneous Because of the sudden traumatic nature of the injury the patient may not be able to give a clear or exact description of the stresses applied to the joint.

Objective Findings

Observation In first- and second-degree strains, the amount of swelling can be directly related to the degree of injury. However, as stated under third-degree injuries, with tearing of the joint capsule there may be less swelling than would be expected considering the degree of injury. The patient should be questioned about how soon after injury the swelling developed. In a severe injury where bleeding occurs within the tissues, the

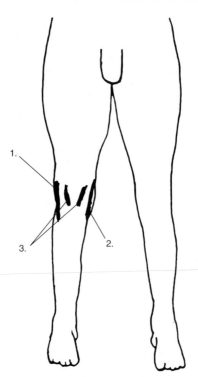

FIG. 6.24   Area of symptoms for a collateral ligament strain of the right knee at either: 1–the lateral aspect of the knee or 2–the medial aspect of the knee. Symptoms may also possibly occur concurrently at 3–the borders of the patella.

swelling would normally appear within 30 minutes. On the other hand, where there is a lesser degree of injury it may take several hours for swelling to occur in the overstrained joint (4–6, 8, 23).

Active Movements   Pain is usually felt at end range of both flexion and extension, but these movements should still be of nearly full range, although flexion in particular may be limited by the joint effusion. In acute second-degree injuries there can be 20 to 30% loss of flexion and 10 to 15% loss of extension (4, 8, 15, 19, 23, 24).

Passive Movements The pattern for loss of range of motion on passive testing will be the same as seen in active testing. Pain will be produced on overpressure at end range of available flexion or extension, and will usually be in the region of the injury, but not necessarily clearly localized to it. Pain will be present on either valgus or varus stress of the knee and on testing of medial or lateral rotation of the knee. Any excessive play found in the joint compared to the unaffected leg would indicate a complete rupture of the ligament and subsequent joint instability, necessitating a referral to an orthopaedic surgeon (4, 10, 15, 19, 23, 24).

Resisted Movements Normally good strength is demonstrated in the muscles of the knee, although pain is usually produced by strongly resisted movements of either flexion or extension. Particular pain can be produced on isometric resisted rotation if carried out at the end of available range (10, 15, 19, 24).

Palpation Tenderness will be elicited at either the medial or lateral knee joint line and will often extend along the length of the affected ligament to some degree or another (Fig. 6.10 and 6.11). Tenderness may also be elicited distally from and to the sides of the patella if the quadriceps expansion is affected, and also towards the anterior of the knee joint line, medially and laterally, if the coronary ligaments are involved in the injury (Fig. 6.6) (1, 2, 22, 26).

Specific Tests Appley's distraction test will produce discomfort on combined rotation and distraction of the knee with the patient tested in prone lying. The menisci should be tested to rule out injury and anterior and posterior drawer tests should be used to assess the stability of the cruciate ligaments. Varus and valgus stresses with the knee extended and then repeated with the knee slightly flexed should produce pain at the site of injury (18, 22, 27).

Treatment Ideas
(1, 3–6, 8, 12, 15, 18–20, 23, 26)

If seen in the first few days following injury, the PRICE formula should be followed; protection (P) of the joint using a splint if necessary and crutches for weight bearing, rest (R) from any pain-producing activities, ice (I) around the affected area for 15–30 minutes every 1 to 2 hours (as allowed by the patient's daily schedule), compression (C) of the joint (provided this is applied in an effective manner using a compression bandage), and elevation (E) of the leg, which is the most important element to reduce swelling in the joint.

The use of a brace or crutches may be required for 1 to 2 weeks, depending on the degree of injury. During this time the patient should maintain active movements of the affected joint in mid-range, with the use of isometric quadriceps and hamstrings exercises to maintain muscle strength and bulk. Active straight leg hip exercises for flexion, abduction, and extension can also be employed to maintain general function of the lower extremity. The patient should remain on crutches until able to complete a straight leg raise with no quadriceps lag (i.e., the patient should be able to straighten the leg fully on the bed and then lift the leg off the bed without the knee flexing at all).

Approximately 4 days postinjury, heat can be applied to the affected joint and active hip and knee exercises can be progressed to full available range. Neuromuscular stimulation can be used to enhance isometric quadriceps and hamstrings muscle work. Interferential therapy applied around the knee can be helpful in reducing discomfort due to swelling, and pulsed doses of ultrasound or laser can be applied over the injured ligament. At this time the patient can also start work on an exercise bike with minimal resistance. It is usually easier for the patient to initially peddle backwards, once the patient starts peddling forwards the seat should be adjusted so that the movement is as comfortable as possible, avoiding any extremes of flexion or extension at the knee. The patient can be progressed to resisted straight leg exercises using light weights or a light exercise band. These exercises can be further progressed to isotonic resisted knee exercises with ankle weights, while continuing with neuromuscular stimulation for the quadriceps and hamstrings. The correct ratio of quadriceps to hamstrings strength should be borne in mind during resistance training; that is, the hamstring resistance should be approximately 65% of that applied to the quadriceps. Proprioceptive neuromuscular facilitation techniques can be used with combined patterns aimed at strengthening rotation of the knee.

At this time, as active movements are becoming less uncomfortable, the patient can start to apply overpressure into extension using his hands placed over the anterior of the knee to straighten it as fully as possible while resting on the bed. While lying prone with the ankle of the affected leg crossed over the back of the ankle of the unaffected leg, the patient can push the joint into further flexion by simply bending the unaffected knee. When non-weight–bearing resisted exercises are being carried out with a reasonable degree of comfort, the patient is progressed to weight-bearing resisted exercises using a step machine, step ups, lateral step ups, and 50% squats. At the same time the patient can start a resisted exercise program on weight-training equipment to strengthen all movements of the hip, knee, and ankle. Proprioceptive training will also be necessary using a balance board and single-leg stance exercises.

The patient can finally be eased back into training or daily activities with gentle running, initially in straight lines and at a jog, then progressing to sudden starts and stops, corners, then lateral gliding, lateral bounding, and eventually a full workout including plyometrics such as jump-ups, jump-downs, and stepping back and forth over a stool. In these final stages the patient should also be given a general stretching and flexibility exercise program for all the major musculature of the lower extremities. These exercises can be carried out during rest breaks in the strengthening and conditioning programs.

Restrictions Initially the patient should avoid squatting for lifting or sustained squatting or kneeling for any activity. They should also not carry heavy loads or push and pull heavy weights. Walking should be restricted to an amount that does not produce any marked discomfort on rest afterwards. Initially the patient should refrain from running, at least until able to demonstrate the correct gait pattern at a walk. Twisting motions of the knee should be avoided, with the patient taught to move his feet instead of twisting the torso, and hence the knees. Weight-bearing activities in either static or dynamic standing should be broken up by sitting for short periods of time.

The patient will have to be kept out of any competitive activities, particularly contact sports, until coping with a vigorous weight-bearing exercise routine in the clinic. Progression should then be made through light training to regular training, and finally to competition once the patient is able to complete normal training without any obvious discomfort. The length of time for which the patient will be unable to compete will depend entirely upon the degree of injury and the speed of recovery. Return to normal activity can only be decided by the absence of typical discomfort on stress testing of the ligaments or on vigorous weight-bearing activities.

Patella Femoral Syndrome (PFS)

Overview

The term "patella femoral syndrome" covers several different possible conditions, such as chondromalacia patella, patella femoral osteoarthritis (PFOA), and maltracking of the patella. However, the symptoms and treatment are similar in most of these cases, with the problem occurring in the articulation between the patella and the femur.

Subjective Findings

Onset The condition occurs gradually after overuse or is due to no known cause. Although initial onset may be for no known cause, certain activities, or one specific activity, will increase symptoms, and may often be incriminated by the patient as being the initial cause, as well as the cause of exacerbation, of the symptoms. Patella femoral syndrome occurs quite often in teenagers, in which case it is almost always idiopathic in origin. In adults it occurs in those from 20 to 50 years of age (1, 2, 12, 18).

Duration Because of the gradual nature of onset, with gradually increasing symptoms over time, the patient does not normally present for treatment until at least 6 to 12 weeks after onset, and often longer.

Frequency The patient may be able to recall recurrent episodes of knee problems going back to their teens. In teenage patients this may be the first time they have had the condition, but even in these cases there will usually have been one or two previous episodes of mild symptoms before the patient sought medical attention for the present episode (8, 14, 20).

Area of Symptoms   Symptoms are poorly localized, but are found mainly at the anterior aspect of the knee and to a lesser extent at the sides of the knee or distally over the anterolateral or anteromedial aspects of the tibia (Fig. 6.25) (2, 4, 7, 12, 18, 20,).

Type of Symptoms   The patient's most common complaint is of an ache either during or after activity. The patient may complain that the knee felt as if it would give way, and in rare cases it does, but the patient is usually able to catch himself before falling to the ground (4, 6, 18, 20).

Miscellaneous   Some patients may complain that they are unable to rise from the full squat position without using their hands for assistance. Patients may also complain of pain and stiffness in the affected joint after sitting for

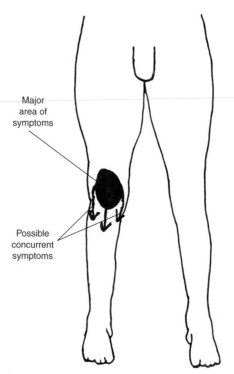

FIG. 6.25   Area of symptoms for patella femoral syndrome at the right knee.

an extended period of time, such as in a theatre, on a plane, or at a meeting. Another common complaint is of pain on going up and down stairs, with more particular discomfort felt on descending (2, 4, 6, 19, 20, 23).

Objective Findings

Observation There is usually nil of note to be observed in or around the affected knee; however, if the patient has a markedly acute episode on top of a very chronic condition, there may be a mild degree of swelling visible over the distal half of the patella. In long-standing cases there may also be observable soft-tissue thickening around the patella femoral joint (2, 4, 8, 23).

Active Movements There is usually no discomfort or restriction in range of motion experienced on testing of active movements of the hip, knee, or ankle (1, 2, 6, 9, 12).

Passive Movements Overpressure at end range of available flexion may produce mild discomfort around the patella, or the patient may complain of a sensation of unpleasant pressure on the same maneuver. Passive movements of the patella are usually painful, particularly proximal to distal gliding of the patella. This is more marked if pressure is applied over the patella to approximate the joint surfaces during the movement. Fine crepitation is usually felt during passive movements of the patella and again is more marked if pressure is applied downwards on the patella (2, 6, 12, 18).

Resisted Movements Isometric testing of the musculature of the hip, knee, and ankle will demonstrate full strength and will elicit no discomfort (2, 6, 18, 23).

Palpation Occasionally tenderness can be felt around the sides or at the upper or lower poles of the patella (Fig. 6.6). The undersurface of the patella may be tender and can be palpated on the medial side with the patella pushed passively medially and on the lateral side with the patella pushed laterally. Approximately one-third to one-half of the undersurface of the patella can be palpated in this manner. Soft-tissue thickening may be palpable around the region of the patella tendon and around the patella femoral joint in chronic cases (6, 18, 22, 26,).

Specific Tests Clark's sign is positive for PFS if the patient complains of discomfort in the patella region when an isometric quadriceps contraction is resisted by the examiner pushing down on the upper pole of the patella. The patient should be instructed to carry out this maneuver slowly, as in more acute cases the amount of discomfort produced can be intense; vigorous resistance, if applied, can produce results that severely strain the trust built up between patient and therapist. The Q angle (or patella femoral angle) between the quadriceps and the patella tendon should be measured as this may give an indication of the degree to which a patient is susceptible to this syndrome.

McConnell's test is carried out by the examiner resisting an isometric quadriceps contraction in varying degrees of flexion. If pain is felt at one particular angle then the patient's leg is straightened and the patella is moved passively medially. With the patella kept in this position the quadriceps contraction is retested at the same angle. If there was decreased pain on retesting, the patella-femoral joint would probably be indicated as the source of the discomfort (1, 4, 22, 27).

Treatment Ideas

Where the patient is suffering an acute episode of pain he should be advised to rest for a short period of time and to apply ice on a regular basis for 2 to 3 days. Rest means avoiding any activity that the patient finds produces the symptoms, either during, or within a few hours following, the activity. After an initial period of rest the patient can start isometric resisted quadriceps exercises, assisted by neuromuscular electrical stimulation, with the exercises carried out with a straight leg at all times. The patient can then move into hip extension and abduction exercises, initially actively and then resisted using ankle weights or a resistance band.

Laser or ultrasound can be applied to the undersurfaces of the patella by gliding it medially or laterally as required. Laser is often the easier application in this position. Ultrasound can also be used around the patella margins, particularly if there is any degree of soft-tissue thickening present. Interferential therapy and transcutaneous electrical nerve stimulation can help to decrease discomfort when applied around the patella femoral joint. At this stage heat should be used before exercises and ice after the exercises.

The patient is progressed to isometric quadriceps contractions at different angles of flexion; once he can cope with this exercise without exacerbating the knee symptoms, he can be progressed to isotonic strengthening exercises for the quadriceps, hamstrings, and hip abductors. Ice should still be applied around the patella following any treatment session in which progression of the exercises was made. Neuromuscular electrical stimulation can be effective when applied to the vastus medialus muscle, as the position of the muscle fibers of this particular muscle apply the only truly medial force on the patella during muscle contraction. The vastus intermedius, vastus lateralis, and rectus femoris all pull the patella laterally to some degree or another. It is not uncommon to find patients with marked patella femoral syndrome who have poor definition of the vastus medialis compared to the other muscles of the quadriceps group, or compared to the vastus medialis on the opposite leg, if the syndrome is confined to only one of the lower extremities. Once muscle strengthening has begun, the quadriceps to hamstrings muscle strength ratio should always be kept in mind, with the resistance applied to the hamstrings being some 30–35% less than that applied to the quadriceps.

For may years the primary approach to this condition has been the use of straight leg exercises to strengthen the musculature of the hip and knee;

however, a newer approach is to work towards normal weightbearing and functional activities in an attempt to return patients to a more functionally efficient lifestyle, especially in sports or work activities. The patient is started on mini-squats to approximately 30–40% of range and a wall slide, holding the flexed knee position initially at 30–40 degrees, and progressing to 60 or even 90 degrees. Weightbearing lunges, lateral stepups, stepdowns, and use of an exercise bike should all be progressed in small doses, with ice used following each progression to reduce the possibility of an inflammatory reaction at the affected joint. The patient can further progress to jumpdowns, lateral bounding, hopping, skipping, and running, again with gradual progression of any weight-bearing exercises involving repeated knee flexion and extension.

Restrictions Initially there should be a blanket restriction on all symptom-producing activities, at least for a short period of time. Activities that are particularly likely to produce symptoms are steps and stairs, repetitive or sustained squatting, kneeling, and crawling, although any weight-bearing activity that involves repeated flexion and extension of the knee is a possible source of symptom exacerbation. A gradual return to these activities can be made, but each activity should be tackled separately, as patients react differently to different stresses and that which may be safe for one patient may prove disastrous for another. Exacerbation of symptoms through specific activity does not necessarily mean that the activity must be avoided indefinitely. It simply means that progression should be made through other activities before this activity is attempted again.

A systematic approach to recording of symptoms related to time and activity will allow patients to progress themselves effectively and painlessly. However, in younger patients this may need closer supervision by the therapist, as they may tend to downplay their symptoms when the activity is one that they are particularly keen to participate in. It is the therapist's job to council both patience and perseverance as the patient tries to regain as near-normal function as possible. This is the type of advice that it is particularly hard to impart with any degree of success to the teenage patient, particularly one who is good at, and keen to, participate in a specific sport. In these cases a clear timetable for recovery should be discussed with the patient so that alternative activities can be viewed as a means to an end, rather than as a meaningless exercise.

Osteoarthritis (OA) of the Knee

Overview

The knee appears to be prone to arthritis with common predisposing factors being previous trauma (miniscal injuries, fractures into the joint surfaces of the tibia or femur, and fractures of the femur or tibia producing biomechanical changes in the lower extremity), ligamentous instability, obesity, knee joint deformities, and a family history of arthritis. The pain in arthritis does not arise directly from the eroded cartilage or bone, which have no nerve endings, instead it is produced by tight periarticular structures. The aim of treatment for relief of symptoms is to stretch this tight tissue and then to strengthen the muscles about the knee in order to support the joint, thus placing less strain on the sensitive passive supporting elements (1–3, 18).

Subjective Findings

Onset   This is gradual either with no cause or possibly due to a previous injury, which may occur many years prior to onset of symptoms. The condition is most common in older patients, usually over the age of 50, although if there has been marked trauma affecting the joint it can occur at any age (3, 14, 18, 20).

Duration   The patient will normally have been suffering symptoms of increasing intensity over a period of months or even years.

Frequency   The patient's history should indicate one long ongoing episode, with exacerbation and remission of symptoms usually associated with increase or decrease in weight-bearing activities (2, 3, 18, 20).

Area of Symptoms   These are general around the knee, although there may be one area of the knee that is more uncomfortable than the rest. In order of frequency this area is commonly the medial side, the anterior of the knee, the lateral side, and finally the posterior of the knee (Fig. 6.26) (1, 2, 18, 23).

Type of Symptoms   The patient will complain of an aching pain and stiffness, which is particularly noticeable in the morning upon rising or after sitting in one position for a period of time. Swelling of varying degrees may be present from time to time or may steadily increase over time. The patient may also have noticed that some deformity of the knee has developed, most typically genu varum (1, 2, 18, 23, 24).

Miscellaneous   Arthritis of the knee is often associated with degenerative changes in other weight-bearing joints, particularly the other knee, the hips, or the low back.

Objective Findings

Observation   Soft-tissue thickening as well as swelling may be noted around the knee-joint line. There may be visible deformity, which may be very noticeable in comparison to the other knee if the arthritis is unilateral in nature. In cases seen in the early stages, there may be minimal observable changes (2, 3, 20, 23).

Active Movements   There will be a mild to moderate degrees of limitation of both flexion and extension of the knee. In the early stages the patient will complain of stiffness, rather than discomfort, at end range of

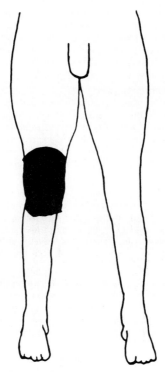

FIG. 6.26 Area of symptoms for osteoarthritis at the right knee. Symptoms may also occur in a similar distribution at the posterior aspect of the joint concurrently with those shown in the diagram.

motion. Loss of range of motion is progressively greater as the condition progresses and coarse crepitation may be felt during movement in more severe cases (3, 9, 18, 24).

Passive Movements The limitation of range of motion on passive testing will be the same pattern as that found on active testing, with pain produced on overpressure at end of available range for each movement, and usually experienced at the typical site of maximal discomfort. Pain is often also present on passive patella movements, particularly superior-inferior gliding. Pain may or may not be present on both medial or lateral rotation of the knee, again depending on the severity of the underlying condition. A hand placed on the patella during passive testing should elicit crepitation during movement. Fine crepitation is usually found occurring in the retropatella region, whereas coarser crepitation comes from the knee joint itself. The coarser crepitation may be heard as well as felt, particularly in more chronic cases (2, 3, 9, 23, 24).

Resisted Movements There is often generalized weakness not only in the knee, but also generally in the legs due to the patient's steadily decreasing levels of activity and therefore declining exercise tolerance. No pain is experienced on steady isometric resistance applied to movements, although strongly resisted movements of flexion, extension, or rotation of the knee may produce discomfort due to stress being placed on the ligamentous structures of the joint (1, 2, 23, 24).

Palpation Tenderness is normally elicited around the knee joint line (Fig. 6.9) and it is usually more marked on one side most commonly the medial side, compared to the other. Crepitation may often be felt at the knee joint line during passive or active movements, while soft-tissue thickening may be felt around the knee joint line, around the patella-femoral joint line, and in the region of the patella tendon. Palpation at the posterior aspect of the knee joint may reveal the presence of a Baker's cyst in more chronic cases (3, 4, 22, 26).

Specific Tests X-rays will normally reveal degenerative changes that may be restricted to, or worse in, one compartment, again usually the medial. In comparison to the hip or low back the x-ray findings are often also clearly indicative of the actual severity of the patient's condition and the degree of degenerative changes seen usually correlates well with the clinical picture presented (14, 18, 20).

Treatment Ideas
(1–3, 8, 14, 18, 20, 23, 24)

Most patients find that application of heat to the affected joint helps relieve discomfort and allows for slightly better function. Some patients, (although a minority) prefer ice, and in some cases a judicious mixture of both heat and ice produces the best results. The patient should be started on isometric exercises for the quadriceps, hamstrings, and hip abductors, all done with a straight leg, which can be progressed quite quickly to active straight leg raising, straight leg hip extension, and hip abduction. Manual distraction of the knee, starting gently with small oscillations, will often relieve discomfort for several hours, and the degree of stretch can be progressed as the tissues become more pliable. Thermal doses of ultrasound applied to the joint line can be helpful in producing further stretch and therefore greater relief. At this period a diplomatic suggestion to the overweight patient that less weight placed on the joint will mean less pain produced by the joint may encourage him to decrease his caloric intake.

Neuromuscular electrical stimulation can be used to enhance the straight leg muscle work. The patient can progress to isometric resisted work for the quadriceps and hamstrings in differing degrees of flexion. Further progression is made to straight leg exercises using ankle weights or a resistance band, initially, through mid-range working into inner and outer range as the patient tolerates the exercise. Passive patella mobilizations should be used if any degree of stiffness is encountered in the patella-femoral articulation during examination. The patient can also attempt distraction of his own knee using progressively increased weights in high sitting over the edge of a treatment table. Initially the patient simply allows the weight to hang, when this is well tolerated a small swinging motion of approximately 10–15 degrees range will help to loosen the joint and release stiff periarticular structures. Application of heat prior to distraction and exercise often allows the patient to perform more effectively. Heat with transcutaneous electrical nerve stimulation or interferential therapy after exercises can help to diminish discomfort produced by the exercises.

Resisted exercises can be progressed to quite significant weights, but should be attempted with a straight leg only. Resisted exercises involving active flexion and extension of the knee should be limited to lighter weights and should be monitored closely to ensure that the patient is not exacerbating the symptoms unduly, as the often quoted "no pain, no gain" really does not apply to discomfort felt at an arthritic joint during or after exercise. I tell patients that discomfort felt in the muscles of the thigh is acceptable, but that the area for 2 to 3 inches above and below the knee is a "no-go zone" as far as pain is concerned, either during or after treatment.

Weight-bearing exercises are never a good idea in OA of the knee; however, hydrotherapy can produce excellent results because strong resistance can be applied to movements while a significant degree of body weight is taken off the affected joint by the effects of buoyancy. A recumbent cycle is also usually well tolerated by the majority of patients. The long-term prognosis for many patients is joint replacement surgery, but the longer this can be postponed, the less likely they are to require revision surgery, as in general joint replacement surgery becomes less effective and efficient the more often it is performed on one joint.

Restrictions The patient should be advised to reduce weight-bearing activities whenever possible, particularly walking. Patients can be advised to try swimming instead of walking as part of a fitness routine. Steps and stairs will always prove problematic in an arthritic knee, as will squatting, kneeling, and crawling, so these are best avoided if at all possible. Standing for prolonged periods, particularly on concrete floors, will be uncomfortable. The provision of rubber mats should be considered if a patient has to stand in one place for a period of time, and can be effective in the reducing the stresses placed on the joint. If only one knee is affected, then the leg can be rested in standing by placing the foot on a small step (6–8 inches high). However, if there are any indications of OA in the knee or hip of the unaffected leg, this should be avoided, as the increased stress on the other joints may precipitate the underlying condition.

There is really no likelihood for return to repetitive or sustained weight-bearing activities for these patients, so at best they will have to make a compromise between their symptoms, the progressive joint degeneration, and the activities that they enjoy. This also applies following a total knee replacement, as the length of time for which the replacement remains functional depends on the degree of wear and tear to which it is subjected. The greater the amount of weight-bearing activities, the shorter the life of the prosthesis.

REFERENCES

1. Mercier, L.R.: Practical Orthopaedics (4th ed). Mosby Yearbook, St Louis, 1991
2. Dandy D.J., Edwards D.J.: Essential Orthopaedics and Trauma (3rd ed). Churchill Livingston, New York, 1998
3. Crowther C.L.: Primary Orthopaedic Care. Mosby, St. Louis, 1999
4. Skinner H.B. (ed): Current Diagnosis and Treatment in Orthopaedics. Appleton and Lange, Norwalk, CT, 1995
5. Braddom R.L. (ed): Physical Medicine and Rehabilitation. W.B. Saunders, Philadelphia, 1996
6. Payton O.D. (ed): Manual of Physical Therapy. Churchill Livingston, New York, 1989
7. Donatelli R.A., Wooden M.J. (eds): Orthopaedic Physical Therapy (2nd ed). Churchill Livingston, New York, 1994
8. Snider R.K. (ed): Essential of Musculoskeletal Care. American Academy of Orthopaedic Surgeons, Rosemont, IL, 1997
9. Goldie B.S.: Orthopaedic Diagnosis and Management: A Guide to the Care of Orthopaedic Patients (2nd ed). ISIS Medical Media, Oxford, U.K., 1998
10. Gross J. Feeto J., Rosen E.: Musculoskeletal Examination. Blackwell Science, Cambridge, MA, 1996
11. Echternack J.L. (ed): Physical Therapy of the Hip. Churchill Livingston, New York, 1990
12. Mangine R.E. (ed): Physical Therapy of the Knee (2nd ed). Churchill Livingston, New York, 1995
13. Fagerson T.L. (ed): The Hip Handbook. Butterworth Heinemann, Boston, 1998
14. Hadler N.M.: Occupational Musculoskeletal Disorders (2nd ed). Lippincott, Williams and Wilkins, Philadelphia, 1999
15. Kesson M. Atkins E.: Orthopaedic Medicine: A Practical Approach. Butterworth Heinemann, Oxford, U.K., 1998
16. Subotnick S.I. (ed): Sports Medicine of the Lower Extremity. Churchill Livingston, New York, 1989
17. Steinburg M.E. (ed): The Hip and its Disorders. WB Saunders, Philadelphia, 1991
18. Apley A.G., Solomon L.: Apley's System of Orthopaedics and Fractures (6th ed). Butterworth, London, 1983
19. Prentice W.E.: Rehabilitation Techniques in Sports Medicine. WCB/McGraw Hill, New York, 1999
20. Anderson B.C.: Office Orthopaedics for Primary Care: Diagnosis and Treatment (2nd ed). W.B. Saunders, Philadelphia, 1999

21. Corrigan B., Maitland G.D.: Vertebral Musculoskeletal Disorders. Butterworth, Oxford, U.K., 1998
22. Magee D.J.: Orthopaedic Physical Assessment (2nd ed). W.B. Saunders, Philadelphia, 1992
23. Corrigan B., Maitland G.D.: Practical Orthopaedic Medicine. Butterworth, London, 1983
24. Cyriax J.: Textbook of Orthopaedic Medicine: Vol.1, Diagnosis of Soft Tissue Lesions (8th ed). Bailliere Tindall, Eastbourne, U.K., 1982
25. Malone T.R., McPoil T.G., Nitz A.J. (eds): Orthopaedic and Sports Physical Therapy (3rd ed). Mosby, St. Louis, 1997
26. Field D.: Anatomy: Palpation and Surface Markings (2nd ed). Butterworth Heinemann, Oxford, U.K., 1997
27. Konin J.G., Wilksten D.L., Isear J.A.: Special Tests for Orthopaedic Examination. Slack, New Jersey, 1997

The following tables contain test movements for examination of the lower leg and foot. The starting positions and a description of each movement are given. These would be considered the optimal test positions in each case and must be modified for individual patients who are unable to achieve or sustain a described position.

Active Movements of the Foot and Ankle

Name of Movement	Starting Position	Movement
Dorsiflexion	The movement is tested with the patient sitting on the treatment table with his leg hanging over the side of the table and the foot dependent.	The patient is instructed to pull the foot upwards, approximating the dorsum of the foot to the anterior of the tibia. Average range of motion: 20°
Dorsiflexion (with calf muscle stretch)	The movement is tested in supine lying or long sitting with the knees straight and the toes pointed upwards.	The patient is instructed to pull the foot up toward himself, approximating the dorsum of the foot to the anterior tibia. The patient must keep the knee straight throughout the movement. This tests tension in the gastrocnemius muscle. Average range of motion: 20°
Plantar flexion	The patient sits over the edge of the treatment table with the foot dependent.	The patient is instructed to push the foot down towards the floor. Average range of motion: 50°
Inversion	The patient sits over the edge of the treatment table with the foot dependent.	The patient is instructed to turn the foot inwards so that the sole of the foot is turned towards the other foot. Average range of motion: 35°
Eversion	The patient sits over the edge of a treatment table with the foot dependent.	The patient is instructed to turn the foot so that the sole of the foot faces outwards away from the other leg. Average range of motion: 20°
Toe Flexion	The movement can be tested in sitting or supine lying with the foot clear of the support.	The patient is instructed to curl his toes over. The movement can be facilitated by placing an object (such as a pencil) under the plantar

Active Movements of the Foot and Ankle (*continued*)

Name of Movement	Starting Position	Movement
		aspect of the toes and asking the patient to grip the object.
		Average range of motion: 40° at the MTP joints and 60° at the IP joints (slightly more range is usually found in the great toe).
Toe Extension	The movement can be tested in sitting or supine lying with the foot clear of support.	The patient is instructed to straighten his toe as much as possible.
		Average range of motion: 70° at the great toe, 90° at the other four toes
Lumbrical Action	The patient sits with the foot resting on the floor.	The patient is instructed to draw the foot backwards, raising the medial arch while keeping the toes extended (tell the patient that he must be able to see his toenails throughout the movement so as to avoid flexion of the IP joints).

Movements of inversion and eversion are often difficult for the patient to grasp initially. The movement should be demonstrated by the therapist and repeated by the patient to ensure that any lack of range is due to pathology and not misunderstanding.

Passive Movements of the Foot and Ankle

Name of Movement	Starting Position	Movement
Ankle Dorsiflexion	With the patient placed in supine lying, cup the patient's heel with your forearm placed along the sole of the patient's foot. The other hand is placed over the anterior tibia just above the ankle joint to stabilize the lower leg.	Apply pressure with the forearm to the heads of the metatarsals to push the foot upwards approximating the dorsum of the foot to the anterior tibia. The movement is initially tested with the knee slightly flexed and then repeated with the knee fully extended.

(continued)

Passive Movements of the Foot and Ankle

Name of Movement	Starting Position	Movement
Plantarflexion	The movement is tested with the patient in supine lying. Support the patient's heel with one hand and place the other hand over the dorsum of the foot.	Pressure is applied to the dorsum of the patient's foot with one hand, while the other hand pulls up on the heel, approximating the calcaneus to the posterior tibia.
Inversion	The movement is tested in supine lying or sitting. Support the patient's heel with one hand and place the other hand on the lateral aspect of their foot.	Pressure is applied to the lateral calcaneus and the lateral aspect of the foot to turn the patient's foot inwards so that the sole of the foot faces towards the other leg.
Eversion	The patient is placed in supine lying or sitting. Support the patient's heel with one hand and place the other hand on the medial aspect of the patient's foot.	Pressure is applied to the medial aspect of the calcaneus and the medial forefoot to turn the sole of the foot outwards away from the other leg.
Abduction at the Mid-tarsal Articulation	The movement is tested in supine lying or sitting. Grasp the patient's foot with both hands placed over the dorsal surface of the foot with the hands meeting at the level of the tarsal–metatarsal articulation.	The proximal hand stabilizes the proximal part of the patient's foot while the distal hand pulls the forefoot outwards.
Adduction at the Mid-tarsal Articulation	The movement is tested in supine lying or sitting. Grasp the patient's foot with both hands placed over the dorsal surface of the foot with the hands meeting at the level of the tarsal–metatarsal articulation.	The proximal hand stabilizes the proximal part of the foot while the distal hand pushes the forefoot inwards.
Flexion of the Toes	The movement is tested in sitting or supine lying. Grasp the dorsal aspect of the foot at the level of the mid-tarsal joint to stabilize the foot. The other hand is placed with the	Flex the wrist in order to curl the toes over, bringing the tips of the toes into approximation with the metatarsal heads.

Passive Movements of the Foot and Ankle (*continued*)

Name of Movement	Starting Position	Movement
Flexion of the Toes (*cont*)	heel of the hand over the dorsum of the patient's toes with the fingertips placed on the plantar aspect of the foot at the level of the metacarpal phalangeal joint.	
Extension	The movement is tested in supine lying or sitting. One hand is placed over the dorsum of the foot at the mid-tarsal level in order to stabilize the foot. The heel of the other hand is applied to the plantar aspect of the toes.	Pressure is applied to the plantar aspect of the toes, raising them upward so as to straighten all five toes simultaneously.
Abduction/ Adduction of Toes	The movement is tested in supine lying or sitting. Grip the tips of two adjacent toes with the index finger and thumb of each hand.	Draw the patient's toes apart and then bring them together again. Movement is tested for every pair of toes (i.e., first and second, second and third, etc.).

Resisted Movements of the Foot and Ankle

Name of Movement	Starting Position	Movement
Plantarflexion	The movement is tested in standing with the patient standing on the leg to be tested with the other foot raised off the ground.	The patient is instructed to go up onto his toes, raising his heels off the ground (if necessary the patient may place his fingers on your hands to maintain balance during the test).
Dorsiflexion	The movement is tested in supine lying. Grip the dorsal aspect of the patient's foot with both hands.	The patient is instructed to draw the foot upwards at the ankle (dorsiflexion) and hold it there. Attempt to pull the patient down the treatment table by applying pressure to

(*continued*)

Resisted Movements of the Foot and Ankle (*continued*)

Name of Movement	Starting Position	Movement
Dorsiflexion (*cont*)		the dorsal aspect of the foot with both hands. The patient should be able to sustain dorsiflexion throughout this test.
Eversion	The movement can be tested in supine lying or sitting with the foot in the neutral position (i.e., relaxed). Grip the lower leg just above the ankle joint with one hand, with the other hand placed over the lateral aspect of the forefoot.	While the patient holds the foot in the neutral position, attempt to push the foot inwards to turn the sole of the foot to face the other leg.
Inversion	The movement can be tested in sitting or supine lying. Grip the lower leg just above the ankle with one hand, with the other hand placed over the medial aspect of the forefoot.	While the patient holds the foot in the neutral position, apply pressure to the medial aspect of the foot to try and turn the sole of the foot outwards.
Toe Flexion	The movement can be tested in sitting or supine lying. Place your fingertips over the tips of the patient's toes with the heel of the hand resting on the dorsum of the foot.	Apply pressure to the tips of the toes and attempt to straighten them while the patient resists the movement.
Toe Extension	The movement is tested in sitting or supine lying. Place the heel of one hand over the dorsal aspect of the patient's toes.	Apply pressure to the dorsal aspect of the toes with the heel of the hand and attempt to bend them as the patient resists the movement.

Examination Findings Related to Specific Conditions

	Onset				
Sudden Due to Trauma	Sudden Due to Overuse	Gradual Due to Trauma	Gradual Due to Overuse	Gradual with No Known Cause	
Ankle Ligament Strain Gastrocnemius Muscle/Tendon Tear Plantar Fasciitis	Shin Splints Plantar Fasciitis	Recurrent Ankle Instability Peroneal Tenosynovitis	Achilles Tendonitis Peroneal Tenosynovitis Posterior Tibial Tendonitis Anterior Tibial Tendonitis Morton's Neuroma Tarsal Tunnel Syndrome	Recurrent Ankle Instability Plantar Fasciitis Morton's Neuroma Tarsal Tunnel Syndrome	

Typical Age Ranges

15–30 Years	15–45 Years	20–40 Years	25–50 Years	35–55 Years	40–60 Years
Shin Splints	Ankle Ligament Strain Recurrent Ankle Instability Peroneal Tenosynovitis Anterior Tibial Tendonitis	Gastrocnemius Muscle/Tendon Tear (Myotendinous Junction) Achilles Tendonitis Plantar Fasciitis (in Athletes) Posterior Tibial Tendonitis Morton's Neuroma (in Runners)	Tarsal Tunnel Syndrome	Gastrocnemius Muscle/Tendon Tear (in Muscle Belly)	Plantar Fasciitis (Non-Athlete) Morton's Neuroma (in Women)

(continued)

Examination Findings Related to Specific Conditions (continued)

Duration

2 Days–2 Weeks	1–3 Weeks	3–6 Weeks	6 Weeks–3 Months	3–6 Months	6 Months to 2 Years +
Gastrocnemius Muscle/Tendon Tear	Ankle Ligament Strain/Tear (Active Person) Shin Splints	Ankle Ligament Strain/Tear (Less Active Person)	Achilles Tendonitis Peroneal Tenosynovitis Posterior Tibial Tenosynovitis Anterior Tibial Tendonitis	Plantar Fasciitis Morton's Neuroma Tarsal Tunnel Syndrome	Recurrent Ankle Instability Plantar Fasciitis

Frequency

First Time with These Symptoms	Several Episodes over the Years	Recurrent Problem following Injury	Recurrent (Seasonal) Symptoms	One Continuous Episode with Remissions/Exacerbations
Ankle Ligament Strain/Tear Gastrocnemius Muscle/Tendon Tear Posterior Tibial Tenosynovitis Anterior Tibial Tendonitis Shin Splints	Recurrent Ankle Instability	Ankle Ligament Strain/Tear Recurrent Ankle Instability	Shin Splints Achilles Tendonitis	Achilles Tendonitis Plantar Fasciitis Peroneal Tenosynovitis Morton's Neuroma Tarsal Tunnel Syndrome

Area of Symptoms

Both Sides of Ankle	Medial Ankle	Lateral Ankle	Posterior Ankle	General Around the Ankle	Upper Calf	Lower Calf	Anterior of Lower Leg	Posterior Medial Lower Leg	Sole of Foot
Ankle Ligament Tear/ Strain	Ankle Ligament Tear/ Strain Posterior Tibial Tenosynovitis	Ankle Ligament Tear/ Strain Peroneal Tenosynovitis	Achilles Tendonitis	Recurrent Instability	Gastrocnemius Muscle Tear	Gastrocnemius Tendon Tear	Anterior Tibial Tendonitis Shin Splints	Shin Splints	Plantar Fasciitis Morton's Neuroma Tarsal Tunnel Syndrome

(continued)

Examination Findings Related to Specific Conditions (*continued*)

| | Type of Symptoms | | | | | | |
Sharp Pain On Weight-Bearing	Pain on Rest after Weight-Bearing Activity	Nagging Ache on Activity	Ill Defined Ache at Rest	Pain on Weight-Bearing following Rest	Stiffness following Rest	Foot Giving Way	Paraesthesia and Numbness in Foot
Ankle Ligament Tear/Strain	Recurrent Ankle Instability	Achilles Tendonitis	Gastrocnemius Muscle/Tendon Tear	Plantar Fasciitis	Ankle Ligament Tear/Strain	Recurrent Ankle Instability	Morton's Neuroma
Gastrocnemius Muscle/Tendon Tear	Plantar Fasciitis	Anterior Tibial Tendonitis		Peroneal Tenosynovitis	Achilles Tendonitis		Tarsal Tunnel Syndrome
Peroneal Tenosynovitis	Posterior Tibial Tenosynovitis	Shin Splints					
Posterior Tibial Tenosynovitis	Anterior Tibial Tendonitis						
Shin Splints	Shin Splints						

Observation

Obvious Limp	Swelling Around Ankle	Swelling at Medial Ankle	Swelling Lateral Ankle	Swelling Posterior Ankle	Swelling in Calf	Bruising in Ankle or Foot
Ankle Ligament Strain/Tear	Ankle Ligament Strain/Tear	Ankle Ligament Strain/Tear	Ankle Ligament Tear/Strain	Gastrocnemius/Tendon Tear	Gastrocnemius Muscle/Tendon Tear	Ankle Ligament Strain/Tear
Anterior Tibial Tendonitis	Recurrent Ankle Instability	Posterior Tibial Tenosynovitis	Peroneal Tenosynovitis	Achilles Tendonitis		Gastrocnemius Muscle/Tendon Tear
Gastrocnemius Muscle/Tendon Tear						

Uneven Wear Outer Edge of Shoe	Uneven Wear Inner Edge of Shoe	Pronation of Foot	Supination of Foot	Flattening of Arches in Foot	Calluses around Heel	Nothing Unusual To Observe
Recurrent Ankle Instability	Posterior Tibial Tenosynovitis	Plantar Fasciitis	Peroneal Tenosynovitis	Plantar Fasciitis	Posterior Tibial Tenosynovitis	Plantar Fasciitis
Plantar Fasciitis	Tarsal Tunnel Syndrome	Posterior Tibial Tenosynovitis		Posterior Tibial Tenosynovitis	Peroneal Tenosynovitis	Anterior Tibial Tendonitis
Excessive Supination of Foot	Morton's Neuroma	Morton's Neuroma		Morton's Neuroma	Achilles Tendonitis	Shin Splints
	Excessive Pronation of Foot	Tarsal Tunnel Syndrome				

(continued)

Examination Findings Related to Specific Conditions (*continued*)

				Active Movements						
Inversion, Painful and Limited	Eversion, Painful and Limited	Pain on Inversion	Pain on Eversion	Inversion and Eversion Both Limited	Dorsiflexion Painful and Limited	Pain on Plantarflexion	Pain on Combined Plantarflexion and Inversion	Pain on Combined Dorsiflexion with Eversion	All Movements Full Range	All Movement Pain Free
Lateral Ligament Tear of Ankle Peroneal Tenosynovitis	Medial Ligament Tear of Ankle	Ankle Ligament Tear/Strain	Ankle Ligament Tear/Strain Posterior Tibial Tendonitis	Ankle Ligament Tear/Strain	Gastrocnemius Muscle/Tendon Tear Achilles Tendonitis	Peroneal Tenosynovitis Posterior Tibial Tenosynovitis	Shin Splints Anterior Tibial Tendonitis	Shin Splints Peroneal Tenosynovitis	Recurrent Ankle Instability Achilles Tendonitis Plantar Fasciitis Posterior Tibial Tendonitis Anterior Tibial Tendonitis Morton's Neuroma Tarsal Tunnel Syndrome	Recurrent Ankle Instability Morton's Neuroma Plantar Fasciitis Tarsal Tunnel Syndrome

Passive Movements

Pain with Overpressure into Inversion	Pain with Overpressure into Eversion	Pain with Overpressure into Plantarflexion	Pain With Overpressure Into Dorsiflexion	Restricted Range of Inversion or Eversion	Pain with Overpressure into Extension of Toes	Restricted Range of Dorsiflexion with Knee Extended	Excessive Play in Ankle Joint	All Movements Full and Pain Free
Ankle Ligament Tear/Strain	Ankle Ligament Tear/Strain	Peroneal Tenosynovitis	Gastrocnemius Muscle/Tendon Tear	Ankle Ligament Tear/Strain	Morton's Neuroma	Gastrocnemius Muscle/Tendon Tear	Recurrent Ankle Instability	Plantar Fasciitis
Recurrent Ankle Instability	Posterior Tibial Tenosynovitis	Posterior Tibial Tenosynovitis	Achilles Tendonitis				Severe Ligament Tear	Tarsal Tunnel Syndrome
Peroneal Tenosynovitis		Anterior Tibial Tendonitis						Morton's Neuroma

(continued)

Examination Findings Related to Specific Conditions (*continued*)

| | | | | Resisted Movements | | | | |
Pain on Plantar-flexion	Pain on Eversion	Pain on Inversion	Pain on Dorsiflexion	Pain on Repeated Weight-Bearing Plantarflexion	Poor Intrinsic Muscle Action in Foot	Weak Toe Flexion	No Pain and Good Strength	Difficulty with Weight-Bearing Plantarflexion
Gastroc-nemius Muscle Tear Shin Splints	Peroneal Teno-synovitis Shin Splints	Posterior Tibial Teno-synovitis	Anterior Tibial Tendonitis Shin Splints	Achilles Tendonitis	Plantar Fasciitis	Tarsal Tunnel Syndrome (Late Stages)	Ankle Ligament Strain Recurrent Ankle Instability Achilles Tendonitis Morton's Neuroma	Gastrocnemius Muscle/Tendon Tear

Palpation

Tenderness in Medial Ankle	Tenderness in Lateral Ankle	Posterior Tender Ankle	Tender Posterior Calf	Tender Plantar Aspect of Heel	Tender in Sole of Foot	Tender Lateral Aspect of Foot
Ankle Ligament Tear/Strain	Ankle Ligament Tear/Strain	Gastrocnemius Tendon Tear	Gastrocnemius Muscle/Tendon Tear	Plantar Fasciitis	Plantar Fasciitis	Peroneal Tenosynovitis
Posterior Tibial Tenosynovitis	Recurrent Ankle Instability	Achilles Tendonitis				
Recurrent Ankle Instability (Uncommon)	Peroneal Tenosynovitis					

Tender Anterolateral Lower Leg	Tender Posteromedial Calf	Tender Web Space of Toes	Crepitation Felt at Anterior Ankle	Crepitation Felt at Lateral Ankle	Crepitation Felt at Medial Ankle
Anterior Tibial Tendonitis	Shin Splints	Morton's Neuroma	Anterior Tibial Tendonitis	Peroneal Tenosynovitis	Posterior Tibial Tenosynovitis
Shin Splints					

PALPATION OF THE LOWER LEG AND FOOT

In this section a description is given of the method of palpating each structure referred to in relation to the following conditions:

- Ankle Ligament Strain/Tear
- Recurrent Ankle Instability
- Gastrocnemius Muscle/Tendon Tear
- Achilles Tendonitis
- Plantar Fasciitis
- Peroneal Tenosynovitis
- Posterior Tibial Tenosynovitis
- Anterior Tibial Tendonitis
- Shin Splints
- Morton's Neuroma
- Tarsal Tunnel Syndrome

The following structures must be identified in the lower leg and foot:

Medial Malleolus

The anterior border of the tibia is easily identified as a sharp ridge at the front of the lower leg (the shin). Run a finger down the anterior border of the tibia and it comes naturally onto a flattened bony area at the medial aspect of the ankle, which has a palpable tip. This is the medial malleolus (Fig. 7.1 and 7.3).

Lateral Malleolus

On the opposite side of the ankle joint there is a rounded bony protuberance, which also has an easily palpated tip and lies slightly lower than that of the medial malleolus. This is the lateral malleolus (Fig. 7.2 and 7.4).

Ankle Joint Line

A line drawn from a point a thumb's breadth above the tip of the medial malleolus (Fig. 7.3) across to a point one and a half thumb's breadth above the lateral malleolus (Fig. 7.2) marks the anterior of the ankle joint line. This is most easily palpated while the foot is moved passively between plantarflexion and dorsiflexion. The joint line can then be further palpated as it continues around the front of the medial and lateral malleolii. There are a great many extensor tendons that cover the front of the ankle joint; however, when these muscles are relaxed and the foot supported in slight dorsiflexion, it is relatively easy to palpate the lower border of the tibia.

Medial (Deltoid) Ligament (see Fig. 7.1)

Approximately one finger's breadth below the medial malleolus an indistinct bony ridge can be palpated. This is the sustentaculum tali, which is more pronounced when the foot is placed into full eversion. If a finger is

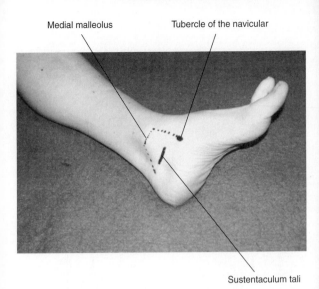

Medial malleolus   Tubercle of the navicular

Sustentaculum tali

FIG. 7.1 The extent of the medial collateral ligament of the right ankle (depicted by the dotted line) from its attachment on the medial malleolus passing to the navicular, talus and calcaneus.

moved anteriorly away from this ridge it will cross a small gap, which is the site of the spring ligament. The next bony protuberance encountered is the tubercle of the navicular. The various spans of the medial ligament pass from the medial malleolus anteriorly to the tubercle of the navicular, along the extent of the sustentaculum tali, and then to the medial tubercle on the talus posteriorly, which lies approximately one finger's breadth posterior to the sustentaculum tali.

Lateral Ligament (see Fig. 7.2)

There are two parts of the lateral ligament that are both relatively weak and prone to injury, particularly the anterior portion. The anterior talofibular ligament passes from the tip of the lateral malleolus almost horizontally towards the head of the talus. The head of the talus can be palpated just distal to, and slightly in front of, the two malleoli. The second part of the lateral ligament passes down and posteriorly from the tip of the malleolus to the lateral aspect of the calcaneus, approximately a finger's breadth posterior to the tip of the lateral malleolus.

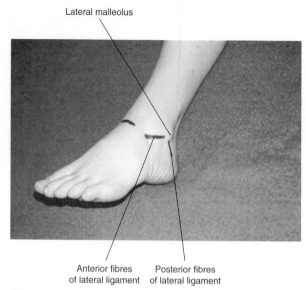

Lateral malleolus

Anterior fibres of lateral ligament   Posterior fibres of lateral ligament

FIG. 7.2   The lateral malleolus of the left ankle and surface marking of the fibers of the lateral collateral ligament.

Achilles Tendon

The Achilles tendon is an easily identifiable soft tissue band found at the posterior of the ankle. (see Fig. 7.4). It can be palpated from its attachment into the posterior aspect of the calcaneus and can be felt to narrow initially approximately two to three inches above the heel. It then broadens into an aponeurosis. As palpation is continued further up the calf the hand passes onto the medial and lateral bellies of the gastrocnemius muscle, which are easily palpated as the distinct rounded soft-tissue bulks that give the typical contour to the posterior aspect of the lower leg (Fig. 7.5).

Peroneal Tendons

The tendons of the peroneus longus and brevis pass behind and below the lateral malleolus and can be easily palpated when the foot is actively everted (Fig. 7.6). As they pass around the posterior aspect of the lateral malleolus they are enclosed in a common synovial sheath, which divides into individual sheaths as the tendons pass under the lateral malleolus. Just below and anterior to the lateral malleolus a small bony point can be

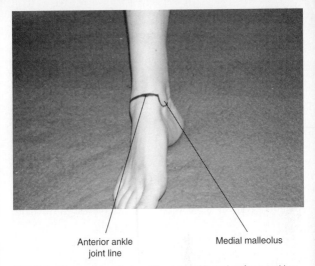

Anterior ankle
joint line   Medial malleolus

FIG. 7.3 The medial malleolus of the right ankle and surface marking of the ankle joint line.

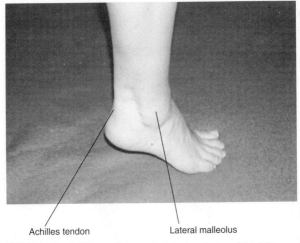

Achilles tendon   Lateral malleolus

FIG. 7.4 The Achilles tendon and the lateral malleolus of the right ankle.

Gastrocnemius muscle

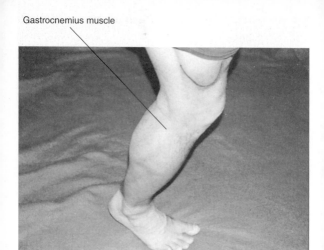

FIG. 7.5 The right calf muscle bulk.

Peroneus longus

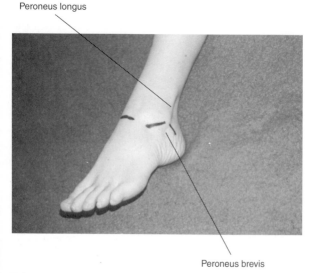

Peroneus brevis

FIG. 7.6 Tendons of the peroneus longus and peroneus brevis muscles at the left ankle.

palpated, called the peroneal tubercle. The peroneus brevis tendon passes above this point and the peroneus longus tendon passes below it. The peroneal tubercle should not be confused with another small bony point lying below and posterior to the lateral malleolus, which is the tubercle marking the distal attachment of the calcaneofibular ligament, the posterior part of the lateral ligament. Passing forward along the lateral aspect of the foot approximately two finger's breadth in front of the lateral malleolus is a rounded bony protuberance, which is the tuberosity at the base of the fifth metatarsal (Fig. 7.7). With the foot placed in active eversion the tendon of the peroneus brevis can be palpated from the tip of the lateral malleolus to its attachment on this tuberosity.

The peroneus longus tendon passes below the peroneus brevis tendon approximately halfway along its extent between the lateral malleolus and the base of the fifth metatarsal. It passes along a groove in the cuboid and then medially across the foot to attach into the lateral aspect of the base of the first metatarsal. This structure can most easily be identified by returning to the medial aspect of the foot and the tubercle of the navicular. Passing carefully forward from that point, the first bone to be palpated is the

Shaft of 5th metatarsal

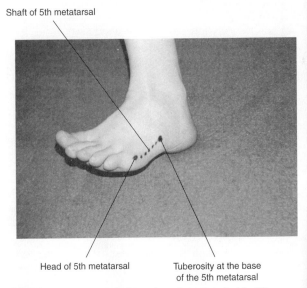

Head of 5th metatarsal   Tuberosity at the base
                                of the 5th metatarsal

FIG. 7.7 Surface marking of the tuberosity and shaft of the fifth metatarsal in the left foot.

medial cuneiform. Just distal to it is the base of the first metatarsal. Further palpation anteriorly, with the finger and thumb placed on the plantar and dorsal aspects of the foot respectively, will reveal the shaft of the first metatarsal ending in its rounded head (Fig. 7.8), which is easily palpable as the pad at the base of the great toe.

Returning to the lateral aspect of the foot and the tuberosity at the base of the fifth metatarsal moving forward along the lateral aspect of the foot, again using finger and thumb, the shaft of the fifth metatarsal can just be palpated and leads onto the head of the fifth metatarsal. This is easily palpated at the broadest point of the foot on the lateral aspect (see Fig. 7.7). The head of the first metatarsal marks the broadest part of the foot on the medial side.

Metatarsals

The heads of the first and fifth metatarsals are common sites of calluses occurring due to ill-fitting shoes. The head of the first metatarsal may be quite pronounced if there is a tendency towards a hallux valgus deformity.

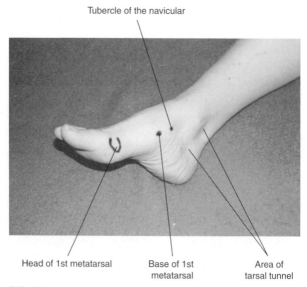

Tubercle of the navicular

Head of 1st metatarsal   Base of 1st
metatarsal   Area of
tarsal tunnel

FIG. 7.8 Surface marking of the tubercle of the navicular, the base and head of the first metatarsal and area of the tarsal tunnel in the right foot and ankle.

This often leads to the presence of a bunion at the site of the head of the first metatarsal.

The Mid-Tarsal Joint

The level of this joint can be marked by a line passing from a point just proximal to the tuberosity of the navicular on the medial side of the foot to a point approximately half an inch proximal to the tubercle of the fifth metatarsal on the lateral side of the foot (Fig. 7.9).

Subtalar Joint (Talocalcaneal Joint)

This can be represented by a line drawn from a point approximately half an inch below the lateral malleolus to a point just above the sustentaculumtali on the medial side of the ankle. This line is slightly concave proximally in its middle extent (Fig. 7.10).

Medial Aspect of the Ankle

The tendons of the tibialis posterior and flexor digitorum longus muscles can be palpated as they pass around the posterior aspect of the medial malleolus in separate osseofibrous tunnels. They are more easily palpated when the ankle is dorsiflexed while the foot is inverted and the toes flexed

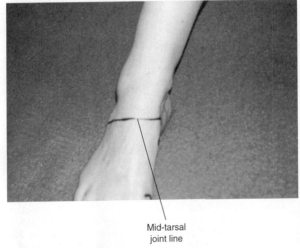

Mid-tarsal
joint line

FIG. 7.9   Surface marking of the mid tarsal joint in the right foot.

Lateral
malleolus

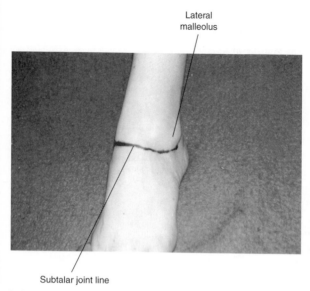

Subtalar joint line

FIG. 7.10 The lateral malleolus and surface marking of the subtalar joint line in the left foot.

simultaneously. This movement should be repeated several times and the tendons can then be felt to tighten up and relax successively. This region from the posterior of the medial malleolus to the sustentaculum talii is the area of the tarsal tunnel (See Fig. 7.8).

Anterior Ankle (Fig. 7.11)

With the foot actively dorsiflexed and inverted, the most medial and most easily observed tendon at the anterior of the ankle is the tendon of the tibialis anterior muscle. It can be palpated from the front of the ankle to its insertion into the base of the first metatarsal and the medial cuneiform. If the ankle is dorsiflexed repeatedly it is possible to palpate the bulk of the anterior tibial muscles at the anterolateral aspect of the proximal half of the lower leg just lateral to the anterior border of the tibia.

As described, just distally and anterior to the malleolii, the head of the talus can be palpated. When the foot is fully plantarflexed the neck of the talus can be palpated just proximal to the head. Distally and slightly medial to this point is the dorsal surface of the navicular. Moving to its medial side the finger lies on the tubercle of the navicular (Fig. 7.8).

Tendon of tibialis anterior

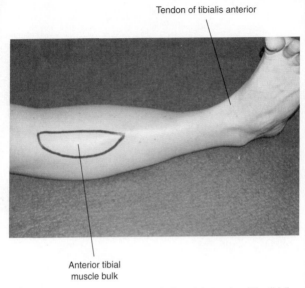

Anterior tibial
muscle bulk

FIG. 7.11 The anterior tibial muscle bulk and the tendon of the tibialis anterior in the right lower leg and ankle.

Metatarsal Heads

If the toes are fully flexed the heads of the metatarsals can be palpated on the dorsum of the foot at the base of the toes (Fig. 7.12.) If the toes are placed in full extension the metatarsal heads can be felt on the plantar surface.

Palpation of the plantar aspect of the heel reveals the presence of a thick pad of fat. This develops over the years from the first days of weight bearing, but it can decrease noticeably in size when the patient has been non weight bearing for a period of time. If this occurs the patient can develop discomfort when returning to weight-bearing activity; in such cases the lack of a plantar pad can be noted on palpation. It should also be noted that the attachment of the Achilles tendon passes onto the plantar aspect of the heel at this point and may be tender in cases of chronic Achilles tendonitis.

Plantar Fascia

With the toes taken into full extension and held there it is possible to palpate the plantar fascia as it passes from its attachments to the medial and

Head of 1st metatarsal

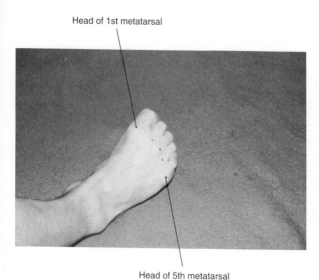

Head of 5th metatarsal

FIG. 7.12 The heads of the metatarsal on the dorsum of the right foot.

lateral tubercles on the proximal plantar aspect of the calcaneus (these are palpable but hard to identify). From there a taut band, the plantar aponeurosis, can normally be palpated along the sole of the foot, which broadens as it passes to its attachment into the soft tissue at the base of the toes (Fig. 7.13).

SPECIFIC TESTS FOR THE LOWER LEG AND FOOT

Anterior Drawer Sign

With the patient placed in the supine lying position with the knee flexed to approximately 90 degrees and the foot placed flat on the treatment table, hold the dorsum of the foot to fix it. With the other hand apply pressure to the anterior of the lower third of the tibia and fibula and attempt to push them backwards at the talocrural articulation. This should then be compared with the same movement on the opposite side. Excessive posterior translation of the tibia and fibula on the talus is considered positive for a tear of the medial and lateral collateral ligaments.

This test can also be done in the supine lying position with the patient's foot placed over the end of the examination table. Push down on the anterior tibia and fibula with one hand and with the other hand grip the dorsum of the foot and attempt to draw it forwards. The test should be repeated in

Head of 1st metatarsal

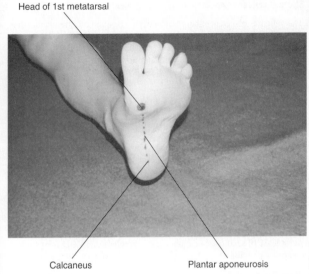

Calcaneus   Plantar aponeurosis

FIG. 7.13 Surface marking of the left plantar aponeurosis.

varying degrees of plantarflexion and dorsiflexion. If excessive translation of the foot is present then the test is considered positive for medial and lateral ligament tears. If there is a significant tear on only one side then the foot will carry forward on that side but not on the other, producing a noticeable rotation of the talus.

Lateral Ligament Stability

With the patient lying supine and the foot relaxed in a neutral position grasp the patient's heel and draw the foot into full inversion. Excessive play compared to the opposite ankle suggests a tear or insufficiency of the lateral ligament.

Kleiger Test

With the patient sitting with his lower legs hanging over the edge of the treatment table and the feet unsupported, support the leg below the knee with one hand and with the other hand laterally rotate the foot. Pain felt medially and laterally suggests a tear of the medial collateral ligament. This can be considered definite if the talus can be felt to displace from the medial malleolus during the maneuver.

Thompson Test (Achilles Tendon Rupture)

The patient is placed in either the prone lying position on a treatment table or kneeling on a chair with the feet positioned over the edge of the support. Squeeze the calf muscle firmly and the patient's foot should plantarflex slightly. If no movement of the foot is observed the test is considered positive for complete rupture of the Achilles tendon.

Balance Tests

The patient is first instructed to stand on the unaffected leg with the foot of the other leg clear of the ground with the knee flexed ("stork standing"). The patient then has to remain in this position for as long as possible without putting the other leg to the ground. This test is then repeated with the patient standing on their affected leg. The amount of time for which a patient can maintain this position varies greatly from person to person and decreases with age. There has to be an obvious difference in the time achieved for the affected leg compared to the unaffected leg for the finding to be significant, such as a discrepancy of 30 seconds or more. The test is again repeated but this time the patient is instructed to close his eyes while standing on one leg. Most normal subjects should be able to balance for at least 10 seconds, but again comparison between the two legs is the clearest indication of a balance problem with the one leg.

Tinnell's Sign

The posterior tibial nerve is percussed with a reflex hammer or finger where it passes in the area behind the medial malleolus. Paraesthesia or tingling felt at the plantar aspect of the foot and toes is considered a positive sign for tarsal tunnel syndrome.

Hoffman's Sign

With the patient lying supine, place the patient's heel in one hand and apply pressure to the sole of the foot with the forearm to bring the ankle into dorsiflexion. Sharp pain produced in the calf may indicate the presence of a deep vein thrombosis. There should also be marked tenderness on palpation of the calf and swelling, which can vary in degree, but is usually very tight and noticeable throughout the calf and into the ankle and foot. There may also be observable redness in the area of the calf muscle or pallor of the foot and lower leg.

LOWER LEG AND FOOT CONDITIONS

Ankle Ligament Strain/Tear

Overview

This is a very common sports injury, but can also be found occurring frequently in the general population. It is a condition that appears to be very poorly treated, particularly in young sports participants who are not competing at the higher levels. In most of these cases the advice given to the patient is to rest the ankle until it feels better and then go back to whatever was being done before. This is unfortunate because it is a condition that responds well to active treatment; lack of treatment or poor treatment predisposes the person to ankle laxity and recurrent problems. Either the medial ligament, lateral ligament, or both can be affected, but injuries of the lateral ligament are the most common (1, 2, 4).

Subjective Findings

Onset This is sudden due to trauma in patients commonly between 15 and 45 years of age, although the condition can occur at any age. The patient's typical history is one of going over onto the outside of the foot (an inversion sprain). Less commonly the patient may have gone over onto the inside of the foot (an eversion sprain), particularly when other people are involved in the incident, either landing on the patient's leg or the patient landing on them (2, 4, 9, 10).

Duration It may be just a matter of days, but may be up to six weeks before the patient presents for treatment, depending on the degree of injury and how much the patient is affected by it functionally. The more sedentary the patient's lifestyle, the more likely he is to think that the ankle will get better with time. On the other hand, if the patient is actively involved in a particular sport, then he will usually seek treatment quite quickly after onset.

Frequency There are two fairly distinct types of history. The first is a one-time problem with the patient having no history of ankle problems. The other is a history of recurrent injuries, usually with one major incident starting the problem—as the injury recurs over time the degree of force required to produce the injury steadily decreases (2, 9, 10, 15).

Area of Symptoms The symptoms are quite well localized to the sides of the ankle, usually more to the lateral than the medial, although this can be reversed. The patient may present with entirely unilateral pain, but it is not uncommon to have marked symptoms on one side and mild symptoms on the other. Patients may also experience discomfort either at the anterior of the ankle or over the dorsal aspect of the foot (Fig. 7.14) (2, 4, 7, 10).

Type of Symptoms The patient's pain is sharp at the time of injury and will continue to be sharp in twinges on weight-bearing activities for an indefinite period of time following the injury. Patients may also complain of stiffness and discomfort after resting following activity (2–4).

Miscellaneous Patients will complain of difficulty going over rough or uneven surfaces and possibly when climbing steps or ladders.

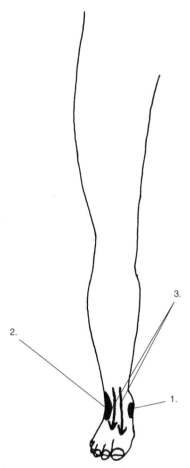

FIG. 7.14 Area of symptoms for ligament sprain at the right ankle either: 1–medially or 2–laterally, and possibly concurrently at: 3–the anterior ankle and dorsum of the foot.

Objective Findings

Observation The patient will usually walk into the examination room demonstrating a limp, caused by a shortened stance phase on the affected leg. Swelling may be observed, which may be localized to the site of injury either medially or laterally around the malleolus, or more general within the ankle itself. There may be a combination of these two forms, with some swelling around the ankle and more specific swelling below one of the malleolii. Bruising may be observed at the medial or lateral aspect of the ankle, spreading into the lateral or medial border of the foot (4, 10, 11, 13).

Active Movements There is usually a mild degree of limitation of both plantarflexion and dorsiflexion, with pain felt at end range of plantarflexion. There will be a moderate degree of limitation of either inversion or eversion depending on the site of the injury, with little or no limitation of the opposite movement. Both movements may be limited if both the medial and lateral ligaments are injured, but usually the limitation will still be greater to one side than the other. Pain will be experienced at end range of the limited movement or movements (1, 4, 6, 8, 10, 14, 27).

Passive Movements The pattern of restriction of motion will be the same on passive testing as on active testing, with pain produced at the site of injury on overpressure at end range of either inversion, eversion, or both movements, depending on the site of injury. It is most common to find lateral ankle pain on pressure at end range of passive inversion and medial ankle pain on overpressure on end range of eversion. However, in some cases pain may be produced at the same side as the one to which the foot is moved (i.e., on the medial side during inversion). This discomfort is produced by pinching of an injured ligament between the bony surfaces of the medial malleolus and the sustentaculum tali on the medial side, and the lateral malleolus and the lateral surface of the calcaneus on the lateral side (1, 4, 6, 10, 14).

Resisted Movements With the foot tested in the neutral position, isometric testing does not produce any definite discomfort. With the foot placed in full inversion, resisted eversion may produce some discomfort due to stress placed on the injured soft tissue when there is a lateral ligament injury. Pain will be felt on resisted inversion from full eversion when the medial ligament is injured (1, 6, 8, 10).

Palpation Tenderness should be marked over either the lateral or medial ligaments or both, depending on the site of injury (Fig 7.1 and 7.2). The most common site of discomfort is over the anterior fibers of the lateral ligament. If there is a local swelling in the area it may have the boggy feel of a hematoma (1, 4, 8, 19, 20).

Specific Tests The anterior drawer sign will be positive if the medial ligament is completely ruptured or if there is major insufficiency of both the lateral and medial ligaments. Lateral instability of the ankle will also be present in the case of a complete rupture of the lateral ligament. Klieger's test will be positive if there is a complete rupture of the medial ligament. In any of these cases the patient is a candidate for orthopaedic surgical intervention and should be referred to the orthopaedic surgeon (4, 19, 21).

Treatment Ideas
(1, 2, 4, 6, 8–10, 12–15, 27, 32)

Initial Stages If the patient is seen in the first few days following injury he should be advised to follow the PRICE formula, protecting the injury using a suitable brace or bandaging, and resting it by either using crutches for non weight-bearing activities or a cane if the injury is not too great. This is relative rest, the patient should still be able to carry out active movements of the ankle within pain-free ranges, not attempting to force into any greater range. The patient should also be advised to ice the ankle as often as possible; in the first few days the ideal would be 15 to 20 minutes of icing every hour. This is seldom possible for the aver-age patient because of work constraints, but application of ice for 10 to 15 minutes five or six times per day will often be effective enough.

Compression may be useful and can be applied in the form of a compression bandage or using a compression pump. For reduction of swelling the most important part of the program is elevation of the leg; again, the more often the patient can get the injured ankle above the level of the heart (being careful to avoid too acute an angle at the hip), then the greater the likelihood of reduction in the volume of swelling. This author advises patients to place a firm pillow under their mattresses so that their legs will be effectively elevated during the time they are asleep. The crutches or cane should be used for as long as required in order for the patient to maintain a correct gait pattern. The patient should be taught active exercises for all movements of the foot and ankle using pain as a guide, always moving within ranges that are comfortable.

Progression Three to four days following injury, or after a shorter period of time if the patient is seen longer than a week after injury, the patient can progress onto light resisted plantarflexion using an exercise band. The active exercises can be progressed by stretching into greater range of dorsiflexion. Pulsed ultrasound or laser applied over the injury may help to promote healing. Once the danger of any further bleeding occurring in the area has passed, heat in the form of hot packs or radiation will help to increase blood flow. Interferential therapy can help to alleviate discomfort, particularly when applied with the leg elevated. A balance board can be used to assist in plantarflexion, dorsiflexion, inversion, and eversion exercises, with the patient sitting then placing minimal pressure on the foot. The patient can also practice heel and toe raises in the same sitting position, applying pressure to his knee with his hands to supply resistance to the movement as tolerated. This will allow the patient to assimilate the heel-toe action required in normal gait. The patient can also progress onto passive stretches for all movements of the injured foot, with the therapist and patient being guided by discomfort in order to prevent further injury.

If a great deal of movement restriction is encountered at this time, then gentle posterior/anterior glides of the tibia and fibula on the talus may help to promote further mobility. Passive mobilizations can also be used for the forefoot to increase flexibility in the joints at which the inversion and eversion movements occur. At this time the patient can also be progressed onto the use of neuromuscular stimulation, particularly for the evertor muscles in the case of a lateral ligament injury, to assist in achieving full-range active movements.

Once the patient is comfortable with the above exercises, he can be progressed to weight-bearing exercises including heel raises, squats, walking forwards, backwards, and sideways (with as much support as needed). Balance board exercises can initially be done with the patient grasping wall bars or a wall to support himself, progressing as possible to free-standing exercises. Eversion of the foot can be manually resisted or the patient can work against a resistance band or dead weights while in the side lying position. This can be combined with the continued use of neuromuscular stimulation. Inversion can be resisted by having the patient squeeze his feet together against a rubber ball. Proprioceptive neuromuscular facilitation techniques for combined resistance of foot, ankle and knee movements can be very helpful. The patient will also need to work on weight-bearing stretches for the gastrocnemius and soleus muscles. If there is still definite restriction of movement around the ankle, passive distraction of the joint may help to free up the movements more quickly.

Once the patient is comfortable with weight-bearing exercises, he can be progressed to a step machine and exercise bike, and from there to running, jumping, skipping, and hopping exercises involving both single- and double-leg work. Plyometrics for the knee, foot, and ankle and single-leg balance exercise, initially on the floor and then on the balance board, will round out the exercise program. Further progression of exercises should then be sports or work oriented as required.

Restrictions   Initially the patient should be advised to walk only short distances with short rests as required. The patient should also avoid going up or down stairs while taking weight through the affected leg, that is, tackling one step at a time, always going up with the unaffected leg leading and down with the affected leg leading. At this time the patient should also avoid uneven surfaces or standing for long periods of time, particularly on hard surfaces such as cement floors. As the condition improves the patient can start increasing the walking distance and can also attempt slopes and hills, then steps and stairs. The patient should still be cautious about sudden turns and quick stop-and-go activities until well into the weight-bearing stage of exercises in the clinic. Activities such as side stepping, sudden stops, and turns, should all be tested in the clinic before the patient attempts them in daily activities. Return to any form of competition should only be started when the patient is coping well with these normal practice activities and is completely clear of discomfort in clinical testing.

Recurrent Ankle Instability

Overview

As stated for ankle ligament strain/tear, poorly treated ankle sprains may lead to recurrent problems due to laxity of the ligamentous support of the ankle joint. Problems may also occur if there was a previously undiagnosed complete ligament rupture, congenital or acquired foot deformities. On occasions the problem can arise with no predisposing factors, which is particularly true in the case of teenage girls during a growth spurt (2, 10, 22, 24).

Subjective Findings

Onset This is gradual in nature, usually with a previous history of trauma, although occasionally there may be no known cause of onset. Where there is a history of previous trauma check with the patient as regards what degree of force was required to produce the injury, as a major force may have seriously disrupted the joint leading to the present instability. Whereas if only minor force was required to produce injury then the joint may always have been unstable. If this is the first injury the patient has had there will usually have been only minor forces involved and relatively minor trauma, but there has been poor recovery of function (3, 10, 15).

Duration The patient will give a history of ankle problems going back over several months or even years, although the history should be concurrent. An original high school injury followed by ankle problems when the patient is in their 30s or 40s, with no history of problems during the intervening years is *not* an example (2, 10).

Frequency The condition is recurrent by name and nature and consists of a series of minor injuries that are typically associated with going over rough ground or stepping awkwardly down from a step or curb. Each episode of symptoms is usually related to a trivial cause or simply to an increase in the amount of weight-bearing activities (2, 10).

Area of Symptoms This is in a general area around the ankle, and in different patients may be more anterior, more lateral, or more medial. The most common site of the problem is, however, lateral (Fig. 7.15) (2, 7, 15).

Type of Symptoms The patient usually complains of the foot giving way, with pain in and around the ankle following trauma or on vigorous weight-bearing, but no discomfort at other times. The patient may also complain of recurrent swelling, particularly after walking or standing for an extended period of time (2, 10, 15).

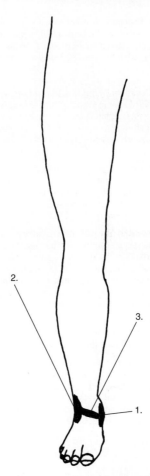

FIG. 7.15 Area of symptoms for recurrent right ankle instability at either: 1–the medial aspect of the ankle, 2–the lateral aspect of the ankle or 3–the anterior aspect of the ankle (or can occur in two or all three areas).

Miscellaneous The patient may have a history of congenital foot problems, the degree of which should be thoroughly explored. In some cases this will require confirmation from the patient's parents, as the patient may have been too young when the problem began to remember exact details.

Objective Findings

Observation Occasionally mild swelling may be seen, particularly if the patient is examined later in the day. This swelling is usually in an arc around the whole ankle, although more often there is nothing of note to be seen either in or around the ankle region. Observation of the patient's shoes may reveal uneven wear, especially on the outer aspect of the heel and sole (6, 10).

Active Movements All movements of the foot and ankle are normally of full range and pain free, although if there was a major ligament injury causing onset of the condition then there may be a variable degree of discomfort at end range of either inversion or eversion. There should be no obvious limitation of movement (2, 6, 7, 10).

Passive Movements The patient's typical pain is often produced on overpressure at end range of inversion, and more rarely at end range of eversion or plantarflexion. As in testing of the active movements, there will be full range of movement present; in fact, there may be relatively greater range of motion present compared to normal for the patient's sex and age. There may also be excessive play on testing of posterior/anterior gliding of the talus at the talocrural articulation (2, 6, 7, 10).

Resisted Movements Strength is usually within normal limits on both non weight-bearing and weight-bearing testing of all movements, with no discomfort found on testing (6, 7, 10).

Palpation There may be a degree of residual tenderness, particularly at the anterolateral aspect of the ankle below and anterior to the lateral malleolus, or less commonly below the medial malleolus (Fig. 7.1 and 7.2). There may also be some discomfort elicited posterior to one of the malleoli if there is an associated tendonitis of either the peroneal muscles or the posterior tibial muscles (2, 6, 19, 20).

Specific Tests Balance tests may reveal poor performance on the affected leg with the eyes either open or closed.

Treatment Ideas
(2, 6, 7, 10, 15, 18, 23, 25–27)

The patient can be started on a program of non-weight–bearing strengthening exercises for all the muscles of the foot and ankle, with particular attention paid to strengthening of the evertors of the foot, particularly if tenderness has been elicited on palpation around the lateral malleolus. The use of neuromuscular electrical stimulation for the anterior tibial muscle, the peroneii, and the calf muscles may help to promote strength. The patient should also be instructed in isometric resisted exercises with the foot and ankle placed in different positions using a large exercise ball or strong resistance band to work against. If discomfort is felt around the sites of the medial or lateral ligaments, the use of ultrasound and laser are indicated and may help to reduce discomfort. In rare cases there may be some decreased mobility on gliding movements of the joints of the foot or ankle, in which case oscillatory mobilizations can be effective.

The patient is progressed to weight-bearing strengthening exercises. These should be done gradually and in a controlled manner so that the patient is always able to support himself with his hands, as these are the types of activities that would typically produce the patient's symptoms on an ongoing basis. A balance board can be used for stop/go balance re-education exercises, with the patient asked to move the board and then hold different positions of the foot and ankle at different times. Single-leg balance exercise should be taught, as these can easily be done at home, work, or school. Muscle stimulation can be combined with exercises such as heel raises to improve calf muscle strength.

Further progression can be made with the patient standing at the bars, jumping using a two-legged stance for take off and landing, and jumping from one leg onto the other. In order to gain good control of the joint via the musculature, the patient should be instructed to land making as little noise as possible (i.e., a soft landing), which can be attempted from varying heights. Step-ups, lateral step-ups, and stepping back and forth over a stool (initially leading with the unaffected leg and then with the affected leg) will all help to promote strength and balance. Again, with activities such as step-ups and step-downs, the patient should be instructed to hold different positions during the exercise. Stabilizations can be used in both double- and single-leg stances so as to promote further muscle control and better balance reactions.

Finally the patient should be started on short distance running, incorporating steadily increasing degrees of turns, stops, and starts all carried out at steadily increasing speeds. Lateral bounds and lateral glides, running sideways and backwards, and jumping over obstacles are further final-stage weight-bearing exercises.

Restrictions The patient should initially avoid any sports or other activities that have been shown to put him at risk of injury, particularly basketball, football, soccer, volleyball, and sprinting. Jogging can be continued on even surfaces, but should be avoided on the road (particularly on the side of the road), and must be completely avoided over uneven surfaces. Jumping down from any height should not be attempted until the patient is able to complete jumps in the clinic with no symptoms. Return to running on the road can be attempted once the patient is coping with significant weight-bearing exercises without requiring any support from his hands and arms. Return to high-risk sporting activities can only be made on completion of the treatment program; the patient must first be progressed through light training to normal practice, then into full competition only as long as there is no indication of recurrence of their symptoms. Use of a custom-made-brace for one or both ankles should be a definite consideration, even after successful completion of a course of treatment, as an added protection against further injury.

Gastrocnemius Muscle/Tendon Tear

Overview

The gastrocnemius muscle is susceptible to injury at two sites. In middle-aged patients the more common site of injury is in the upper medial muscle belly, while in younger patients the site of injury is more likely to be at the distal myotendinous junction between the muscle belly and the Achilles tendon. Patients often say that they were too old for the sport that they were attempting. The truth of the matter is that usually they were too lazy to do the warm up and stretch routine that can keep the muscle flexible enough to avoid injury, or to keep fit enough so as not to fatigue enough to lose coordination. Another common problem is competing at too high a level relative to their level of physical fitness. Effective treatment, particularly in the early stages following injury, will prevent future problems from arising, such as a complete rupture of the Achilles tendon (1, 3, 6).

Subjective Findings

Onset Onset is sudden due to trauma and is usually found in 35 to 55 year olds when the lesion is in the muscle, and in 20 to 40 year olds when the lesion is at the myotendinous junction between the muscle and the Achilles tendon. Classic sports likely to cause the injury are squash or tennis, where deceleration forces produce the injury (1, 3, 4).

Duration The patient normally presents for treatment within a matter of days or at most 1 to 2 weeks following onset, as the condition will affect walking, usually to quite a marked extent. Patients therefore present for treatment quickly.

Frequency Usually there will be only one episode per patient, although the patient may state that he has had tight calf muscles with twinges of discomfort from time to time, particularly in the weeks preceding onset of the present episode.

Area of Symptoms The symptoms are typically felt at one of two sites either in the upper calf medially, just below the knee (in the medial muscle belly of the gastrocnemius), or at the myotendinous junction of the gastrocnemius with the Achilles tendon, approximately at the junction of the middle and distal thirds of the calf (Fig. 7.16) (1, 6, 7, 10).

Type of Symptoms The patient will complain of a sharp pain at the time of injury. Sometimes it may feel as if someone kicked him or threw something at his leg. There will also be a deep ill-defined ache at rest,

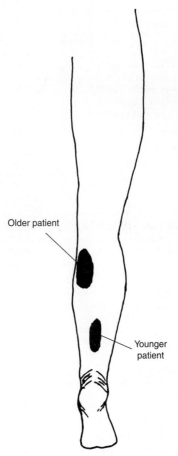

FIG. 7.16 Two possible sites of symptoms in a tear of the right gastrocnemius muscle or tendon, at either the upper calf or the distal myo-tendinous junction.

with further sharp pain on contraction or stretch of the muscle, such as occurs during walking (6, 7, 10).

Miscellaneous The typical mechanism of injury is a strong weight-bearing stress applied with the knee extended and the ankle dorsiflexed while the muscle is simultaneously required to contract, as in pushing into a group of players in a football game. It can also be due to a sudden deceleration force with the ankle being forcefully dorsiflexed as the gastrocnemius muscle contracts, as in trying to stop oneself from hitting the wall during a game of squash.

Objective Findings

Observation There may be observable swelling in the muscle belly of the gastrocnemius when compared with the other side, or there may be localized swelling at the base of the muscle around the region of the Achilles tendon. Bruising may occur, but is usually not marked in nature and is more often found at the sides of the ankle or even tracking into the sides of the foot (3, 6, 15).

Active Movements Mild limitation of dorsiflexion with pain may be found when the movement is tested with the knee flexed. This limitation and discomfort will become more marked if the knee is then fully extended. Pain may also be present at end range of plantarflexion, but there will be no limitation in range of this movement (6, 10, 15, 16).

Passive Movements Pain and possibly muscle spasm will be produced on overpressure into the restricted range of dorsiflexion. There will be a noticeable difference between the range of motion for dorsiflexion when the knee is extended as compared to when it is flexed. All other passive movements of the foot and ankle will be of full range and pain free (6, 10, 16).

Resisted Movements Pain is produced at the site of injury on resisted plantarflexion, particularly when tested from the position of full dorsiflexion. The patient will also have some degree of difficulty achieving a heel raise when in a single-leg stance on the affected leg (1, 3, 7, 10).

Palpation Tenderness will be elicited on palpation at the site of injury, either at the proximal and medial part of the gastrocnemius muscle belly or at the myotendinous junction in the lower third of the calf centrally. There may be a small gap palpable in the proximal part of the Achilles tendon with a small soft-tissue lump of rolled-up fibers palpable just above the gap (1, 6, 20).

Specific Tests In case of complete rupture, Thompson's test will reveal loss of plantarflexion when the calf muscle is squeezed. There may also be no Achilles tendon observable at the heel. However, the patient will still be able to actively plantarflex the foot in non-weight bearing through the action of the posterior tibial muscles. This author has seen patients who have raised their heels slightly off the ground in the weight-bearing single-leg stance, even with a complete rupture of the Achilles tendon, but the amount of movement achieved is minimal in each case. If a complete rupture is detected the patient will require an orthopaedic consultation and will need surgery or casting, following which the treatment regime will be very similar to that following a partial tear. The hamstring muscles should be checked through isometric resisted contraction and passive stretching if the pain is high in the calf, as occasionally a hamstring tendon tear can masquerade as a calf muscle tendon tear (3, 6, 19).

Treatment Ideas
(1, 3, 4, 6, 7, 10, 15)

Patients should be supplied with a heel raise. This can be something as simple as a one-quarter–inch thickness of foam cut out in the shape of the patient's heel and placed in his shoe. This will take the strain off the gastrocnemius muscle during walking and will enable the patient to walk more comfortably and with a less pronounced limp. In the early stages following injury, ice and rest can be effective in reducing discomfort, with elevation of the lower leg whenever possible for drainage of effusion, if it is present. The degree of discomfort is usually fairly self-limiting as regards activities for patients in the early stages of the condition, but they should be advised to maintain active range of motion as available in the foot and ankle, both with the knee flexed and with the knee extended, and always within pain-free range. Interferential therapy and transcutaneous electrical nerve stimulation may prove useful for relief of discomfort.

Three or four days following the injury the patient can be progressed to the use of heat over the injured tissues, with active exercises enhanced by the use of a neuromuscular stimulator for the calf muscles. The patient should quickly be able to progress to plantarflexion and dorsiflexion exercises in sitting, with pressure applied to the foot via the knee by the patient's hand. Balance-board exercises can also be carried out in sitting for plantarflexion, dorsiflexion, inversion, and eversion. Patients can also attempt the use of an exercise bike (with a low resistance) in order to maintain cardiovascular fitness, and should experience no discomfort at the site of injury while completing this exercise. The patient can also start to gently stretch the gastrocnemius muscle using a towel or a belt wrapped around the foot with the exercise carried out with the knee fully extended. Pulsed ultrasound and laser can be applied to the site of injury to promote repair. Treatment sessions should still end with the application of ice to the injured area.

Further progression can be made to resisted inversion and eversion exercises using a ball and exercise band as resistance, respectively, and at the same time the patient can start attempting resisted plantarflexion against the exercise band. The band can also be used to assist in stretching the muscle into dorsiflexion. Neuromuscular electrical nerve stimulation can be employed to produce a contraction of the calf muscle, against which the patient holds the ankle statically in a mild degree of dorsiflexion, the amount of dorsiflexion being increased as the patient is able to tolerate the stretch. Supported walking can be introduced, with the patient being instructed in

the proper heel/toe gait. At this time the size of the heel raise can be reduced or the patient can spend part of the day, particularly when around
the house, not using the raise. At this time the patient can also be progressed
onto weight-bearing balance-board exercises initially using the support of
wall bars or a wall, progressing to unsupported double-leg work, then to
single-leg balance exercises.

As the weight-bearing exercise program is progressed, the patient should
always have a 5 to 10 minute warm up and stretch period before the exercises. The exercise sessions can now include activities such as double-heel
raises, weight-bearing gastrocnemius and soleus stretches, step-ups, step-
downs, the use of a step machine, and progression of resistance on the exercise bike. Final progression is to single-leg balance exercises on a balance
board, plyometrics, straight line running, skipping, and hopping, with progression to lateral bounding and lateral glides, sharp turns, and quick starting and stopping activities. Exercise sessions should always finish with
thorough stretching of the calf musculature. At this time the use of physical
agents and electrical modalities should no longer be required. The patient
can then make a graduated return to normal daily activities; if involved in a
particular sport there should be progress through light to normal training
and then to competition. However, competition should only be attempted
once the patient is pain free both throughout the exercise program and on
isometric resisted and stretch testing of the affected muscle in the clinic.

Restrictions As noted, the condition is normally initially self-limiting,
however, the patient must be advised to attempt no running, jumping, or
going down stairs while taking weight on the affected leg. The full-squat
position should also be avoided particularly for lifting weights. The patient
may also have difficulty on ladders, which may be a high-risk situation as
a slip on a ladder will cause sharp pain, and the muscle will give way as
pressure is put on the forefoot. Once the patient can complete a full-stride
length with no discomfort, he can discard the heel raise. At this time the
patient can ease himself back into running activities, but with no sudden
starting and stopping and no hill running. Progression must be made slowly
in all activities, particularly explosive activities of the lower extremity. The
classic re-injury occurs just a few weeks after onset when the amount of
discomfort the patient is experiencing is minimal, but when the scar tissue
has not yet consolidated and, therefore, the repair is weak. At this stage
something as simple as an unthinking jump into the air off both feet may
well set the patient back another 2 weeks. Patients need to be informed of
this discrepancy between the state of repair and degree of pain relief before
they injure themselves, not as a lecture after the fact.

Achilles Tendonitis

Overview

This is an inflammation of the Achilles tendon and its paratenon, which is
occasionally incorrectly described as a tenosynovitis, however, there is no

synovial lining around the tendon. The tendon is susceptible to friction forces and attrition at the point where it winds around the posterior and inferior surfaces of the calcaneus. This condition can severely limit performance in athletes if left untreated. Since the tendon has a poor vascular supply in this area there is a tendency towards poor healing and slow recovery (9, 10, 12, 17).

Subjective Findings

Onset Patients are typically between 20 and 40 years of age. Onset is gradual in nature usually due to overuse, most commonly on running or jumping activities and particularly following running on hard surfaces or uphill. They then most commonly occur during a switch to these activities from other, less demanding, activities (2, 4, 6, 12).

Duration Symptoms usually develop over several weeks, but it is often 1 to 2 months before the patient is referred for treatment, with the length of time often depending on the demands of sport or daily activities. The condition is chronic by nature (2, 9, 17).

Frequency This will normally be the first time that the patient has had these symptoms. There usually has been one long continuous episode, with exacerbations and remissions depending on the degree of activity. However, if the patient participates in an intermittent training program or only occasional bouts of the given activity, then the exacerbations may appear as separate episodes. However, on further investigation during the assessment it will come to light that if particular activities are attempted, then the underlying symptoms always appear to be present (2, 4, 9).

Area of Symptoms Symptoms are normally felt in the Achilles tendon, most noticeably at the sides of the tendon and often most marked at its calcaneal attachments (Fig. 7.17) (3–6, 9).

Type of Symptoms The patient will complain of a deep nagging ache that occurs during running or other specific weight-bearing activities. If the condition is acute enough, symptoms will also occur on walking, particularly uphill. The patient will also complain of stiffness after rest felt in the area of the Achilles tendon and around the heel, or on rising first thing in the morning (2, 4–6, 9).

Miscellaneous The presence of a posterior heel spur (exostosis) shown to be present on x-ray may be the cause, or may possibly aggravate the condition. Running shoes with low heels will tend to exacerbate the condition and the patient should be asked if he has recently changed shoes for any particular activity or simply changed the shoes that he wears most often throughout the day (3, 6, 10, 11).

Objective Finding

Observation Mild swelling may be noted at the sides of the Achilles tendon if the paratenon is also inflamed. In very chronic cases soft-tissue

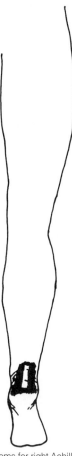

FIG. 7.17 Area of symptoms for right Achilles tendonitis, mainly at the sides of the tendon and occasionally over the calcaneal attachments.

thickening may be observed when comparing one Achilles tendon to the other (6, 9, 10, 12).

Active Movements There should be no limitation of movement, although dorsiflexion may be slightly limited compared to the other side when tested with the knee fully extended. No pain will be present on any of the active movements (1, 2, 10, 12).

Passive Movements Overpressure into end range of dorsiflexion with the knee extended, may produce local discomfort in the area of the Achilles tendon or at the heel. However this will usually only happen in the acute stage, otherwise there is usually nothing of note to be found as all movements are normally of full range and pain free (2, 6, 12, 13).

Resisted Movements These are most typically pain free with good strength. However if plantar flexion is tested in standing on one leg and from the position of full dorsiflexion (as in standing on the edge of a stool with the heel dropped below the top), then the patient may experience some discomfort when raising the heel from that fully dorsiflexed position. Also if weight-bearing plantarflexion is carried out repeatedly there may be some pain produced and the patient may demonstrate a lack of endurance for this activity compared to single-leg activities on the unaffected side (6, 9, 12).

Palpation Pain is normally elicited on palpation around the posterior of the calcaneus and on pressure applied with the finger and thumb along the sides of the Achilles tendon. This palpation should be done gently, as any strong pressure applied in this way is uncomfortable, even in the normal subject. There must be a noticeable difference between the amount of discomfort produced over the affected tendon as compared to the unaffected side for the finding to be significant (4, 6, 19, 20).

Treatment Ideas
(1–4, 6, 9, 10, 12, 13, 15, 17)

The patient is placed on a regime of ice and rest, with a small heel raise placed in the shoe to be used at all times. The patient should discontinue running or any other weight-bearing activity that produces symptoms for a period of 1 to 2 weeks, depending on the severity of the condition. A stationary bike can be used with low to medium resistance as tolerated to maintain strength and cardiovascular fitness as required.

After a few days of rest the patient can be progressed to active foot and ankle exercises and passive stretches of the Achilles tendon. Heat and ultrasound should be applied before stretch and ice afterwards. One form of stretch that this author has found useful is the use of a neuromuscular stimulator to produce a contraction of the calf muscle, with the patient instructed to hold the foot in dorsiflexion against the contractions each time they occur. The patient can then be further progressed to weight-bearing exercises such as double-heel raises and step-ups, followed by passive weight-bearing stretches aimed at gaining further mobility of the tendon, to which end contract/relax and hold/relax techniques can also be employed. The patient can then progress to the use of neuromuscular electrical stimulation for the calf muscle, with active dorsiflexion carried out against the contraction as it occurs. Ultrasound or laser may be helpful in reducing discomfort and thermal doses of ultrasound may help to increase the degree of stretch obtained.

Once the patient is able to cope with weight-bearing exercises and vigorous stretches without any discomfort then the weight-bearing activities can be progressed to include using a step machine, an exercise bike with strong resistance, plyometrics such as jump-downs or jump-ups, and strong plantarflexion/dorsiflexion exercises, such as heel raises over the edge of a step or stool. Heat may be used before exercise and ice after exercise, but the use of these agents and the electrical modalities should be steadily decreased as the exercises are progressed. Neuromuscular stimulation can still be used in combination with weight-bearing stretches of the Achilles tendon. The patient can finally progress onto strong single-leg workout activities, such as the use of a balance board or mini-trampoline, again with stretching exercise both before and after the resisted exercise program

Restriction As stated, the patient should initially be advised to stop running. This may be difficult to achieve as the patient often seeks treatment when the symptoms appear just as a progression in training has begun. The author has found that a compromise in this situation never works. The longer the patient is allowed to carry on attempting activities that produce the symptoms, the worse the condition becomes, and the less likely it is to clear completely. A firm approach, with the patient clearly informed about the recovery process, will avoid a great deal of frustration on the part of both the patient and the therapist. The patient should also be advised to restrict the amount of repetitive activity done involving stairs, prolonged squatting, and walking up and down hills or slopes. Return to running should first be attempted on a forgiving surface, such as a treadmill or on grass, with progression to track and then road as the patient shows an ability to tolerate these activities without exacerbating the symptoms. Orthotics, particularly in the form of a permanent heel raise, may be necessary, particularly in the distance runner.

Plantar Fasciitis

Overview

The plantar fascia extends from the tubercles at the medial and lateral aspects of the inferior surface of the calcaneus to the level of the metatarsal-phalangeal joints, where it blends with the capsular ligaments. It is the strongest single ligament in the human body and helps to maintain the medial longitudinal arch of the foot. Flattening of the arch of the foot places a strain on the plantar fascia, as does extension of the toes. Both collapse of the arches (pes planus) or excessive arching of the foot (pes cavus) can predispose towards this condition. The aim of treatment is to stretch the fascia, which is usually tight, and to promote strength in the intrinsic muscles of the foot, particularly the lumbrical muscles, which act to produce flexion at the metatarsalphalangeal joints and extension at the interphalangeal joints, helping to relieve strain on the plantar fascia (9, 10, 11, 17).

Subjective Findings

Onset This is typically gradual with no known cause, although on occasions it may be sudden due to trauma. However, the patient in these cases will usually indicate some signs existing prior to the date of injury. The patient is typically over 40, although in running athletes the age range is 20 to 40, and some may even present with problems in their teens (1, 2, 9, 11).

Duration The patient will typically report a history of weeks or more commonly months of steadily increasing symptoms before attending for treatment. In the case of trauma the patient may present within 1 to 2 weeks, but this is unusual.

Frequency The typical history is of one long episode with the condition aggravated by weight-bearing activities, particularly running. However if the patient attempts strenuous weight-bearing activities only on an occasional basis, then the history may appear as a series of recurrent episodes (2, 4, 5, 10).

Area of Symptoms Symptoms start in, and are at that time localized to, the distal aspect of the inferior surface of the calcaneus, most commonly to the medial side. With time symptoms will spread along the sole of the foot and will also do so if at any time the patient continues with an activity that is provoking the symptoms (4, 9–11).

Type of Symptoms The patient will complain of sharp pain on rising in the morning, which normally lasts for 10 to 20 minutes until it can be walked off. The patient will also complain of a pulling- or tearing-type pain in the sole of the foot if an activity that provokes the symptoms is continued. The patient will also state that there is tenderness in the bottom of the foot around the heel (Fig. 7.18) (2, 3, 5).

Miscellaneous This condition can often be bilateral in nature and can be found in patients who have to stand for prolonged periods of time. The condition was once known as policemen's heel, back in the time when most policemen still "walked the beat" (1, 3, 7).

Objective Findings

Observation There is usually little to be observed, although patients may present with flattening of the arches or pronation of the foot, both of which can predispose to this condition (1, 3, 10).

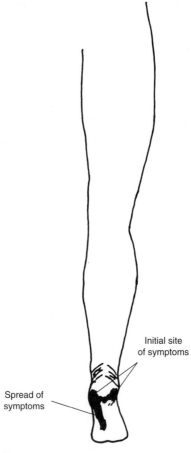

Initial site
of symptoms

Spread of
symptoms

FIG. 7.18   Area of symptoms for plantar fasciitis in the right foot.

Active Movements There is normally full active range of motion at the foot, ankle, and toes. Intrinsic action of the lumbricals may be poor, but this is always difficult to ascertain as the patient may not understand the requirements of the movement and will therefore curl the toes into flexion using the long flexors, rather than the lumbricals. There should be no pain present on any active movement of the foot, ankle, or toes (5, 10, 11, 17).

Passive Movements Normal range of motion should be found on all movements, with no pain in the foot or ankle. Extension of the toes, particularly when combined with dorsiflexion of the ankle, will help with visualization of the plantar fascia and may in acute cases produce discomfort. Passive gliding movements carried out in the mid-tarsal region and forefoot may reveal general stiffness, but again no pain should be produced during testing (10, 11, 17).

Resisted Movements All resisted movements of the ankle, foot, and toes should be of good strength and will produce no discomfort. It is virtually impossible to effectively resist the action of the lumbricals.

Palpation Tenderness will usually be elicited at the distal plantar aspect of the calcaneus over the medial and lateral tuberosities, particularly the medial tuberosity, and also for a varying distance along the extent of the plantar fascia. There may also be occasional associated tenderness at the insertion of the Achilles tendon at the plantar and posterior aspects of the calcaneus (6, 11, 12, 20).

Specific Tests X-rays may reveal the presence of a calcaneal spur. However, the significance of this finding is questionable because these spurs may also be found in the asymptomatic subject (3, 9, 10, 15).

Treatment Ideas
(1, 2, 4, 6, 9, 11–13, 15, 17, 31)

If the patient is a runner and running produces the symptoms, he should be advised to stop running for 2 to 3 weeks. Treatment then commences with the use of heat and ultrasound along the extent of the plantar fascia and muscle stimulation to facilitate lumbrical muscle action, which is combined with active lumbrical exercises. These exercises should be done in sitting with pressure applied to the foot through the knee using the hand. The patient should continue doing active lumbrical exercises at home, completing 40 to 50 repetitions eight to ten times per day, as the lumbricals are not a muscle group that will work for three sets of 20 repetitions twice per day. They are required to contract every time weight is transferred to the foot, which should be explained to the patient.

The heat, ultrasound, and muscle stimulation are continued as before and may be alternated with the use of laser, particularly for any tender areas on the plantar aspect of the calcaneus. Passive stretch of the fascia can be applied by fully extending the toes, with pressure on the inferior surface of the calcaneus to push it up and backwards. This should, in turn, be combined with weight-bearing calf muscle stretches. The patient can be advised to roll a cold can under the foot at home after completing the exercises at the end of a day. This helps to decrease discomfort felt in the plantar fascia and helps the patient to mold the foot to a surface, hence enhancing the natural arch of the foot. Ice should be applied at the end of the treatment sessions, as this will help to lessen any exercise-induced discomfort. Muscle stimulation for the lumbricals can be progressed to the full weight-bearing standing position, with weight transferred onto the affected leg during stimulation and the patient simultaneously producing an active lumbrical contraction. This can be further progressed by the patient gripping a support such as wall bars and applying upward pressure with the hand (as if trying to lift the wall bars off the floor), which will place greater pressure on the feet. Patients often feel some benefits from a general program of weight-bearing foot and ankle exercises, including step-ups and balance-board exercises starting in a two-leg stance and progressing to single-leg work.

As the patient's discomfort decreases, particularly in the early morning, he can start attempting running and static standing activities as tolerated. The use of orthotics may be required for either work or specific sports activities, although on occasion patients can return to the previous level of activity without any form of external support.

Restrictions   As noted previously, the patient should be advised to rest from any weight-bearing activities that produce discomfort in particular running, but also standing or walking on hard surfaces such as concrete floors. A 2-week rest period is usually sufficient to allow treatment to progress effectively. Return to these activities can be attempted on a graduated basis as tolerated by the patient. Climbing steps, stairs, or ladders, and jumping down from any height are activities that should be limited and are not recommended until the patient is showing definite improvement of the condition. Again, the "acid test" is less discomfort felt in the foot on rising in the morning.

Peroneal Tenosynovitis

Overview

The tendons of the peroneus longus and peroneus brevis muscles can become inflamed within their synovial sheaths in their course behind and below the lateral malleolus. The symptoms arising from this condition can be confused with those caused by a previous or underlying lateral ligament injury of the ankle, but the symptoms persist far longer or tend to recur (1, 10, 17).

Subjective Findings

Onset   This is typically gradual after trauma or overuse and occurs most commonly in those 15 to 45 years of age, although it can occur at any age (1, 6, 10).

Duration The patient will normally be able to tolerate the symptoms for weeks or even months, before seeking treatment.

Frequency There may be a previous history of trauma involving the ankle joint; however, this episode of symptoms is usually one long episode with increasing pain on activity, which therefore may mimic recurrent episodes of discomfort. However, the patient will usually have some degree of discomfort on a daily basis felt in the area of the tendon sheaths (1, 7, 10).

Area of Symptoms Symptoms should be fairly well localized to the lateral aspect of the ankle and foot at a point behind the lateral malleolus, with some symptoms also referred into the lateral aspect of the foot (Fig. 7.19) (1, 2, 6).

Type of Symptoms The patient will usually complain of a sharp or burning pain on certain activities, particularly walking or running over uneven ground, walking long distances, and going up and down stairs or ladders. There will also be very marked pain on first getting out of bed, which will take anything from 10 to 30 minutes to ease as the patient walks around (1, 2, 10).

Miscellaneous This condition may be associated with systemic inflammatory conditions such as rheumatoid arthritis. The patient may find that certain boots or shoes worn cause pain at the lateral ankle due to pressure on the tendons. During assessment it is important to observe the shoes, particularly how they fit in relation to the peroneal tendons; if the ridge of the shoe lies at that particular level, the patient should use boots that lace above the malleoli (2, 6, 10).

Objective Findings

Observation There may be a sausagelike swelling behind and below the lateral malleolus in the region of the tendon sheaths. Observe the patient's shoes for uneven wear, as supination of the foot, shown by excessive wear at the outer aspect of the heel and sole, may predispose the patient to this condition (1, 2, 6).

Active Movements There is usually pain associated with mild limitation of inversion of the foot, with pain also produced at end range of active eversion on occasions, and sometimes at end range of plantarflexion. All other movements will be of full range and pain free (1, 6, 7).

Passive Movements The pattern of limitation and discomfort on passive testing is the same as that found on active testing, with more marked pain felt at the site of the peroneal tendons when overpressure is applied at end range of inversion or plantarflexion (1, 6, 7).

Resisted Movements The patient will often have discomfort on resisted eversion, which is worse if the movement is resisted through range

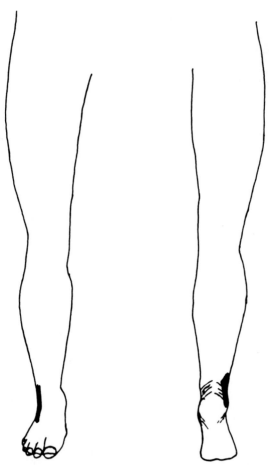

FIG. 7.19   Area of symptoms for peroneal tenosynovitis at the right ankle.

(isotonically) as compared to isometric testing in any given position of the foot (1, 7, 10).

Palpation Tenderness will be elicited posterior to and just below the lateral malleolus. Occasionally there may also be pain at the lateral aspect of the foot as far as the base of the fifth metatarsal. Crepitation may be felt over the offending tendons on both active and passive movements of the ankle if a finger is placed posterior and inferior to the malleolus during the movement (Fig. 7.6) (1, 2, 19, 21).

Specific Tests The patient may have decreased balance ability on the affected leg; balance testing may recreate the patient's typical symptoms at the lateral aspects of the ankle.

Treatment Ideas
(2, 6, 7, 10)

Patients can gain benefit from regularly performed ice massage over the affected tendon sheaths in the area behind and below the lateral malleolus, particularly when combined with rest from all pain-producing activities over a 2–3-day period. A simple crepe bandage can also help to reduce discomfort. The patient should be advised to elevate the foot above the level of the heart for periods during the day, but being careful not to overflex the hip greater than 70 degrees. Non-weight–bearing foot and ankle exercises should be encouraged using a pumping action, which can help to disperse fluid in the region of the ankle. Pulsed ultrasound may also be effective and can be combined with interferential therapy to the foot and calf, particularly to the gastrocnemius muscle.

Pumping-type passive movements can be used for both dorsiflexion, plantarflexion, and eversion. This can be followed by passive stretches into end range of all movements, particularly inversion. The patient can be taught to stretch the foot and ankle into dorsiflexion and inversion using a towel, with greater pressure applied to the medial side of the foot compared to the lateral. The patient can also be shown how to roll a large can under the foot to produce an inversion and eversion movement of the foot. At this time the patient may benefit from the application of heat prior to exercise and the use of ice at the end of a treatment session.

The dosage of ultrasound can be steadily increased and can be replaced or can be alternated with the use of laser over the affected tendons and tendon sheaths. Manually resisted foot and ankle exercises, again using a pumping action, may help to disperse fluid from the area. Proprioceptive neuromuscular facilitation techniques, such as hold/relax and contract/relax, used to gain further stretch into eversion, may also prove to be beneficial. The patient can then progress to balance exercises using both feet on a balance-board and progressing to single-leg work. The patient should be advised to take rests for as long as necessary and as often as required in order to prevent any symptoms occurring during this treatment. Ice should still be applied at the end of the treatment session. If recalcitrant swelling is noted at the posterior or inferior aspects of the lateral malleolus, then contrast bathing can be used, with the patient placing the foot into very cold water for 1 minute, followed by immersion in warm water for 3 minutes. This process is then repeated three times, once or twice a day.

As pain and swelling decreases at the site of inflammation the patient can be progressed to further weight-bearing single- and double-leg exercises including heel raises, step-ups, lateral step-ups, use of a step machine, and an exercise bike. They should continue with rests as required; ice applied at the end of treatment will help in avoiding exacerbation of symptoms. The degree of vigor with which the exercises are done can be steadily increased as the patient demonstrates no tendency towards recurrence of symptoms.

The final stages of treatment should include hopping, skipping, jumping, and short runs with quick stops and starts. Once these exercises are being attempted the use of heat and ice should be discontinued, with the patient still advised to use ice at home if any symptoms recur. Once no symptoms are found on either passive, active, or resisted testing in the clinic, or following weight-bearing exercises, then the patient can progress gradually back to normal weight-bearing activities such as running. The patient should start with straight running on smooth and even surfaces, then banked surfaces, uneven surfaces, and finally sprints with quick turns.

Restrictions   The patient should be advised not to use any footwear that irritates the condition and to restrict weight-bearing activities, particularly walking over uneven surfaces. Standing for long periods, particularly on hard surfaces, and the use of steps, stairs, or ladders should also be limited as required. The patient may also have some difficulty kneeling with the foot fully plantarflexed, as in sitting back on the heels; again, this should be avoided or the kneeling position altered so as to apply less pressure to the irritated tendons. The patient can make a graduated return to these activities, but only when showing signs of improvement during treatment in the clinic and only as long as the activity does not produce any of the typical symptoms at the lateral aspect of the foot or ankle.

Posterior Tibial Tenosynovitis

Overview

This is an overuse problem associated with increased friction of the posterior tibial tendons in their sheaths behind and below the medial malleolus, which produces an inflammatory reaction within the tendon sheath. The condition may be associated with congenital or acquired foot deformities, particularly excessive pronation of the foot. Flattening of the arches of the foot and general obesity can also contribute to the onset of this condition (13, 15, 17, 29).

Subjective Findings

Onset   This is gradual due to overuse, although on rare occasions it may occur following trauma. If this is the case the symptoms often do not occur for quite some time after the original trauma. Patients are typically 20 to 40 years of age (2, 4, 13).

Duration The patient is usually able to tolerate the symptoms for an extended period of time and will not present for treatment until several weeks have passed, or more commonly, 2 or more months.

Frequency This is usually the first time that the patient has experienced these symptoms, although there may be a history of some previous foot and ankle problems or possibly recurrent calf muscle strains (2, 4, 5).

Area of Symptoms These are fairly well localized to the medial aspect of the ankle posterior to and just below the medial malleolus (Fig. 7.20) (2, 4, 5).

Type of Symptoms The patient will usually complain of pain and swelling. The pain is usually burning in nature with sharp twinges experienced if the ankle is stressed in any way. The swelling usually occurs during or immediately following weight-bearing activities. The patient may also experience a general aching discomfort in the ankle on rest following activity (4, 5, 6, 15).

Miscellaneous In severe cases this condition can be accompanied by compression of the posterior tibial nerve in the tarsal tunnel (tarsal tunnel syndrome). The patient may also state that a particular type of footwear tends to produce the condition, when the shoes or boots are examined it is usually found that the cuff of the shoe is pressing on the area behind the medial malleolus (2, 6).

Objective Findings

Observation Swelling may be found localized to the area of the tendon sheaths posterior to the medial malleolus. The patient may have flattening of the arches of the foot, particularly the medial longitudinal arch, and there may be excessive pronation of the foot, seen as relative eversion of the calcaneus. The patient's shoes should be checked for uneven wear, which would tend to be on the inner aspect of the heel and sole. The patient may also have calluses in the skin around the heel if pressure from footwear is a problem (5, 6, 13).

Active Movements Pain is usually experienced at end range of eversion and occasionally at end range of inversion, although there is normally no loss of range of motion of the foot and ankle and all other movements will be pain free (2, 4, 6, 7).

Passive Movements Pain will be produced at the posteromedial aspect of the ankle on overpressure applied at end range of eversion and possibly end range of plantarflexion (2, 4, 6).

Resisted Movements Resisted inversion is usually painful, particularly if tested at the point of full eversion or if resisted through range

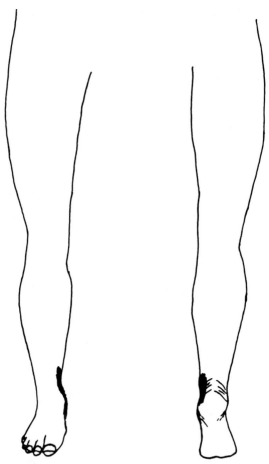

FIG. 7.20   Area of symptoms for posterior tibial tenosynovitis at the right ankle.

(i.e., isotonically), while all other movements should be pain free. All movements should demonstrate good strength (4, 6, 7).

Palpation Tenderness is usually elicited over the offending tendon sheaths behind and below the medial malleolus. Fine crepitation will often be felt on palpation over the tendon sheaths during either passive or active testing of movements, particularly the movements of inversion and eversion (Fig. 7.8) (2, 6, 19, 20).

Treatment Ideas
(2, 4–7, 13, 15, 30)

Corrective orthotics may be required if there are obvious deformities or abnormalities of the foot. Ice and rest, particularly ice massage over the affected tendons and their sheaths carried out for 5 to 10 minutes every 2 hours for 2 to 3 days, may help to resolve the initial problem. The patient can also be advised to soak the foot in an ice bath for 5 to 10 minutes at a time. Active exercises for the foot and ankle should be carried out in elevation with the foot placed higher than the patient's heart and the hip flexed to no greater than 60 to 70 degrees. The patient may use either a crepe bandage or a sleeve-type bandage, or can simply wear high-top shoes or boots to support the ankle.

Progression The patient can be progressed onto eversion and dorsiflexion exercises using an exercise band with passive stretches into eversion. Rhythmic passive movements of the foot and ankle for the movement of plantarflexion, dorsiflexion, inversion, and eversion may help to reduce the amount of swelling and will mobilize the tendons within their sheaths. Isometric resisted exercises can begin for all movements of the foot and ankle, and again can be executed in a rhythmical manner so as to promote a muscle-pumping action. Pulsed ultrasound or laser can be combined with heat application and interferential therapy for the ankle and calf, again applied with the leg in elevation. Ice should be used post-exercise in order to minimize any inflammatory response.

The patient can be taught to passively evert the foot at home using a towel wrapped around it, with pressure applied to the lateral side by pulling up more strongly on that side of the towel, bringing the foot into plantarflexion and eversion. The patient can be progressed onto isometric resisted inversion exercises using pressure against a rubber ball or similar object and resisted plantarflexion against resistance band. The patient can be taught to roll a can under the foot at home to produce plantarflexion/dorsiflexion and inversion/eversion movements of the foot. While in the clinic the patient can be progressed to the use of a balance board, initially done in sitting, both double and single leg, and then progressed to weight-bearing balance-board exercises.

As swelling and discomfort decreases (and is not provoked by the present exercises), the patient can be progressed to further weight-bearing exercises, initially attempting step-ups, heel-raises, heel-raises over the edge of a step, lateral step-ups and step-downs, and stepping over and back on a stool, initially with the affected leg remaining on the stool and then standing on the unaffected leg using the affected leg for propulsion. Ice should still be applied after the exercises, but its use can be steadily reduced and eventually eliminated as the patient's symptoms ease. The use of all other modalities should also be steadily reduced as the patient's symptoms decrease.

The patient can progress onto running, jumping, skipping, and hopping exercises; then onto lateral glides; lateral bounding; walking sideways, backwards, and forwards; and plyometric exercises such as jump-ups, jump-downs, and vertical jumps, concentrating on soft, light landings. The patient must be advised to rest whenever required throughout the exercise program at the first indication of any symptoms arising in the affected area, but at the same time to push himself to this limit unless the symptoms are threatening.

Restrictions   Initially the patient should avoid walking or running over rough or uneven surfaces and should also limit climbing of steps, stairs, and ladders, or standing on hard surfaces for prolonged periods of time. Running on hard surfaces should be avoided until the patient is pain free during and after the exercises in the clinic. The patient should also avoid the use of high-heeled footwear and will benefit from wearing a "sensible shoe" that laces quite high on the ankle, above the malleoli. Return to weight-bearing activities can be attempted once the patient is pain free on all exercises carried out in the clinic, and even then return to activity must be made in a graduated manner, with the final progression being to walking and running over uneven surfaces. If the patient is going to be returning to work with severe ankle strain, such as in construction or in specific sports such as soccer or football, the use of a custom-made ankle brace should be seriously considered.

Anterior Tibial Tendonitis

Overview

The tendon of the tibialis anterior muscle can be become irritated and inflamed with unaccustomed walking (particularly up and down hills) or running, as this muscle decelerates the foot as weight is taken on the foot at each stride. This condition can also occur when the patient's gait is affected by a knee condition as more strain may then be placed on the muscle during the weight-bearing phase of walking (2, 6, 7).

Subjective Findings

Onset   This is gradual due to overuse, particularly unaccustomed activity or increase in the level of a particular weight-bearing activity such as walking or running. The majority of patients are young to middle aged (2, 4).

Duration The patient will present for treatment typically some 6 to 12 weeks after onset as the symptoms tend to be irritating, rather than functionally limiting.

Frequency Normally this is a condition that only occurs once, although it may be associated with previous ankle and foot conditions, or knee problems that may still be ongoing.

Area of Symptoms Symptoms are usually felt at the distal third of the anterior of the lower leg. On continued activity symptoms will spread across the anterior of the ankle and possibly into the dorsum of the foot (Fig. 7.21) (2, 4, 6).

Type of Symptoms The patient will complain of a burning pain occurring after a period of weight bearing. This pain will become sharp if the patient continues with the causative activity. After activity there will be a persistent ache that will remain for a variable amount of time (2, 6).

Miscellaneous A common history is that of a patient who is un-accustomed to hiking and then attempts that activity. Patients appear to be particularly prone if they happen to have been wearing heavier boots than they are used to. Change of footwear may also produce onset of this problem in a patient who is accustomed to walking or running.

Objective Findings

Observation Upon entering the clinic the patient will often be observed to walk with a slight limp, caused by decreased force taken on the affected leg at initial weight bearing during each stride.

Active Movements Active movements are usually full, but with pain experienced at end range of both plantarflexion and dorsiflexion. All other movements of the foot and knee will be pain free (2, 6, 7).

Passive Movements Pain in usually produced on passive plantar-flexion and is experienced at the distal musculotendinous junction of the tibialis anterior muscle. This pain will increase appreciably if over-pressure is applied to the movement, but the pain will not increase if passive flexion of the toes is carried out with the ankle positioned at the point in plantarflexion at which the pain is produced (4, 7).

Resisted Movements Pain will normally be felt on isometric resisted dorsiflexion, particularly when the foot is held in a position of dorsiflexion and inversion. Testing of all other movements will be pain free and none of the movements will be weak (4, 6, 7).

Palpation Pain will be elicited at the myotendinous junction of the tibialis anterior muscle and for a variable distance both proximally and distally along the tendon. Crepitus may be felt over the area of the tendon if it is palpated during either passive or active movements of the foot and ankle (Fig. 7.11).

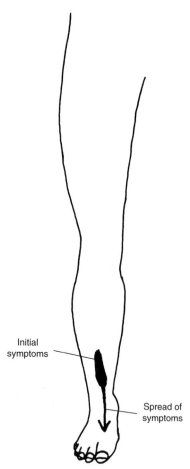

Initial symptoms

Spread of symptoms

FIG. 7.21 Area of symptoms for anterior tibial tendonitis at the right ankle.

Treatment Ideas
(2, 4, 6, 7)

The patient must be advised initially to rest from walking or running activities, particularly when the patient himself can identify these activities as causative factors in either onset or exacerbation of the symptoms. The patient should also be advised to wear light shoes with low heels. Ice packs, ice massage, or emersion of the lower leg in an ice bath may all help to relieve symptoms. The ice pack and ice massage should be applied directly to the anterior aspect of the tibia over the area of the muscle belly and tendon of the tibialis anterior muscle. Pulsed ultrasound may also help; interferential therapy or transcutaneous electrical nerve stimulation can assist in relieving discomfort. The patient should be taught to elevate the leg while carrying out mid-range active exercises, followed by two or three full-range movements at the end of the exercise.

The patient is progressed onto resisted plantarflexion and eversion of the foot and ankle using a resistance band. The patient can also be taught to stretch into plantarflexion by rolling a can under the foot while in the sitting position. The can should be placed a reasonable distance from the chair so that as the can is rolled forward the foot is taken into full plantarflexion, thus stretching the anterior tibial muscles. A balance board can also be used in sitting to achieve the same effect, with the patient repetitively plantarflexing and dorsiflexing the ankle with the board moved progressively further away from the patient so that the degree of plantarflexion stretch applied is steadily increased. Rhythmical manually resisted plantarflexion and eversion exercises can help to reduce pooling of fluid in the lower leg by promoting a muscle-pumping action.

Further progression is made by application of heat to the lower leg. The patient can then start weight-bearing exercises such as the balance-board in standing using hand support, step-ups, and heel-raises. Neuromuscular electrical stimulation can be given to the anterior tibial muscles, accompanied by active dorsiflexion in early to mid range. This can be progressed by the patient holding the foot in mid range of dorsiflexion against the contractions of the muscle produced by the neuromuscular stimulator. Once this is well tolerated, the patient can be progressed onto resisted isometric dorsiflexion, initially done in mid range, then into varying degrees of inner and outer range of dorsiflexion.

The patient can continue isometric resisted dorsiflexion at home using an exercise band attached to a suitably heavy stationary support with the band looped over the anterior aspect of the foot. The patient then holds the foot in dorsiflexion while actively flexing the knee, thus isometrically working the anterior tibial muscles. These exercises should be carried out in short bursts with long rest periods, incorporating gentle stretches into both plantarflexion and dorsiflexion. Weight-bearing activities can be further progressed to step-downs and balance-board exercises with no hand support, followed by static balancing on the board. The patient can also start walking on a treadmill, initially with the walking surface flat and then steadily increasing the degree of elevation. The patient should also be able to tolerate single-leg balance exercises at this time.

The patient can be progressed onto a general lower extremity weight-bearing exercise program including, walking up slopes, running, jumping, skipping, and balance-board exercises on one leg. The rest and stretch breaks should be continued, but should be steadily decreased in both frequency and duration until the patient is able to cope with a normal degree of daily activities without any rests being taken.

Restrictions The patient should be advised to initially walk only short distances and will also benefit from taking smaller steps and walking more slowly, thus creating less momentum and therefore less force required to decelerate the body. Walking down hills or slopes is particularly provocative and will be made worse if the patient is carrying any weight in his arms. The patient may also find it difficult to drive a car, particularly over long distances, if the right leg is affected, as there may be some difficulty holding the foot steady on the gas pedal over a prolonged period of time. In this case car trips should be broken up into manageable time periods, (although this will not be a problem if the car has cruise control). Return to all these activities can be made in short bursts, with appropriate rests taken before onset of symptoms, and with progression made only as tolerated without aggravation of symptoms. Any aggravation of symptoms should be treated with ice and rest for 1 to 2 days as required, then followed by a slower and more cautious return to the offending activities.

Shin Splints

Overview

This diagnosis is by no means clearcut. This is an overuse injury associated with inflammation of the bellies of the posterior tibial or anterior tibial muscles, which is always associated with a degree of increase in, or resumption of, training activities. It is easy to relieve this condition, but takes patience on the patient's part to prevent recurrence (3, 10, 11).

Onset This is sudden due to overuse, usually at the beginning of the training season for a particular sport, or on marked increase in training, or other specific weight-bearing activities, and occurs mainly in younger patients (6, 10, 11).

Duration The patient usually presents within 2 to 3 weeks of onset as the symptoms are not usually too restricting; however, they will prevent progression of training, which is what usually brings the patient into the clinic.

Frequency This is commonly a one-time occurrence as the patient is either cured or stops the progression of activity that caused the condition. However, occasionally patients may relieve their symptoms by rest and slowing the progression of training, but will then return to the increased level of training, once again producing the symptoms.

Area of Symptoms These are fairly well localized to the postero-medial aspect of the middle third of the tibia or in the anterior compartment at the area of the mid shin (Fig. 7.22) (6, 10, 11).

Type of Symptoms The patient complains of a burning pain during activity, a residual ache following activity, and sharp pain if trying to re-start a weight-bearing activity once the pain is present (6, 11).

Miscellaneous This condition may be associated with injuries or other conditions affecting the knee, ankle, or foot in a "domino" effect.

Objective Finding

Observation There will be nothing out of the ordinary observed in the area of the lower leg.

Active Movements These are normally full, but with some pain on combined dorsiflexion and eversion, or at end range of plantarflexion when combined with inversion (3, 6, 11).

Passive Movements These will be of full range but with discomfort at end range of either dorsiflexion or eversion. This pain is worse when the two movements are combined and overpressure is applied at end of available range (6, 11).

Resisted Movements Good strength is found on testing of all movements of the foot and ankle. Pain may be produced on isometric plantarflexion and eversion and is felt at the posterolateral aspect of the lower leg. Pain may also be produced on resisted dorsiflexion, in which case it is felt in the anterolateral aspect of the lower leg. Each of these movements will be more uncomfortable if tested with the muscle on stretch (e.g., dorsiflexion is more painful when the movement is tested with the ankle in full plantar flexion) (3, 6, 11).

Palpation If the patient is seen during an acute episode then pain is normally produced on palpation around the posteromedial aspect of the lower half of the middle third of the tibia, just in front of the bulk of the calf muscles, or over the anterior tibial muscle mass at the anterolateral aspect of the lower leg (Fig. 7.11) (6, 11, 20).

Treatment Ideas
(3, 6, 10, 11)

The first stage of treatment is immediate suspension of weight-bearing training activities for a short period of time (3 to 5 days). The patient is then instructed to resume training in a very graduated manner, starting at approximately one quarter of the training schedule attempted at the time of onset of symptoms. Ice can help to relieve discomfort, as can transcutaneous electrical nerve stimulation and pulsed ultrasound. Patients

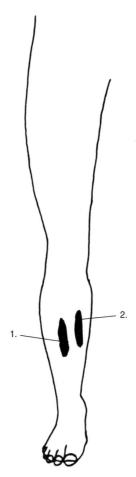

FIG. 7.22   Two possible sites of symptoms for shin splints at either:
1–the anterolateral aspect of the lower leg or 2–the posteromedial aspect
of the lower leg.

may get further relief of immediate discomfort by sonation of a topical cortisone cream.

On resuming training activities patients should be taught stretches for all foot and ankle movements. This can be done in two ways: Shorter duration stretches (10 to 15 seconds) repeated for several sets, followed by longer duration stretches (30 to 40 seconds) done individually. The application of heat prior to stretching and ice post stretching may be beneficial. A balance-board can be used in sitting in order to apply a better force to the plantarflexion stretches. The patient can use a towel or strap wrapped around the foot to assist stretching into dorsiflexion, as well as either inversion or eversion. This can be progressed to resisted plantarflexion against the exercise band with the recoil force of the band used to assist in the dorsiflexion stretch.

The patient can then progress onto light weight-bearing exercises and exercises on a static bike or step machine, with heat and stretch applied prior to the exercise and stretch followed by ice after the exercise. The use of modalities can be discontinued at this time and the patient can be progressed onto isometric resisted exercises with holds in various positions for both plantarflexion and dorsiflexion, then inversion and eversion. These exercises should still be followed by rest and stretch breaks. Graduated return to training activities should start with the patient taking many short rest breaks; the number of rest periods can then be steadily decreased while maintaining the level of training, rather than increasing the training activities and maintaining the same amount of rest. Any, even mild, recurrence of symptoms should signal immediate reduction in training. Further icing, followed by heat and stretching, should be done while maintaining the reduced training schedule, which once again must be gradually progressed. It is the therapist's part to continually counsel the patient to be patient and persevering with the reduced activity level, as in the long run this condition is 100% relievable.

Restrictions As stated above the patient must be advised to stop all activities that cause pain. The activities should be resumed only as they are shown to be non-symptom producing; when in doubt the progression of activities should be slower rather than faster.

Morton's Neuroma

Overview

Irritation and inflammation of the digital nerve can occur in the foot and produces increased production of neural tissue in the neural sheath. A common cause can be shoes that are too tight at the forefoot, particularly if they also have a high heel. Foot abnormalities such as flattening of the transverse arch or excessive pronation of the foot may also contribute to the condition. Appropriate conservative treatment can produce permanent relief of symptoms, although in some cases surgery is indicated (4, 9, 11).

Subjective Findings

Onset This is gradual with no known cause or following overuse, mainly walking and running. The typical range is 40 to 60 years of age in women, where the major cause is incorrectly fitting footwear, whereas in runners the age range tends to be 20 to 40 years (2, 4, 9, 14).

Duration Symptoms build gradually; therefore, the patient does not seek treatment for at least several weeks, or more often, months after onset.

Frequency The history is of one long episode with varying degrees of discomfort associated with changes in weight-bearing activity or with wearing one particular pair of shoes, particularly new work boots or new running shoes (2, 4, 14).

Area of Symptoms These are localized to the web between two toes and the adjacent sides of the two toes, most commonly the third and fourth (Fig. 7.23) (9, 11, 12).

Type of Symptoms Pain is felt between the toes and paraesthesia or numbness is felt along the adjacent sides of the toes (4, 9, 12).

Miscellaneous The patient may state that he is comfortable in slippers and may complain of increased pain on squatting, climbing stairs, or pushing an object, such as a wheeled cart, up a slope (6, 14, 15).

Objective Findings

Observation There is generally nothing specific to be noted on examination of the foot; however, there may be some flattening of the transverse arch. The patient may have flat feet overall or there may be noticeable pronation of the foot (4, 6, 11, 14).

Active Movements These are full and pain free for all movements of the ankle, foot, and toes (11, 12, 14, 16).

Passive Movements Passive movements will be of full range and pain free, however, pain may be experienced on forceful extension of the toes. Posterior/anterior gliding of one metatarsal on the other at the tarsal-metatarsal level may produce localized discomfort (6, 11, 12, 14, 16).

Resisted Movements All movements will be of full strength and no pain will be elicited on isometric muscle testing (6, 12, 14).

Palpation Tenderness is often felt on deep pressure in the offending web space between the toes (i.e., between the metatarsals), particularly when compared to the same point on the other foot (4, 6, 11, 12).

Specific Tests Pressure applied simultaneously to the sides of the foot at the level of the base of the metatarsals may reproduce the patient's typical pain in the web space, paraesthesia in the toes, or both. The pressure may have to be applied for 30 to 40 seconds before any noticeable symptoms appear (9, 11, 20).

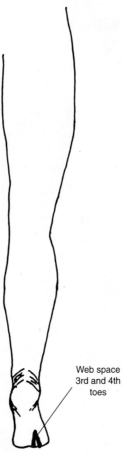

Web space
3rd and 4th
toes

FIG. 7.23   Area of symptoms for Morton's Neuroma in the right foot showing the commonest distribution.

*Treatment Ideas
(2, 4–6, 9, 11, 12, 14, 15)*

If particular footwear is a problem the patient must stop using that footwear for several weeks. If the symptoms are coupled with specific weight-bearing activities then these should be stopped. The patient should also be tested to see if orthotics are needed. A pad can be placed between adjacent toes so as to spread them at the level of the metatarsals. Passive mobilizations of the forefoot may be helpful and can be taught to the patient or a relative, friend, or trainer. Weight-bearing exercises can be attempted with a pad placed across the metatarsals using exercises such as rolling a can under the foot or using a balance board in sitting. Contrast bathing or ice baths following activity may help reduce discomfort. The application of heat before mobilizations can make them more tolerable to the patient. Ultrasound or laser applied around the heads of the metatarsals may also be helpful in this way.

Neuromuscular electrical stimulation with active lumbrical exercises should be instigated if the patient is seen to have a flat foot with loss of the natural arches. Initial weight-bearing exercises should be done in bare feet and progressed to the patient working in shoes, particularly those that they will use on a daily basis, such as work shoes or running shoes. The patient should also be advised to investigate the purchase of shoes with a greater width.

Restrictions The patient has to limit weight-bearing activities on hard surfaces, as well as climbing steps and stairs if this is identified as a problem. Initially the patient should stop running on any surface, then should return to running on soft surfaces in bare feet, then to running in the chosen footwear on soft surfaces, then on progressively harder surfaces, such as going from a treadmill to grass, to track, and then to road. If necessary the patient should also purchase orthotics, which may have to be worn in all the patient's shoes, or only in those used for a specific purpose, such as running, if this is the only time the problem is experienced.

Tarsal Tunnel Syndrome

Overview

The tarsal tunnel is formed between the medial malleolus and the flexor retinaculum. It contains the posterior tibial nerve plus the tendons and tendon sheaths of the tibialis posterior, flexor digitorum longus, and flexor hallucis longus muscles. Irritation of the tendons and their sheaths can produce an inflammatory reaction, which in turn produces compression of the nerve. This can also occur following soft tissue injury in the area. The condition may also be associated with congenital or acquired foot abnormalities (4, 13, 15, 17).

Subjective Findings

Onset This is either gradual with no known cause or is due to overuse. It occurs typically in 25 to 50 year-olds. There may be a history of trauma, although this is much less common; the symptoms of tarsal tunnel compression will normally occur a good while after the initial trauma (11, 13, 17).

Duration This is always a period of weeks or months as the condition is innocuous in its early symptoms and not functionally limiting to any particular extent (2, 4, 6).

Frequency The patient's history will be of one long episode of symptoms, with occasional remissions, but with the symptoms always present to some degree or another (2, 4, 6).

Area of Symptoms These are experienced on the plantar aspect of the foot and toes, usually more pronounced on the medial side. In very severe or chronic cases symptoms may also spread into the calf (Fig. 7.24) (2, 6, 11, 17).

Type of Symptoms Patients will complain of a burning or throbbing sensation, usually brought on initially by walking or standing for lengthy periods of time. Later on these symptoms may be present at rest, particularly during the night. The patient may state that he gets up during the night to walk around or stamp the foot to alleviate symptoms (2, 6, 11, 17).

Objective Findings

Observation There may be nothing out of the ordinary to be observed, although flattening of the arches (pes planus) or over pronation of the foot may occur concurrently with this condition (4, 6, 9).

Active Movements These are typically full and pain free, although there could be mild limitation or mild discomfort on full dorsiflexion of the ankle when combined with eversion of the foot, if there is an associated posterior tibial tendonitis (2, 6, 10).

Passive Movements These are of full range and pain free for all movements of the foot and ankle (2, 6).

Resisted Movements Normal strength will be found on testing of the movements of the foot and ankle with no discomfort elicited, although in prolonged cases there may be some weakness of flexion of the toes at the interphalangeal joints as in the action of trying to pick something up using the toes (2, 4, 6, 10).

Palpation Tenderness is usually elicited over the area of the tarsal tunnel posterior and distal to the medial malleolus (Fig. 7.8) (4, 6, 20).

Specific Tests Pressure or percussion over the region of the tarsal tunnel may elicit paraesthesia in the typical distribution of symptoms described above (Tinnell's sign). Nerve conduction studies can help to specifically pinpoint the diagnosis (4, 6, 19, 21).

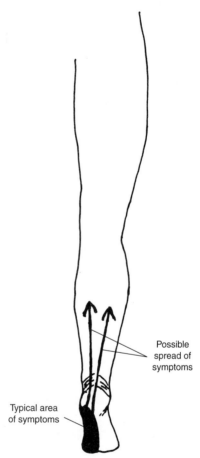

Possible
spread of
symptoms

Typical area
of symptoms

FIG. 7.24   Area of symptoms in tarsal tunnel syndrome at the right ankle/foot.

Treatment Ideas
(2–6, 9, 10, 11, 13, 14, 17)

The patient should be advised to rest the foot and stop any activity that obviously irritates the nerve and produces the symptoms. Ice baths or ice massage to the area of the tarsal tunnel may help to decrease symptoms when they are present, particularly in the earlier stages of the condition. Orthotics should be a consideration if there is an obvious foot deformity present. In more chronic cases contrast bathing with the foot placed in ice-cold water for 1 minute and warm water for 3 minutes, repeated three times, can again help to decrease symptoms. This can be combined with short bursts of rhythmical foot exercises, done in mid range with the leg placed in elevation, with the patient advised to take appropriate rests as required so as not to provoke onset of symptoms.

Once the patient's typical symptoms decrease, either in intensity or frequency of occurrence, the exercises can be progressed by increased range of motion and decreased rest periods. Passive stretches of the ankle and foot can also be attempted using rhythmical passive movements, with the length of time for which the stretches are applied steadily progressed as the patient shows no tendency towards onset of symptoms. Where pes planus is present the patient should be taught exercises such as active lumbricals to attempt to restore some strength to the arches of the foot. This can be combined with neuromuscular electrical stimulation for the intrinsic muscles of the foot. The patient can also be taught gripping exercises with the toes, these should be alternated with extension exercises done both actively and passively.

Gait and balance exercises present a further progression and should be carried out in short bursts with long rests, and are, in turn, progressed by increasing the length of time for which the exercise is carried out and decreasing the rest time between exercises. Stabilizations in double-leg stance, progressing to single-leg stance, will help to improve general foot function; these types of weight-bearing activities should be progressed as tolerated by the patient with the foot elevated when necessary.

Restrictions Any weight-bearing activity that provokes symptoms should be modified by introducing a reasonable amount of rest. Where the patient has to stand for extended periods of time it should not be on a hard surface; where possible, correct flooring, such as rubber mats, should be used. Repetitive use of peddles or other foot controls should be avoided until symptoms are abating. Kneeling with the toes extended, as in activities such as carpet laying, should either be done in short bursts or avoided altogether in the early stages.

Care should be taken when ascending and descending ladders, breaking up this activity as often as possible by sitting or standing with the affected leg resting on a small stool or step. This position can also be adopted if the patient normally has to stand for extended periods of time in work or other daily activities. However, the patient should be advised not to constantly remain with the foot up in order to prevent irritating the other foot and leg. Typically, alternating periods with the foot resting on the support for 15 minutes and then 15 minutes standing on both feet would be a reasonable protocol.

REFERENCES

1. Kesson M, Atkins E.: Orthopaedic Medicine: A Practical Approach. Butterworth Heinemann, Oxford, U.K., 1998
2. Subotnick S.I. (ed): Sports Medicine of the Lower Extremity. Churchill Livingston, New York, 1989
3. Apley G.A., Solomon L.: Apley's System of Orthopaedics and Fractures (6th ed). Butterworth, London, 1982
4. Prentice W.E. (ed): Rehabilitation Techniques in Sports Medicine. New York, W.C.B./McGraw Hill, 1994
5. Anderson B.C.: Office Orthopaedics for Primary Care: Diagnosis and Treatment (2nd ed). W.B. Saunders, Philadelphia, 1999
6. Corrigan B., Maitland G.D.: Practical Orthopaedic Medicine. Butterworth, London, 1983
7. Cyriax J.: Textbook of Orthopaedic Medicine, Vol. 1, Diagnosis of Soft Tissue Lesions (8th ed). Bailliere Tindall, Eastbourne, U.K., 1982
8. Malone T.R., McPoil T.G., Nitz A.J. (eds): Orthopaedic and Sports Physical Therapy (3rd ed), Mosby, St. Louis 1997
9. Mercier, L.R.: Practical Orthopaedics (4th ed). St. Louis, Mosby Yearbook, 1991
10. Crowther C.L.: Primary Orthopaedic Care. Mosby, St. Louis, 1999
11. Skinner H.B. (ed): Current Diagnosis and Treatment in Orthopaedics. Appleton and Lange, Norwalk, CT, 1995
12. Braddom R.L. (ed): Physical Medicine and Rehabilitation. W.B. Saunders, Philadelphia, 1996
13. Payton O.D. (ed): Manual of Physical Therapy—Churchill Livingston, New York, 1989
14. Donatelli R.A., Wooden M.J. (eds): Orthopaedic Physical Therapy (2nd ed). Churchill Livingston, New York, 1994
15. Snider R.K. (ed): Essential of Musculoskeletal Care. American Academy of Orthopaedic Surgeons, Rosemont, IL, 1997
16. Goldie B.S.: Orthopaedic Diagnosis and Management: A Guide to the Care of Orthopaedic Patients (2nd ed). ISIS Medical Media, Oxford, U.K., 1998
17. Dandy D.J., Edwards D.J.: Essential Orthopaedics and Trauma (3rd ed). Churchill Livingston, New York, 1998
18. Bernier J.N., Perrin D.H.: Effect of Coordination Training on Proprioception of the Functionally Unstable Ankle. J. Orthop. Sports Phys. Ther., 27 (4):262–275, 1998
19. Magee D.J.: Orthopaedic Physical Assessment (2nd ed). W.B. Saunders, Philadelphia, 1992
20. Field D.: Anatomy: Palpation and Surface Marking. Butterworth-Heinemann, Oxford, U.K., 1997
21. Konin J.G., Wilksten D.L., Isear J.A.: Special Tests for Orthopaedic Examination. Slack, New Jersey, 1997
22. Waddington G., Adams R..: Discrimination of Active Plantar Flexion and Inversion Movements after an Ankle Injury. Aus. J. Physiother. 45:7–13, 1999
23. Ebig M., et al.: The Effect of Sudden Inversion Stress on EMG Activity of The Peroneal and Tibialis Anterior Muscles In the Chronically Unstable Ankle. J. Orthop. Sports Phys. Ther., 26 (2):73–77, 1997

24. Lofenberg R., et al.: Prolonged Reaction Time In Patients With Chronic Lateral Instability of the Ankle—Am. J. Sports Med., 23 (4):414–417, 1995
25. Roebroek M.E., et al.: Physiotherapy for Patients with Lateral Ankle Sprains, Physiother., 84 (9):421–432, 1998
26. Simpson P.E.: Management of Sprained Ankles Referred for Physiotherapy, Physiotherapy. 77:314–316, 1991
27. Reynolds J.C.: Functional Examination of the Foot and Ankle. In Sammarco J.G., Rehabilitation of the Foot and Ankle, p. 57–75, St. Louis, Mosby Yearbook, 1995
28. Gross J, Feeto J., Rosen E.: Musculoskeletal Examination. Blackwell Science, Cambridge, MA, 1996
29. Mosier S.M., Pomeroy G., Manoli II A.: Pathoanatomy and Etiology of Posterior Tibial Tendon Dysfunction. Clin. Orthop., 365:12–22, 1999
30. Wapner K.L., Chao W.: Non-Operative Treatment of Posterior Tibial Tendon Dysfunction. Clin. Orthop., 365:39–45, 1999
31. Geppert M.J., Mizel M.S.: Management of Heel Pain in the Inflammatory Arthritides. Clin. Orthop., 349:93–99, 1998
32. Waddington G., Adams R.: Wobble Board (Ankle Disc) Training Effects on the Discrimination of Inversion Movement. Aus. J. Physiother., 45:95–101, 1999

Index

A

Abdominal contraction, decreased
    tenderness with, 17
Achilles tendon
    palpation of, 400, 401*f*
    rupture test (Thompson test), 410
Achilles tendonitis
    objective findings, 425, 427
    overview, 424–425
    subjective findings, 425, 426*f*
    treatment, 427–428
        restrictions, 428
Acromial rim, palpation of, 34–35,
    34*f*–35*f*
Acromioclavicular joint
    injury
        objective findings, 63–64
        overview, 62
        subjective findings, 62, 63*f*
        treatment, 64–65
    irritation
        objective findings, 66
        overview, 65
        subjective findings, 63*f*, 65–66
        treatment, 66–67
    palpation of, 36, 38*f*
    shear test, 39
Active movements, 7–8
Adductor tendonitis of the hip
    objective findings, 338–340
    overview, 338
    subjective findings, 338, 339*f*
    treatment, 340–341
        restrictions, 341
Adductor tendons of the thigh,
    palpation of, 316, 318*f*
Adhesive capsulitis
    objective findings, 53–54
    overview, 52
    restrictions, 55
    subjective findings, 52–53, 53*f*
    treatment
        initial treatment, 54
        progression, 55
        restrictions, 55
Anatomical snuff box, 97, 99*f*–100*f*

Ankle assessment. *See* Lower leg and
    foot assessment
Antalgic gait, 13
Anterior drawer test, 327, 408–409
Anterior superior iliac spine (ASIS),
    palpation of, 239*f*, 240
Anterior tibial tendonitis
    objective findings, 441
    overview, 440
    subjective findings, 440–441, 442*f*
    treatment, 443–444
        restrictions, 444
Appley's compression test, 327
Arm. *See* Elbow, wrist, and hand
    assessment; Shoulder
    and upper
arm assessment
ASIS (anterior superior iliac spine),
    palpation of, 239*f*, 240

B

Babinski sign, 17
Back assessment. *See* Low back and
    pelvis assessment
Balance tests, 410
Biceps reflex test, 173
Biceps tendon, palpation of, 35–36,
    37*f*, 96, 98*f*
Bicipital tendonitis
    objective findings, 56–57
    overview, 55
    subjective findings, 56, 57*f*
    treatment
        initial treatment, 57–58
        restrictions, 58
Bladder function changes, 15–16
Bowel incontinence, 15
Brachial plexus tension test, 175–176
Breath, shortness of, 15
Bursitis
    olecranon, 111–114, 113*f*
    psoas, 341–344, 342*f*
    subacromial (shoulder impinge-
        ment syndrome), 70–74, 71*f*
    trochanteric, 329–333, 330*f*
Buttock lesion, sign of, 325

C

Can emptying test, 39
Carpal bones, palpation of, 100, 101*f*
Carpal tunnel syndrome (CTS)
    objective findings, 120–121
    overview, 119
    restrictions, 122
    subjective findings, 120, 121*f*
    tests for, 102, 121
    treatment, 122
Carpometacarpal joint of the thumb
    osteoarthritis
        objective findings, 135
        overview, 133
        subjective findings, 133–135,
            134*f*
        treatment, 135–136
    palpation of, 97, 99*f*
Cervical and thoracic spine assessment
    conditions
        cervical disc (with radicu-
            lopathy), 183–188, 184*f*
        cervical disc signs (with no
            radiculopathy), 178–183, 179*f*
        cervical facet joint irritation
            (no radiculopathy), 188–191,
            189*f*
        cervical facet joint irritation
            (with radiculopathy),
            191–195, 192*f*
        cervical facet joint locking,
            206–209, 207*f*
        cervical postural strain, 195–199,
            197*f*
        cervical spondylosis, 220–224,
            222*f*
        latisimus dorsi muscle strain,
            203–206, 204*f*
        thoracic facet joint locking,
            209–212, 210*f*
        thoracic outlet syndrome,
            212–215, 213*f*
        upper trapezius muscle strain,
            199–203, 201*f*
        whiplash, 215–216, 217*f,*
            218–220

findings related to specific conditions
    active movements, 162*t*–163*t*
    age range, 157*t*
    area of symptoms, 159*t*
    duration, 158*t*
    frequency, 158*t*
    observation, 161*t*
    onset, 157*t*
    palpation, 166*t*
    passive movements, 164*t*
    resisted movements, 165*t*
    type of symptoms, 160*t*
palpation, 167–168, 171–172
    clavicles, 172, 178*f*
    external occipital protuberance,
        168, 169*f*
    facet joints, 168, 171*f*
    iliac crest, 171, 174*f*
    lateral processes, 171–172,
        175*f*–176*f*
    latisimus dorsi muscle, 171, 174*f*
    nuchal line, 168, 169*f*
    paravertebral muscles, 168, 170*f,*
        172, 177*f*
    scapula, medial border of, 168,
        172*f*
    spinous processes, 168, 170*f*
    thoracic spinous processes, 168,
        171, 173*f*
    trapezius, middle fibers of, 168
    trapezius, upper fibers of,
        167–168, 167*f*
specific tests
    dural signs, 176
    myotomes, 177
    reflexes, 173, 175–176
test movements
    cervical spine, active move-
        ments, 151*t*–152*t*
    cervical spine, passive move-
        ments, 153*t*
    cervical spine, resisted move-
        ment, 154*t*
    overview, 151
    shoulder girdle, active move-
        ments, 155*t*

thoracic spine, active movements, 156t
Chest pain on exertion, 16
Clark's sign, 328
Clavicles, palpation of, 172, 178f
Clubbing of nails, 16
Collateral ligament strain of knee
  objective findings, 369–371
  overview, 368–369
  subjective findings, 369, 370f
  treatment, 371–373
    restrictions, 373
Combined disc/facet joint problem
  objective findings, 284
  overview, 282
  subjective findings, 282, 283f, 284
  treatment, 284–286
    restrictions, 286
Crepitation, 36–37
Cross over sign, 246
CTS. *See* Carpal tunnel syndrome
Cubital tunnel syndrome (ulnar nerve entrapment)
  objective findings, 101, 115–116
  overview, 114
  subjective findings, 114–115, 115f
  treatment, 116–117
    restrictions, 117
Cyanosis, 16
Cyriax, James, 8

D

de Quervains tenosynovitis
  objective findings, 101–102, 128
  overview, 126
  subjective findings, 126–127, 127f
  treatment, 128–130
    restrictions, 130
Dupytren's contracture
  objective findings, 143
  overview, 142
  subjective findings, 143, 144f
  treatment, 144–145
    restrictions, 145
Dural signs, 176, 246

E

Elbow, wrist, and hand assessment
  conditions
    carpal tunnel syndrome (CTS), 119–122, 121f
    de Quervains tenosynovitis, 101–102, 126–130, 127f
    Dupytren's contracture, 142–145, 144f
    lateral epicondylitis of the elbow, 102–107, 104f
    medial epicondylitis of the elbow, 107–111, 108f
    median nerve entrapment, 117–119, 118f
    metacarpophalangeal joint injury of the thumb (ulnar collateral ligament injury), 130–133, 132f
    olecranon bursitis, 111–114, 113f
    osteoarthritis of carpometacarpal joint of the thumb, 133–136, 134f
    trigger finger, 136–139, 138f
    ulnar nerve entrapment (cubital tunnel syndrome), 114–117, 115f
    wrist extensor tendonitis, 122–126, 124f
    wrist flexor tendonitis, 139–142, 141f
    wrist sprain, 145–148, 146f
  findings related to specific conditions
    active movements, 90t
    age range, 86t
    area of symptoms, 88t
    duration, 87t
    frequency, 87t
    observation, 89t–90t
    onset, 86t
    palpation, 92t
    passive movements, 91t
    resisted movements, 91t–92t
    type of symptoms, 88t–89t
  palpation
    elbow region, 93, 94f–98f, 95

Elbow, wrist, and hand assessment; palpation (*Continued*)
overview, 93
wrist region, 96–97, 98*f*–101*f*, 100
specific tests
carpal tunnel syndrome, 102
cubital tunnel syndrome, 101
de Quervains syndrome, 101–102
lateral epicondylitis, 100–101
medial epicondylitis, 101
thumb carpometacarpal joint, 102
test movements
elbow, forearm, wrist, and hand, resisted movements, 84*t*–85*t*
elbow and forearm, active movements, 76*t*–77*t*
elbow and forearm, passive movements, 80*t*–81*t*
hand, active movements, 78*t*–80*t*
overview, 76
wrist, active movements, 77*t*–78*t*
wrist and hand, passive movements, 82*t*–83*t*
Emptying can test, 39
End feel of movements, 9
External occipital protuberance, palpation of, 168, 169*f*

F
Facet joints, palpation of, 168, 171*f*
Fatigue and general loss of energy (malaise), 15
Femoral stretch test (prone knee bending), 246
Fever, 15
Fibula, head of, palpation, 321–322, 323*f*
Finkelstein's test, 102, 128
Flexor carpi radialis, palpation of, 97, 100*f*
Foot assessment. *See* Lower leg and foot assessment

G
Gait, 13
abnormalities, 13
footwear, 13
Gastrocnemius muscle/tendon tear
objective findings, 422–423
overview, 420
subjective findings, 420, 421*f*, 422
treatment, 423–424
restrictions, 424
Glenohumeral joint
active movements, 21*t*–22*t*
instability tests, 39
Greater trochanter, palpation of, 315, 316*f*–317*f*
Groin strain
objective findings, 345–346
overview, 344
subjective findings, 344, 345*f*
treatment, 346–347
restrictions, 347

H
Hamstring muscles
palpation of, 317, 319*f*
tear
objective findings, 355–357
overview, 354–355
subjective findings, 355, 356*f*
treatment, 357–358
tension tests, 326
Hamstring tendonitis
objective findings, 360
overview, 358
subjective findings, 358–360, 359*f*
treatment, 360–361
restrictions, 361
Hand assessment. *See* Elbow, wrist, and hand assessment
Health history, 1, 18*t*–19*t*
Hip and knee assessment
conditions
adductor tendonitis of the hip, 338–341, 339*f*
collateral ligament strain of knee, 368–373, 370*f*

groin strain, 344–347, 345*f*

hamstring muscle tear, 354–358, 356*f*

hamstring tendonitis, 358–361, 359*f*

iliotibial band friction syndrome, 351–354, 352*f*

osteoarthritis of the hip, 333–338, 335*f*

osteoarthritis (OA) of the knee, 377–382, 379*f*

patella femoral syndrome (PFS), 373–377, 374*f*

piriformis syndrome, 347–351, 349*f*

psoas bursitis, 341–344, 342*f*

quadriceps muscle tear, 361–365, 363*f*

quadriceps tendon tear, 365–368, 366*f*

trochanteric bursitis, 329–333, 330*f*

findings related to specific conditions

active movements, 311*t*

age range, 306*t*

area of symptoms, 308*t*

duration, 307*t*

frequency, 307*t*

observation, 310*t*

onset, 306*t*

palpation, 314*t*

passive movements, 312*t*

resisted movements, 313*t*

type of symptoms, 309*t*

palpation

adductor tendons of the thigh, 316, 318*f*

greater trochanter, 315, 316*f*–317*f*

hamstring muscles, 317, 319*f*

head of the fibula, 321–322, 323*f*

hip area, 315–317, 316*f*–319*f*

hip joint, 315–316, 318*f*

ischial tuberosity, 315, 317*f*

knee area, 317, 319*f*–325*f*, 320–323

knee joint line, 319*f*, 321, 322*f*

lateral collateral ligament, 322, 323*f*

lateral epicondyle of the femur, 320, 320*f*

medial collateral ligament, 322, 324*f*

medial epicondyle of the femur, 320, 321*f*

overview, 315

patella, 317, 319*f*, 320

patella tendon, 321, 322*f*

piriformis muscles, 316

quadriceps muscles, 322, 325*f*

quadriceps tendon, 323, 325*f*

tibial tubercle, 320, 322*f*

specific tests

hip region, 323–326

knee region, 326

ligament stress tests, 326–329

test movements

hip, active movements, 296*t*–297*t*

hip, passive movements, 298*t*–299*t*

hip, resisted movements, 300*t*–301*t*

knee, active movements, 302*t*

knee, passive movements, 303*t*–304*t*

knee, resisted movements, 305*t*

overview, 296

patella, passive movements, 304*t*

History, 1, 18*t*–19*t*

Hoffman's sign, 410

I

Iliac crest, palpation of, 171, 174*f*, 239, 239*f*

Iliotibial band friction syndrome

objective findings, 352–353

overview, 351

subjective findings, 351–352

treatment, 353–354

restrictions, 354

Impingement tests (shoulder and upper arm), 39

Incontinence, bowel, 15

Ischial tuberosity, 242f–243f, 243, 315, 317f

J

Jaundice, 16

K

Kleiger test, 409

Knee assessment. *See* Hip and knee assessment

L

Lateral collateral ligament
palpation of, 322, 323f
test (varus strain), 327

Lateral epicondyle (elbow), palpation of, 93, 94f

Lateral epicondyle (femur), palpation of, 320, 320f

Lateral epicondylitis (elbow)
objective findings, 100–101, 103–104
overview, 102
subjective findings, 102–103, 104f
treatment, 104–107
restrictions, 106–107

Lateral ligament
palpation of, 399, 400f
stability test, 409

Lateral malleolus, palpation of, 398, 400f–401f

Lateral processes, palpation of, 171–172, 175f–176f

Latisimus dorsi muscle
palpation, 171, 174f
strain
objective findings, 204–205
overview, 203
subjective findings, 203–204, 204f
treatment, 205–206

Leg
length discrepancy, 13, 324–325
lower leg assessment. *See* Lower leg and foot assessment

L4–L5 interspace, 242f, 243

Low back and pelvis assessment
conditions
chronic spinal instability, 290–293, 291f
combined disc/facet joint problem, 282, 283f, 284–286
low back postural sprain, 270, 271f, 272–274
lumbar disc lesion (no radiculopathy), 247–251, 248f
lumbar disc lesion (with radiculopathy), 251–257, 253f
lumbar facet joint irritation (no radiculopathy), 257–261, 258f
lumbar facet joint irritation (with radiculopathy), 274–278, 276f
lumbar facet joint strain, 278, 279f, 280–282
lumbar muscle strain, 266–269, 267f
sacroiliac joint strain, 261–266, 263f
spinal stenosis, 286–290, 288f
findings related to specific conditions
active movements, 235t–236t
age range, 230t
area of symptoms, 232t
duration, 231t
frequency, 231t
observation, 234t
onset, 230t
palpation, 238t
passive movements, 236t–237t
resisted movements, 237t
type of symptoms, 233t
palpation
anterior superior iliac spine (ASIS), 239f, 240
iliac crests, 239, 239f
ischial tuberosity, 242f–243f, 243
L4–L5 interspace, 242f, 243
overview, 239

posterior superior iliac spine (PSIS), 240, 240*f*
sacroiliac joint, 240, 240*f*
sacrospinous ligament, 243*f*, 244
sacrotuberous ligament, 242*f*, 243
skin sensation, 244
spinous processes, 241, 242*f*, 244*f*
thoracolumbar paravertebral muscles, 241, 241*f*
specific tests
ankle reflexes, 245
cross over sign, 246
dural signs, 246
femoral stretch (prone knee bending), 246
knee reflexes, 245
myotomes, 245, 245*t*
straight leg raising, 246
stressing the sacroiliac joint, 246–247
test movements
low back, active movements, 227*t*–228*t*
low back, resisted movements, 228*t*–229*t*
overview, 227
Lower leg and foot assessment
conditions
Achilles tendonitis, 424–425, 426*f*, 427–428
ankle instability, recurrent, 416, 417*f*, 418–420
ankle ligament strain/tear, 410–411, 412*f*, 413–416
anterior tibial tendonitis, 440–441, 442*f*, 443–444
gastrocnemius muscle/tendon tear, 420, 421*f*, 422–424
Morton's neuroma, 447–448, 449*f*, 450
peroneal tenosynovitis, 432–433, 434*f*, 435–436
plantar fasciitis, 428–429, 430*f*, 431–432
posterior tibial tenosynovitis, 436–437, 438*f*, 439–440

shin splints, 444–445, 446*f*, 447
tarsal tunnel syndrome, 450–451, 452*f*, 453–454
findings related to specific conditions
active movements, 394*t*
age range, 389*t*
area of symptoms, 391*t*
duration, 390*t*
frequency, 390*t*
observation, 393*t*
onset, 389*t*
palpation, 397*t*
passive movements, 395*t*
resisted movements, 396*t*
type of symptoms, 392*t*
palpation
Achilles tendon, 400, 401*f*
ankle joint line, 398, 401*f*
anterior ankle, 406, 407*f*
lateral ligament, 399, 400*f*
lateral malleolus, 398, 400*f*–401*f*
medial aspect of the ankle, 404*f*, 405–406
medial (deltoid) ligament, 398–399, 399*f*
medial malleolus, 398, 399*f*, 401*f*
metatarsal heads, 407, 408*f*
metatarsals, 404–405, 404*f*
mid-tarsal joint, 405, 405*f*
overview, 398
peroneal tendons, 400, 402*f*–404*f*, 403–404
plantar fascia, 407–408, 409*f*
subtalar joint (talocalcaneal joint), 405, 406*f*
specific tests
anterior drawer sign, 408–409
balance tests, 410
Hoffman's sign, 410
Kleiger test, 409
lateral ligament stability, 409
Thompson test (Achilles tendon rupture), 410
Tinnell's sign, 410

Lower leg and foot assessment
(*Continued*)
test movements
foot and ankle, active movements, 384*t*–385*t*
foot and ankle, passive movements, 385*t*–387*t*
foot and ankle, resisted movements, 387*t*–388*t*
overview, 384
Lumbar disc lesion (no radiculopathy)
objective findings, 249
overview, 247
subjective findings, 247–249, 248*f*
treatment, 249–251
restrictions, 251
Lumbar disc lesion (with radiculopathy)
objective findings, 252–254
overview, 251–252
subjective findings, 252, 253*f*
treatment
final stages, 256
initial treatment, 254
progression, 255
restrictions, 256–257
Lumbar facet joint irritation (no radiculopathy)
objective findings, 259–260
overview, 257
subjective findings, 257–259, 258*f*
treatment, 260–261
restrictions, 261
Lumbar facet joint irritation (with radiculopathy)
objective findings, 275–276
overview, 274
subjective findings, 274–275, 276*f*
treatment, 277–278
restrictions, 277–278
Lumbar facet joint strain
objective findings, 280
overview, 278
subjective findings, 278, 279*f*, 280
treatment, 280–282
restrictions, 281–282

Lumbar muscle strain
objective findings, 266–268
overview, 266
subjective findings, 266, 267*f*
treatment
initial treatment, 268
latter stages, 269
progression, 268–269
restrictions, 269

M

Malaise, 15
McConnell test, 328–329
McMurray's test, 327–328
Medial collateral ligament
palpation of, 322, 324*f*
test (valgus strain), 316
Medial epicondyle (elbow), palpation of, 93, 95*f*
Medial epicondyle (femur), palpation of, 320, 321*f*
Medial epicondylitis of the elbow
objective findings, 109
overview, 107
subjective findings, 107–109, 108*f*
test for, 101
treatment, 109–111
restrictions, 111
Medial (deltoid) ligament, palpation of, 398–399, 399*f*
Medial malleolus, palpation of, 398, 399*f*, 401*f*
Median nerve entrapment
objective findings, 117–119
overview, 117
subjective findings, 117, 118*f*
treatment, 119
restrictions, 119
Metacarpophalangeal joint injury of the thumb (ulnar collateral ligament injury)
objective findings, 131
overview, 130
subjective findings, 131, 132*f*
treatment, 131–133
restrictions, 133

Metatarsal heads, palpation of, 407, 408f
Metatarsals, palpation of, 404–405, 404f
Mid-tarsal joint, palpation of, 405, 405f
Morton's neuroma
  objective findings, 449
  overview, 447
  subjective findings, 448, 449f
  treatment, 450
    restrictions, 450
Myotomes
  cervical and thoracic spine, 177
  lower extremity, 245, 245t

N

Nail clubbing, 16
Nausea and vomiting, 15
Neurological "red flags," 17
Noble compression test (knee), 326
Nuchal line, palpation of, 168, 169f

O

OA. *See* Osteoarthritis
Objective examination
  active movements, 7–8
  gait, 13
  observation, 6–7
  overview, 5–6
  palpation, 10
  passive movements, 8–9
  posture, 10–13
  resisted movements, 9–10
  specific tests, 10
Observation, 6–7
Olecranon
  bursitis
    objective findings, 112
    overview, 111
    subjective findings, 111–112, 113f
    treatment, 113–114
  palpation of, 95, 96f
Orthopaedic physical therapy assessment
  findings, 17–19

health history, 1, 18t–19t
objective examination
  active movements, 7–8
  gait, 13
  observation, 6–7
  overview, 5–6
  palpation, 10
  passive movements, 8–9
  posture, 10–13
  resisted movements, 9–10
  specific tests, 10
overview, 1–2
subjective examination
  medical history, 1, 5
  overview, 2
  onset, 2–3
  duration, 3
  frequency, 3–4
  area of symptoms, 4
  type of symptoms, 4–5
  question 6: miscellaneous, 5
Osteoarthritis (OA)
  carpometacarpal joint of the thumb, 133–136, 134f
  hip
    objective findings, 334–336
    overview, 333
    subjective findings, 333–334, 335f
    treatment, 336–338
  knee
    objective findings, 378–380
    overview, 377–378
    subjective findings, 378, 379f
    treatment, 380–382
Overuse *versus* trauma, 2–3
Oxford Scale, 9

P

Pain
  abdominal contraction, decreased tenderness with, 17
  chest pain on exertion, 16
  painful arc of movement test (shoulder and upper arm), 37–38

Pain (*Continued*)
    rebound tenderness, 17
    severe incessant, 17
Palpation, 10
Paravertebral muscles, palpation of,
        168, 170*f*, 172, 177*f*
Passive movements, 8–9
    end feel, 9
Patella
    palpation of, 317, 319*f*, 320–321,
        322*f*
    passive movements, 304*t*
Patella-femoral angle (Q angle) test,
        328
Patella femoral syndrome (PFS)
    objective findings, 375–376
    overview, 373
    subjective findings, 373–375, 374*f*
    treatment, 376–377
        restrictions, 377
Pectoral muscle tear
    objective findings, 69
    overview, 67
    subjective findings, 67–68, 68*f*
    treatment, 69–70
        latter stages, 69–70
        progression, 69
        restrictions, 70
Pelvis assessment. *See* Low back and
        pelvis assessment
Peroneal tendons, palpation of, 400,
        402*f*–404*f*, 403–404
Peroneal tenosynovitis
    objective findings, 433, 435
    overview, 432
    subjective findings, 432–433, 434*f*
    treatment, 435–436
        restrictions, 436
PFS. *See* Patella femoral syndrome
Phalen's sign, 102, 121
Piriformis muscles, palpation of, 316
Piriformis syndrome
    objective findings, 348–350
    overview, 347
    subjective findings, 347–348, 349*f*

    treatment, 350–351
        restrictions, 350–351
Piriformis test, 326
Pisiform, palpation of, 96, 99*f*
Plantar fascia, palpation of, 407–408,
        409*f*
Plantar fasciitis
    objective findings, 429, 431
    overview, 428–429
    subjective findings, 429, 430*f*
    treatment, 431–432
        restrictions, 432
Posterior superior iliac spine (PSIS),
        palpation of, 240, 240*f*
Posterior tibial tenosynovitis
    objective findings, 437, 439
    overview, 436
    subjective findings, 436–437, 438*f*
    treatment, 439–440
        restrictions, 440
Posture, 10–13
    abnormalities, 11–13
        viewed from the front, 12
        viewed from the side, 12–13
    good, 10–11
Prone knee bending (femoral stretch
        test), 246
PSIS (posterior superior iliac spine),
        palpation of, 240, 240*f*
Psoas bursitis
    objective findings, 341–343
    overview, 341
    subjective findings, 341, 342*f*
    treatment, 343–344
        restrictions, 344

Q

Q angle (patella-femoral angle) test,
        328
Quadriceps muscles
    palpation of, 322, 325*f*
    tear
        objective findings, 362–363
        overview, 361–362
        restrictions, 364–365

subjective findings, 362, 363f
treatment, 364–365
Quadriceps tendon
palpation of, 323, 325f
tear
objective findings, 365–367
overview, 365
subjective findings, 365, 366f
treatment, 367–368

R
Radial styloid, palpation of, 97, 99f
Radius, head of, palpation, 93, 94f
Rebound tenderness, 17
"Red flags"
abdominal contraction, decreased
tenderness with, 17
bladder function changes, 15–16
chest pain on exertion, 16
clubbing of nails, 16
difficulty passing urine, 15
fatigue and general loss of energy
(malaise), 15
fever, 15
gradual onset with no cause, 14
increased urination with excessive
thirst, 16
mild bowel incontinence, 15
nausea and vomiting, 15
neurological findings, 17
no variation in symptoms with
activities or rest, 14
overview, 14
patient not improving with treatment, 14
rebound tenderness, 17
severe incessant pain, 17
shortness of breath, 15
skin changes, general, 16
skin color, 16
skin lesions, 16
temporary loss of consciousness
(syncope), 15
unexplained weight loss, 14–15
Reflex tests (cervical and thoracic
region), 173, 175–176

Resisted movements, 9–10
Review of systems, 1
Rotator cuff tear
objective findings, 49–50
overview, 48–49
subjective findings, 49, 50f
treatment
initial treatment, 50–51
restrictions, 51–52
Rotator cuff tendonitis, acute
objective findings, 41–42
overview, 40
subjective findings, 40, 41f
treatment
initial treatment, 42–43
progression, 43
restrictions, 43–44
Rotator cuff tendonitis, chronic
objective findings, 45–46
overview, 44–45
subjective findings, 45, 46f
treatment, 46–48
latter stages, 48
restrictions, 48

S
Sacroiliac joint
palpation of, 240, 240f
strain
objective findings, 262–264
overview, 261–262
subjective findings, 262, 263f
treatment, 264–266
tests, 246–247
Sacrospinous ligament, 243f, 244
Sacrotuberous ligament, 242f, 243
Scapula, medial border of, palpation,
168, 172f
Shin splints
objective findings, 445
overview, 444
subjective findings, 444–445, 446f
treatment, 445, 447
restriction-
Shortn-

Shoulder and upper arm assessment
  conditions
    acromioclavicular joint injury,
      62–65, 63f
    acromioclavicular joint irrita-
      tion, 63f, 65–67
    acute rotator cuff tendonitis,
      40–44, 41f
    adhesive capsulitis, 52–55, 53f
    bicipital tendonitis, 55–58, 57f
    chronic instability of shoulder
      joint, 58–62, 60f
    chronic rotator cuff tendonitis,
      44–48, 46f
    pectoral muscle tear, 67–70, 68f
    rotator cuff tear, 48–52, 50f
    subacromial bursitis (shoulder
      impingement syndrome),
      70–74, 71f
  findings related to specific conditions
    active movements, 31t–32t
    age range, 28t
    area of symptoms, 30t
    duration, 29t
    frequency, 29t
    observation, 31t
    onset, 28t
    palpation, 33t
    passive movements, 32t
    resisted movements, 33t
    type of symptoms, 30t
  palpation
    acromial rim, 34–35, 34f–35f
    acromioclavicular joint, 36, 38f
    biceps tendon, 35–36, 37f
    crepitation, 36–37
    overview, 34
    supraspinatus tendon, 35, 36f
  specific tests
    acromioclavicular shear test, 39
    emptying can, 39
    impingement tests, 39
    painful arc of movement, 37–38
    shoulder joint instability, 39
    Speeds test, 38

  Yergason's sign, 38
  test movements
    glenohumeral joint, active
      movements, 21t–22t
    overview, 21
    shoulder, passive movements,
      23t–24t
    shoulder, resisted movements,
      25t–26t
    shoulder girdle, resisted move-
      ments, 27t
Sign of the buttock, 325
Skin
  "red flags"
    color, 16
    general changes, 16
    lesions, 16
    sensation, lower extremities, 244
Speeds test, 38
Spine. See Cervical and thoracic spine
      assessment; Low back and
  pelvis assessment
Spondylosis, cervical, 220–224, 222f
Springy block test, 328
Stiff leg gait, 13
Straight leg raising test, 246
Subacromial bursitis (shoulder
      impingement syndrome)
  objective findings, 72
  overview, 70
  subjective findings, 70–72, 71f
  treatment
    initial treatment, 72–73
    latter stages, 73–74
    progression, 73
    restrictions, 74
Subjective examination
  medical history, 1, 5
  overview, 2
  onset, 2–3
  duration, 3
  frequency, 3–4
  area of symptoms, 4
  type of symptoms, 4–5
  miscellaneous, 5

Subluxation of the shoulder, recurrent, 58–62, 60f

Subtalar joint (talocalcaneal joint), palpation of, 405, 406f

Supraspinatus tendon, palpation of, 35, 36f

Syncope, 15

T

Talocalcaneal joint (subtalar joint), palpation of, 405, 406f

Tarsal tunnel syndrome
objective findings, 451
overview, 450
subjective findings, 450–451, 452f
treatment, 453–454
restrictions, 453–454

Temporary loss of consciousness (syncope), 15

Textbook of Orthopaedic Medicine, 8

Thirst, excessive, 16

Thompson tests
Achilles tendon rupture, 410
hip flexion contracture, 323–324

Thoracic Outlet Syndrome 212–215, 213f

Thoracic spine assessment. *See* Cervical and thoracic spine assessment

Thoracolumbar paravertebral muscles, palpation of, 241, 241f

Thumb
carpometacarpal joint. *See* Carpometacarpal joint of the thumb
metacarpophalangeal joint injury, 130–131, 132f

Tibial tubercle, palpation of, 320, 322f

Tinel's sign, 121, 410

Trapezius
middle, palpation of, 168
upper
palpation of, 167–168, 167f
strain of, 199–203, 201f

Trauma *versus* overuse, 2–3

Trendelenburg gait, 13

Trendelenburg sign, 324

Triceps reflex test, 173

Triceps tendon, palpation of, 95, 97f

Trigger finger
objective findings, 137–138
overview, 136–137
subjective findings, 137, 138f
treatment, 138–139
restrictions, 139

Trochanteric bursitis
objective findings, 331f
overview, 329
subjective findings, 329–331, 330f
treatment
initial treatment, 331–332
progression, 332–333
restrictions, 333

U

Ulna, head of, palpation, 96, 98f

Ulnar collateral ligament injury (metacarpophalangeal joint injury of the thumb), 130–133, 132f

Ulnar groove, palpation of, 95, 95f

Ulnar nerve entrapment (cubital tunnel syndrome)
objective findings, 101, 115–116
overview, 114
subjective findings, 114–115, 115f
treatment, 116–117
restrictions, 117

Upper arm. *See* Shoulder and upper arm assessment

Upper trapezius muscle strain
objective findings, 200–201
overview, 199
subjective findings, 200, 201f
treatment, 202–203
restrictions, 203

Urination
difficulty with, 15
increased, 16

V

Vertebral artery test, 175

W

Warning signs. *See* "Red flags"
Weight loss, unexplained, 14–15
Whiplash
    objective findings, 216, 218
    overview, 215
    subjective findings, 215–216, 217*f*
    treatment, 218–220
        restrictions, 220
Wrist assessment. *See* Elbow, wrist,
        and hand assessment

Y

Yergason's sign, 38

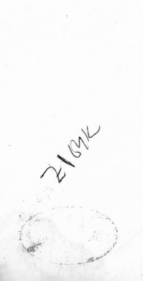